Yearbook of
CRITICAL CARE 2023
HICS Initiative

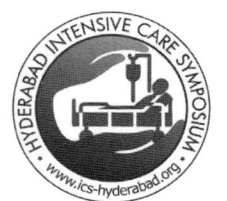

Yearbook of
CRITICAL CARE 2023
HICS Initiative

Editors

Srinivas Samavedam
MD DNB FRCP FNB EDIC FICCM
Chief Intensivist
Ramdev Rao Hospital
Hyderabad, Telangana, India

Ganshyam Jagathkar
MD FNB FICCM
Director (Critical Care)
Medicover Hospitals
Hyderabad, Telangana, India

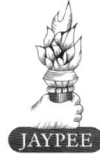

JAYPEE BROTHERS MEDICAL PUBLISHERS
The Health Sciences Publisher
New Delhi | London

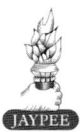
Jaypee Brothers Medical Publishers (P) Ltd

Headquarters
Jaypee Brothers Medical Publishers (P) Ltd
EMCA House, 23/23-B
Ansari Road, Daryaganj
New Delhi 110 002, India
Landline: +91-11-23272143, +91-11-23272703
+91-11-23282021, +91-11-23245672
Email: jaypee@jaypeebrothers.com

Corporate Office
Jaypee Brothers Medical Publishers (P) Ltd
4838/24, Ansari Road, Daryaganj
New Delhi 110 002, India
Phone: +91-11-43574357
Fax: +91-11-43574314
Email: jaypee@jaypeebrothers.com

Overseas Office
JP Medical Ltd.
83, Victoria Street, London
SW1H 0HW (UK)
Phone: +44 20 3170 8910
Fax: +44 (0)20 3008 6180
Email: info@jpmedpub.com

Website: www.jaypeebrothers.com
Website: www.jaypeedigital.com

© 2024, Jaypee Brothers Medical Publishers

The views and opinions expressed in this book are solely those of the original contributor(s)/author(s) and do not necessarily represent those of editor(s) or publisher of the book.

All rights reserved. No part of this publication may be reproduced, stored or transmitted in any form or by any means, electronic, mechanical, photo copying, recording or otherwise, without the prior permission in writing of the publishers.

All brand names and product names used in this book are trade names, service marks, trademarks or registered trademarks of their respective owners. The publisher is not associated with any product or vendor mentioned in this book.

Medical knowledge and practice change constantly. This book is designed to provide accurate, authoritative information about the subject matter in question. However, readers are advised to check the most current information available on procedures included and check information from the manufacturer of each product to be administered, to verify the recommended dose, formula, method and duration of administration, adverse effects and contra indications. It is the responsibility of the practitioner to take all appropriate safety precautions. Neither the publisher nor the author(s)/editor(s) assume any liability for any injury and/or damage to persons or property arising from or related to use of material in this book.

This book is sold on the understanding that the publisher is not engaged in providing professional medical services. If such advice or services are required, the services of a competent medical professional should be sought.

Every effort has been made where necessary to contact holders of copyright to obtain permission to reproduce copyright material. If any have been inadvertently overlooked, the publisher will be pleased to make the necessary arrangements at the first opportunity.

Inquiries for bulk sales may be solicited at: jaypee@jaypeebrothers.com

Yearbook of Critical Care 2023

First Edition: **2024**

ISBN: 978-93-5696-967-4

Printed at: Sterling Graphics Pvt. Ltd. India

Dedication

*This yearbook is dedicated to all the front-line healthcare workers
who put their profession ahead of personal life and strive
to deliver the best to their patients.*

Contributors

SECTION EDITORS

Deven Juneja
DNB FNB EDIC FCCP
Director
Institute of Critical Care Medicine
Max Super Specialty Hospital
New Delhi, India
(Section 8: Hematology)

Gunjan Chanchalani
MD IFCCM FNB EDIC FICCM
Chief Intensivist
KJ Somaiya Hospital and Research Centre
Mumbai, Maharashtra, India
(Section 11: Guidelines)

Jaicob Varghese
MD (General Medicine) DM (Critical Care) EDIC
Senior Consultant and Head
Department of Critical Care
Rajagiri Hospital
Kochi, Kerala, India
(Section 7: Sepsis)

Kanwalpreet Sodhi
DA DNB IDCCM EDIC FICCM
Director and Head
Department of Critical Care
Deep Hospital
Ludhiana, Punjab, India
(Section 5: Nephrology)

Ketan Kargirwar
MD FNB EDIC IDCCM
Senior Consultant
Critical Care Medicine
Sir HN Reliance Foundation Hospital
and Research Centre
Mumbai, Maharashtra, India
(Section 3: Neurocritical Care)

Lalita Gouri Mitra DA MD DNB FICCM
Professor and Officer In-charge
Department of Anesthesia,
Critical Care, and Pain
Homi Bhabha Cancer Hospital and Research Centre
Medicity Mullanpur (New Chandigarh)
Punjab, India
(A Unit of Tata Memorial Centre, Mumbai and
Department of Atomic Energy, Govt of India)
(Section 4: Gastroenterology/Hepatobiliary)

Manoj Y Singh
MD (Med) FNB (Critical Care) EDIC PG Dipl (Peri-op)
AFRACMA FCICM
Clinical Director and Senior
Intensive Care Physician
The Canberra Hospital
Garran, ACT, Australia
*(Section 2: Respiratory/Ventilation/Acute
Respiratory Distress Syndrome)*

Ranajit Chatterjee
MRCP FRCP EDIC DA FIACM CMO SAG
In-charge Intensive Care Unit
Swami Dayanand Hospital
New Delhi, India
(Section 11: Guidelines)

Shrikanth Srinivasan MD DNB FNB EDIC FICCM
Consultant and Head
Department of Critical Care Medicine
Manipal Hospital, New Delhi, India
(Section 9: Sonography/Imaging)

Sivakumar MN DA DNB IDCCM EDIC FICCM
Head
Institute of Critical Care Medicine
Royal Care Super Speciality Hospital
Coimbatore, Tamil Nadu, India
(Section 10: Nutrition and Metabolic)

Sumesh Arora FCICM EDIC MD
Senior Staff Specialist
Intensive Care
Prince of Wales Hospital
Randwick, NSW, Australia
Director: http://www.gotheextramile.com; www.gotheextramile.com MCQ in Critical Care
(Section 6: Infections and Antibiotics)

Supradip Ghosh
DNB (Internal Medicine) MNAMS MRCP (Edinburgh) EDIC FICCM
Director and Head
Department of Critical Care Medicine
Fortis-Escorts Hospital
Faridabad, Haryana, India
(Section 1: Cardiac/Hemodynamics/Fluids)

ASSOCIATE EDITORS

Aditya Lyall
MD (Internal Medicine) IDCCM IFCCM
Consultant
Department of Critical Care Medicine
Fortis-Escorts Hospital
Faridabad, Haryana, India

Amandeep Singh
MD (Internal Medicine) IDCCM
Senior Consultant
Department of Critical Care Medicine
Fortis-Escorts Hospital
Faridabad, Haryana, India

Atul Phillips MD FNB (Critical Care)
Neurocritical Care Fellow
Cummings School of Medicine University of Calgary
Alberta, Canada

Basjinder Kaur DA DNB IDCCM IFCCM
Senior Consultant
SPS Hospital
Ludhiana, Punjab, India

Harsimran Singh Walia MD IDCCM FNB (CCM)
Assistant Professor
Department of Anesthesia, Critical Care, and Pain
Homi Bhabha Cancer Hospital and Research Centre
Medicity Mullanpur (New Chandigarh)
Punjab, India
(A Unit of Tata Memorial Centre, Mumbai and Department of Atomic Energy, Govt of India)

Jagdeep Sharma MD DNB DESAIC
Assistant Professor
Department of Anesthesia, Critical Care, and Pain
Homi Bhabha Cancer Hospital and Research Centre
Medicity Mullanpur (New Chandigarh)
Punjab, India
(A Unit of Tata Memorial Centre, Mumbai and Department of Atomic Energy, Govt of India)

Lakshmikanthcharan S
MD IDCCM EDIC EDAIC
Senior Consultant
Institute of Critical Care Medicine
Royal Care Super Speciality Hospital
Coimbatore, Tamil Nadu, India

Lalit Gupta MD
Associate Professor
Department of Anesthesiology and Critical Care
Maulana Azad Medical College
New Delhi, India

Magesh Parthiban
MD DM (Critical Care Medicine)
Consultant Intensivist
Kovai Medical Center and Hospital
Coimbatore, Tamil Nadu, India

Manu Gupta MD (Medicine) IDCCM
Consutant Intensivist
Department of Critical Care
St Stephen's Hospital
New Delhi, India

Melwin George MD IDCCM EDIC
DrNB Resident
Department of Critical Care
Rajagiri Hospital
Kochi, Kerala, India

Nilanjan Umesh
DNB (Respiratory Medicine) FNB (Critical Care) IFCCM
Consultant
Department of Critical Care
Rajagiri Hospital
Kochi, Kerala, India

NVSN Prasant MD DM (Critical Care Medicine)
Resident
Department of Critical Care
Sri Ramachandra Institute of Higher
Education and Research
Chennai, Tamil Nadu, India

Ripenmeet Salhotra
MD (Anesthesiology) IDCCM IFCCM EDIC
Consultant
Department of Anesthesia and Critical Care
Amrita Hospital
Faridabad, Haryana, India

Sahil Kataria MD DrNB
Associate Consultant
Department of Critical Care Medicine
Holy Family Hospital
New Delhi, India

Sanket Hansora MBBS IDCCM
Associate Consultant
Critical Care Medicine
Sir HN Reliance Foundation Hospital
and Research Centre
Mumbai, Maharashtra, India

Saurabh Kumar Rai
DNB (Emergency Medicine)
2nd Year DrNB Critical Care Medicine Fellow
Fortis-Escorts Hospital
Faridabad, Haryana, India

Seema S Tekwani MD MHA
Assistant Professor of Medicine
Division of Pulmonary, Allergy,
Critical Care, and Sleep Medicine
Emory University School of Medicine
Atlanta, Georgia, USA

Vadhan Prasanna S
MD DM (Critical Care Medicine)
Former Senior Resident
Department of Critical Care
All India Institute of Medical Sciences
Rishikesh, Uttarakhand, India

Velmurugan Selvam
MD DM (Critical Care Medicine)
Assistant Professor
Sri Ramachandra Institute of
Higher Education and Research
Chennai, Tamil Nadu, India

Vetriselvan P
MD DM (Critical Care Medicine)
Consultant
Department of Critical Care
Kauvery Hospital
Chennai, Tamil Nadu, India

Preface

The field of critical care is highly dynamic and rapidly evolving. The pathophysiology of critical illness is also unique and different from the normal pathophysiology of noncritical illnesses. It is therefore essential for astute and committed practitioners of the specialty to keep themselves well informed and up-to-date with the emerging evidence in the field. The recent pandemic has resulted in an explosion of information and has increased the need for rational evaluation of published literature. The usual way for intensivists to keep themselves abreast of recent advances is to engage in continuing medical education (CMEs) and conferences. But the amount of information that can be accessed and assimilated is limited by the agenda that is set out and the finite time everyone has to attend these programs. Moreover, it is also likely that some cutting-edge information has been overlooked by the chosen speaker.

The Hyderabad Intensive Care Symposium (HICS) has been in the forefront of knowledge dissemination for more than one and a half decades. The annual symposium held in June every year has been well received and has become one of the most awaited events in the annual critical care calendar. The content of the symposium is always carefully curated and compiled to encompass recent advances and emerging paradigms. Certain concepts such as mechanical power and point-of-care coagulation testing were discussed in the symposium several years before they became clinical realities. The team therefore felt that it would be appropriate to compile all the interesting practices influencing publications over the year and bring these out in the format of a book. This yearbook is a result of this thought process.

The editorial team identified some of the most academically accomplished teachers and practitioners of intensive care to summarize the best publications of 2022–2023. They were then allocated specific sections and were given a brief to identify the noteworthy publications. Their analysis of the information whetted by their experience is what makes this yearbook unique and worth a read.

We hope you find this publication useful and will recommend it to others. We promise to make this an annual feature with wider scope in the years to come.

Srinivas Samavedam
Ganshyam Jagathkar

Contents

SECTION 1   **Cardiac/Hemodynamics/Fluids** 1
Section Editor: Supradip Ghosh
Associate Editors: Ripenmeet Salhotra, Amandeep Singh,
Aditya Lyall, Saurabh Kumar Rai

SECTION 2   **Respiratory/Ventilation/Acute Respiratory Distress Syndrome** 33
Section Editor: Manoj Y Singh

SECTION 3   **Neurocritical Care**.. 39
Section Editor: Ketan Kargirwar
Associate Editor: Sanket Hansora

SECTION 4   **Gastroenterology/Hepatobiliary** 54
Section Editor: Lalita Gouri Mitra
Associate Editors: Jagdeep Sharma, Harsimran Singh Walia

SECTION 5   **Nephrology**... 79
Section Editor: Kanwalpreet Sodhi
Associate Editors: Manu Gupta, Atul Phillips, Basjinder Kaur

SECTION 6   **Infections and Antibiotics** 116
Section Editor: Sumesh Arora

SECTION 7   **Sepsis** 135
Section Editor: Jaicob Varghese
Associate Editors: Nilanjan Umesh, Melwin George

SECTION 8   **Hematology** 144
Section Editor: Deven Juneja
Associate Editor: Sahil Kataria

SECTION 9   **Sonography/Imaging**... 161
Section Editor: Shrikanth Srinivasan
Associate Editors: NVSN Prasant, Velmurugan Selvam, Magesh Parthiban,
Vetriselvan P, Vadhan Prasanna S

SECTION 10   **Nutrition and Metabolic** 175
Section Editor: Sivakumar MN
Associate Editor: Lakshmikanthcharan S

SECTION 11   **Guidelines**... 195
Section Editors: Gunjan Chanchalani, Ranajit Chatterjee
Associate Editors: Lalit Gupta, Seema S Tekwani

Index *217*

Section 1

Cardiac/Hemodynamics/Fluids

Section Editor: Supradip Ghosh
Associate Editors: Ripenmeet Salhotra, Amandeep Singh, Aditya Lyall, Saurabh Kumar Rai

---

ARTICLE 1

Direct Assessment of Microcirculation in Shock: A Randomized-controlled Multicenter Study

Bruno RR, Wollborn J, Fengler K, Flick M, Wunder C, Allgäuer S, et al. Direct assessment of microcirculation in shock: a randomized-controlled multicenter study.
Intensive Care Med. 2023;49:645-55.

CLINICAL QUESTION

Could the utilization of sublingual microcirculatory perfusion variables in the therapeutic management of patients admitted to the intensive care unit (ICU) with shock reduce 30-day mortality?

WHAT IS ALREADY KNOWN?

- Microcirculation (vessel diameter <100 µm) is responsible for maintaining this supply of oxygen and substrates at tissue level and homeostasis.[1] In circulatory shock, there is impairment at the level of microcirculation leading to tissue hypoperfusion.
- Resuscitation strategies aim to restore microcirculatory function with an ultimate aim to restore tissue perfusion. Currently, several parameters are used to monitor resuscitation strategies that indirectly reflect states of microcirculation, e.g., lactate, mottling score, or capillary refill time (CRT).[2]
- Several image-based direct visualization devices have been developed to assess microcirculation directly such as sidestream dark field (SDF) cameras. Images obtained by these devices from the sublingual mucosa have been suggested as appropriate surrogate parameter for whole body microcirculation.[3] Several studies have clearly established significant correlation between the severity of microcirculatory disturbances observed by these devices and outcome of critically ill patients.[4,5]
- One of the criticisms against the wider use of these devices is lack of standardization in interpreting data obtained. More recently, automated analysis of the video

sequences by the AVA 4.3C software has been developed for quick objectification of microcirculatory variables avoiding any subjectivity.[6]
- Current study aims to assess impact of microcirculatory assessment using this automated algorithm during shock resuscitation on clinical outcome as well as on the decision-making process.

STUDY DESIGN

This study was a randomized prospective, clinical multicenter trial conducted at different hospitals in Germany.

POPULATION STUDIED

- Adult patients (≥18 years) with circulatory shock at ICU admission were enrolled. Shock was defined as requirement of vasopressor despite adequate fluid resuscitation and elevated lactates (>2 mmol/L).
- *Exclusion criteria*:
  - Inaccessibility of sublingual mucosa
  - Lack of consent
  - Impracticality to attain measurements such as uncooperative patients, weakly sedated patients, or infectious reasons like coronavirus.
- Patients were randomized to either "Intervention Group" or "Control Group" based on randomization performed using sealed envelopes by neutral person in blocks of 50 (25 per group).

INTERVENTION GROUP

- Sublingual measurements of microcirculation were done using MicroScan USB3 video microscope at ICU admission (within 4 hours), periodically thereafter and at 24 hours (±4 hours) after ICU admission.
- Four highest quality videos at different location were evaluated using an algorithm and the average was then calculated.
- Percentage of perfused small vessels (sPPV) and others microcirculatory parameters were calculated using automated algorithm. According to protocol, patients were divided into three risk categories on admission based on sPPV values (≤80% red, 81–94%: yellow, and ≥95%: green).
- Recommendations based on microcirculatory assessments were as follows:
  - Resuscitate till sPPV is >80%.
  - If central venous pressure (CVP) is low and sPPV is >80%, be careful in increasing CVP to 12 mm Hg or higher
  - If baseline sPPV <80%, then increase mean arterial pressure (MAP) only
  - If baseline sPPV >80%, then to be careful with increasing MAP >65 mm Hg
  - Consider to increase cardiac output only if baseline sPPV <80%
- Use of inotropes or vasodilator drugs were not restricted as per protocol.
- One hour after first microcirculation-based assessment, dosing data of fluids and vasoactive drugs were obtained from medical records and compared with dosing data at time of first microcirculation assessment, and documented if these were increased, reduced, started, or stopped.

CONTROL GROUP

- Patients in control group were treated as per usual practice including all decisions pertaining to hemodynamic and perfusion-related monitoring.
- Microcirculatory assessments were done in the control group too, but the results were not informed to treating physician.

OUTCOMES
- 987 patients were screened out of which 141 were included in the study, 69 patients in intervention group and 72 patients in the control group.
- There was no significant difference between the two group regarding age, comorbidities, sequential organ failure assessment (SOFA) score at admission and cause of ICU admission. The most common cause of shock was sepsis and cardiogenic in both the group.
- *Primary outcome*: Crude 30-day mortality was not statistically different between the two group [34.7% control group vs. 47.1% intervention group, relative risk (RR) 1.39 (0.91–1.97)]. In Cox regression analysis, 30-day mortality did not differ between the two group [hazard ratio (HR) 1.54, 95% confidence interval (CI) 0.90–2.66, $p = 0.118$]
- *Secondary outcome*: In the interventional group, significantly more patients received an adjustment (increase or decrease) in vasoactive drugs or fluids (66.7% vs. 41.8%, $p = 0.009$) within the next hour.
  - All-cause mortality at 6 months did not differ between the two groups—crude 44.4% control group versus 55.1% intervention group, RR 1.23 (95% CI 0.89–1.71), cox regression analysis (HR 1.38, 95% CI 0.86–2.11, $p = 0.189$).
  - No statistically significant difference between length of ICU stay and length of hospital stay was reported.

AUTHORS' VIEWPOINT
- This study revealed that real-time data on microcirculatory status significantly influenced the management of different kind of shock.
- Authors feel this study generated valuable technical data of real-time microcirculation assessment for management of patients with shock due to various reasons.
- Management of shock aims at normalizing MAP, but a normal MAP may not achieve improved microcirculation, on the other hand elevated surrogate marker of microcirculation, e.g., lactates may not always mean tissue hypoperfusion. Authors feel that real-time microcirculation assessment can aid the clinician by providing important information of tissue perfusion and help them in titration of fluid or vasopressors.
- Authors feel that this study opens the way to further analyze the use of real-time microcirculation assessment in management of shock and further studies may find out best interventions based on different patterns of microcirculatory derangement.

STRENGTHS OF THE STUDY
- This is the first randomized study evaluating the effectiveness of an automated algorithm to assess microcirculation during resuscitation of shock.
- Being a multicenter study, its results may be fairly generalizable.
- All types of shock were included including septic and cariogenic.

DRAWBACKS OF THE STUDY
- Obtaining quality video sequence of sublingual measurements in itself highly subjective. All uncooperative and weakly sedated patients were simply excluded.
- This study was logistically supported by MicroVision medical, although protocol design and data interpretation were independent of the company.

- Different types of shock may have different microcirculatory dysfunctions, this was not addressed.

REVIEWERS' VIEWPOINT

- Sublingual measurements of microcirculation require specialized equipment and software, can be subjective, require time and expertise in interpretation, and may not be an ideal tool while managing patients with shock especially in recourse limited facility.
- Study result does not impact clinical outcome of included patients. This can either be explained by futility of assessing microcirculatory parameters or lack of intervention directly affecting microcirculation or lack of validity of current measurement methods or simply lack of adequate power of the study itself.
- Further studies are required to elucidate impact of microcirculation assessment-based resuscitation of various subset of shock.

ARTICLE 2
Restriction of Intravenous Fluid in ICU Patients with Septic Shock

Meyhoff TS, Hjortrup PB, Wetterslev J, Sivapalan P, Laake JH, Cronhjort M, et al. Restriction of intravenous fluid in ICU patients with septic shock.
N Engl J Med. 2022;386:2459-70.

CLINICAL QUESTION

After initial resuscitation of patients admitted with septic shock in the ICU, does a restrictive fluid approach as compared to standard fluid therapy decrease the all-cause mortality at 90 days?

WHAT IS ALREADY KNOWN?

- In patients with septic shock intravenous (IV) fluid boluses are given with an aim to increase in mean systemic filling pressure and subsequent venous return and cardiac output with the ultimate target of achieving optimal end organ perfusion.
- However, several observational studies have established a clear association between higher cumulative fluid volume and poor patient outcome.[7,8] In a randomized study in pediatric population from resource-limited setting fluid boluses have actually shown to increased mortality.[9]
- With growing concerns about possible harmful effects of fluid overload, there is now an increasing demand for conservative fluid management in patients of septic shock, supported by systematic review and meta-analysis.[10,11]
- In an earlier pilot study by the same research group, confirmed the feasibility of conducting a larger study using restrictive fluid management protocol in septic shock.[12] The protocol was shown to reduce resuscitation volume in adult patients with septic shock compared to standard management. There was also a trend toward improved patient-centered outcome in restrictive group.
- The current study was planned to test the hypothesis whether a restrictive fluid strategy will have impact on meaningful clinical outcome in patients with septic shock.

STUDY DESIGN

- This study was an international, parallel group, stratified, open label, randomized clinical trial conducted in 31 ICUs in Denmark, Norway, Sweden Italy, Switzerland, Belgium, United Kingdom, and Czech republic.
- The study period was from November 2018 to November 2021.

POPULATION STUDIED

- Adult patients (≥18 years) admitted in ICU with septic shock. Septic shock was defined as presence of suspected or confirmed infection with plasma lactate of 2 mmol/L or higher, requirement of vasopressor, or inotropic agent and has received at least 1 liter of IV fluids within 24 hours before screening.
- Onset of shock within 12 hours before screening.
- Following patients were excluded from the study:
  - Shock onset >12 hours
  - Consent not given
  - Patients with life-threatening bleeding
  - Acute burns with >10% body surface area involved
  - Pregnant patients.

INTERVENTION GROUP

In the restrictive fluid group, 250–500 mL fluid boluses (isotonic crystalloids) could be given only under four conditions:
1. If patient had evidence of severe hypoperfusion, defined as plasma lactate of at least 4 mmol/L, MAP <50 mm Hg despite vasopressor support, mottling beyond kneecap (mottling score >2), or urine output <0.1 mL/kg/h in first 2 hours of randomization.
2. To replace documented fluid losses (drains, gastrointestinal)
3. To correct electrolyte abnormalities and dehydration when enteral route was contraindicated.
4. To ensure daily intake of 1 liter (including dilution fluids for medications and nutrition).

CONTROL GROUP

- No upper limit set for the amount of fluids that could be given in this group.
- Intravenous fluids could be given on three conditions:
  1. Intravenous fluids were given till patients had improvement in hemodynamic parameters (as per 2016 surviving sepsis guidelines).
  2. For correction of expected or observed fluid losses and to correct electrolyte abnormalities and dehydration
  3. Maintenance fluids as per admitting ICU's protocol
- Following interventions were common in both groups:
  - Albumin to be given only during abdominal paracentesis
  - Isotonic crystalloids used
  - Other interventions for septic shock as per trial protocol (appropriate antibiotics, source control, norepinephrine as vasopressor, and renal replacement therapy (RRT) as per routine indications)
  - Diuretics were given as per discretion of the treating doctor.

OUTCOMES

- *Study process*: 2,223 patients were screened and 1,554 underwent randomization.
  - Finally, 764 patients were included in the intervention group and 781

patients were included in the control group for primary analysis.
- Others screened were excluded due to exclusion criteria, withdrew consent and loss of follow-up.
- There was no difference in baseline characteristics between the two groups. Most common source of infection was gastrointestinal followed by pulmonary infections.
- *Primary outcome*: Death by day-90 was not statistically different.
  - Intervention group (restrictive fluid group)—42.3% versus control group (standard fluid group—42.1%). Adjusted absolute difference 0.1 (95% CI −4.7–4.9), $p = 0.96$.
- *Secondary outcome*: There was no significant differences observed in:
  - Serious adverse events
  - No of days alive without life support (mechanical ventilation, vasopressors, or RRT)
  - No of days alive and out of hospital.

AUTHORS' VIEWPOINT

- The authors concluded that in adult patients admitted to ICU with septic shock, IV fluid restriction did not result in fewer deaths at 90 days than standard IV fluid therapy.
- Authors admit that the results of this trial are different from some observational studies which have shown harm from higher fluid volumes but they feel that the concerned studies might have been biased by indication and time-dependent exposure.
- The authors also feel that results may differ in settings where comparatively more IV fluids are given in standard care.

STRENGTHS OF THE STUDY

- The fact that trial was conducted in different countries in 31 different ICUs increases validity and generalizability (at least in advanced healthcare settings).
- Good matching of baseline characteristics
- A very important research question raised as the concerned area has lack of evidence.
- Intention to treat analysis
- Loss of follow-up in only 0.6% cases.

DRAWBACKS OF THE STUDY

- One of the drawbacks of such trial is lack of blinding, which is not possible given the nature of the intervention.
- Giving fluid boluses to patients with lactate 4 mmol/L or MAP <50 mm Hg despite vasopressor support or mottling score >2 or urine output <0.1 mL/kg/h without looking for fluid responsiveness or fluid tolerance, as suggested by the intervention protocol, probably lacks scientific rationale.
- Protocol violations were observed in large number of patients in both groups—21.5% patients in restricted group (fluid boluses administered without criteria being fulfilled) and 13% patients in standard fluid group (no IV fluid given on any single day in ICU).
- Majority of patients had gastrointestinal tract as infection source that may have required large fluid volume replacements.
- Both the groups received almost 3 L fluid before randomization (outside volumes specified by trial protocol).
- Authors calculated the power of study based on a 7% absolute difference in mortality between the two groups, which is probably much of an expectation from a single intervention in varied population of patients studied.

- Cumulative fluid difference between both groups on day 5 was only about 890 mL that is not possibly a clinically meaningful difference.

■ REVIEWERS' VIEWPOINT

- Harmful consequences of cumulative fluid volume depend on a large number of factors including severity of illness, nature of the acute conditions (septic shock due to pneumonia versus abdominal sepsis), comorbidities (e.g., chronic kidney disease or chronic heart failure), and amount of fluids administered. Planning a study without taking into consideration, all these factors can make the generalizability of the results doubtful.
- Small difference in cumulative volume between two groups (890 mL at day-5) makes us to consider whether the standard care provided in the control group already conservative in its approach to fluid therapy.
- The debate regarding restrictive versus liberal fluid will still continue to go on. In the meantime, IV fluid should be considered just like any other drug where its use should be justified and should be tailored as per each patient's clinical requirement.

ARTICLE 3

Aggressive or Moderate Fluid Resuscitation in Acute Pancreatitis

de-Madaria E, Buxbaum JL, Maisonneuve P, García García de Paredes A, Zapater P, Guilabert L, et al. Aggressive or moderate fluid resuscitation in acute pancreatitis.
N Engl J Med. 2022;387:989-1000.

■ CLINICAL QUESTION

Is moderate fluid resuscitation safer and more efficacious in preventing development of moderately severe and severe pancreatitis as compared to aggressive fluid resuscitation in a diverse sample of patients with acute pancreatitis?

■ WHAT IS ALREADY KNOWN?

- Early aggressive fluid resuscitation up to 250–500 mL/h or 5–10 mL/kg/h in acute pancreatitis has been recommended by several guidelines.[13] The rationale being presumed hypovolemia due to vomiting, reduced oral intake, and third spacing of fluids. It was hypothesized that hypovolemia may contribute to decreased blood flow to inflamed pancreas and promote development of necrosis.
- Several animal studies and some small human trials have shown that early aggressive fluid resuscitation, either empirically or targeting hematocrit or blood urea reduction, can prevent development of necrosis and improve outcomes.[14,15]
- However, some other studies and a systematic review and meta-analysis have linked aggressive fluid administration with worse outcomes including mortality as compared to moderate fluid resuscitation.[16-18] But these studies include only sicker (severe pancreatitis) patients and did not specifically target early (within 6–12 hours of onset) fluid administration.

- The systematic review included heterogenous and poor-quality studies.
- With this background, the authors planned to test their hypothesis whether less aggressive fluid resuscitation more beneficial in preventing development of severe pancreatitis in patients with acute pancreatitis.

STUDY DESIGN

- Multicenter, open-label, parallel-group, randomized, controlled, and superiority trial
- Included patients from 18 centers from 4 countries including (India, Italy, Mexico, and Spain). Most of the trial subjects, however, were from Spain.

POPULATION STUDIED

- Consecutive patients (≥18 years of age) diagnosed as acute pancreatitis according to the Revised Atlanta Classification.
  - Patients should have presented to the emergency department (ED) no >24 hours after pain onset and should have been diagnosed no >8 hours before enrolment.
- Following patients were excluded from the study:
  - Moderately severe or severe disease at baseline (presence of organ failure at baseline)
  - Who had baseline heart failure (New York Heart Association functional class II, III, or IV).
  - Who had uncontrolled arterial hypertension.
  - Who had hypernatremia, hyponatremia, hyperkalemia, and hypercalcemia.
  - Who had an estimated life expectancy of <1 year.
  - Patients with chronic pancreatitis, chronic renal failure, or decompensated cirrhosis
- Patients were randomly assigned in a 1:1 ratio to receive aggressive fluid resuscitation (aggressive resuscitation group) or moderate fluid resuscitation (moderate-resuscitation group) with the use of a computer-based central randomization system. The random-assignment sequence was concealed from the trial team.
- Randomization was stratified according to trial center, the presence or absence of systemic inflammatory response syndrome (SIRS), and the presence or absence of baseline hypovolemia.

INTERVENTION GROUP

In the moderate-resuscitation group, patients were given lactated Ringer's solution at a dose of 1.5 mL/kg/h (without a bolus in patients without hypovolemia or after receipt of a bolus of 10 mL per kilogram in patients with hypovolemia).

CONTROL GROUP

- In the aggressive-resuscitation group, a bolus of lactated Ringer's solution at a dose of 20 mL/kg of body weight, followed by infusion at a rate of 3 mL/kg/h.
- In both trial groups, an initial and subsequent physical and biochemical assessment was done at 3, 12, 24, 48, and 72 hours and resuscitation were adjusted on the basis of the presence of hypovolemia, normovolemia, or suspicion of fluid overload.
- Oral feeding was attempted at 12 hours in both groups. In case patients were able to tolerate orally, fluid resuscitation was terminated at 20 hours in moderate group but not earlier than 48 hours in aggressive group.

OUTCOMES

- Originally, sample size was calculated as 744. However, the study was terminated after the first interim analysis following enrollment of 249 patients (122 in aggressive-resuscitation group and 127 in moderate-resuscitation group) owing to between-group safety outcome.
- Baseline characteristics were similar in both groups including demographics, comorbidities, BISAP score, urea, creatinine, hematocrit, and percentage of patients with SIRS or hypovolemia.
- Patients in the aggressive-resuscitation group received a median of 7.8 liters (interquartile range, 6.5–9.8) of lactated Ringer's solution during the first 48 hours, as compared with 5.5 liters (interquartile range, 4.0–6.8) in the moderate-resuscitation group. The greatest between-group difference in volume administration occurred during the first 12 hours.
- *Primary outcome*: 22.1% of the patients in the aggressive-resuscitation group and in 17.3% of those in the moderate-resuscitation developed moderately severe or severe acute pancreatitis. The difference was not statistically significant (adjusted RR, 1.30; 95% CI, 0.78–2.18; $p = 0.32$).
- *Secondary outcomes*: Though there was a trend toward higher local complications including necrosis, persistent SIRS, ICU admission, organ failure, duration of hospitalization, and death in aggressive-resuscitation group, none were statistically significant.
- *Safety outcomes*: Significantly higher risk of fluid overload in aggressive-resuscitation group than moderate fluid resuscitation (20.5% vs. 6.3%; adjusted RR, 2.85; 95% CI, 1.36–5.94).
- Fluid overload was diagnosed with signs and symptoms of heart failure or echocardiographic or radiologic evidence of pulmonary congestion or with cardiac catheterization.
- *Subgroup analysis*: Subgroups with baseline hypovolemia and baseline SIRS did not yield findings different from overall analysis.

AUTHORS' VIEWPOINT

- Aggressive fluid resuscitation in patients with acute pancreatitis leads to increased harm (fluid overload) without any decrease in progression to moderately severe or severe pancreatitis, length of hospital stay, or mortality. In their opinion, the trial added to growing evidence of adverse effects of aggressive fluids in acutely ill patients.
- Authors, however, acknowledge several limitations. As trial was prematurely terminated due to safety concerns, it was underpowered to evaluate primary and secondary outcomes.

STRENGTHS OF STUDY

- The trial is first of its kind—multicenter, randomized, and clinical trial on the question of intensity of fluid resuscitation in these patients. Furthermore, intention to treat analysis was performed and there was no loss to follow up. Baseline characteristics were well matched.
- Protocol for fluid administration was well defined in both groups. Clear checkpoints were available for clinicians to detect hypovolemia and fluid overload and modify their prescription accordingly. Both hypovolemia and fluid overload were objectively defined and not based on subjective assessment.

- Furthermore, there were clearly defined primary and secondary outcomes including necrosis on imaging and organ failures.

DRAWBACKS OF STUDY

- Only patients with mild pancreatitis were included (BISAP score 0–1). Patients with organ failure at presentation (even though transient) were excluded. Thus, the trial population does not represent patients with a range of severity of disease.
- Though guidelines recommend aggressive fluid resuscitation even in patients with mild pancreatitis, these patients usually tolerate orally relatively early. Fluid resuscitation continued for 48 hours (as per protocol) even if patients taking oral fluids seems unnecessary.
- Fluid resuscitation was not based on targeting a decrease in biochemical parameters like blood urea or hematocrit which is recommended by several international guidelines but was based on fixed weight-based volumes. There is no mention of hemodynamic monitoring or tests of fluid responsiveness which could be used by clinicians to modify the resuscitation volume.
- The trial was unblinded which might have influenced the credibility of detection of fluid overload or hypovolemia by clinicians. For example, the treating clinician might overdiagnose fluid overload in aggressive-resuscitation group. However, blinding was difficult if not impossible considering the nature of interventions.
- Though trial sites were from three continents most of the patients were from Spain.
- Trial was underpowered to detect significant differences in efficacy outcomes and does not definitely rule out benefits of aggressive resuscitation, because of early termination related to safety concerns including need for mechanical ventilation or death.
- Lastly, no information was provided about the amount of fluid administered before randomization and what effect it had over total fluid difference between groups or outcomes.

REVIEWERS' VIEWPOINT

- Aggressive fluid administered in patients with mild pancreatitis as proposed by several guidelines may lead to increase harm in the form of fluid overload as compared to moderate fluid resuscitation but the fluid requirement of each patient must be reassessed frequently.
- However, results of this trial do not unequivocally exclude proposed benefits of aggressive fluid resuscitation including reduction in development of necrosis or organ failure.
- The reader is cautioned against extrapolating the results to patients with severe pancreatitis. Adequately powered trials which include mild-to-severe pancreatitis are a need of the hour.

ARTICLE 4

A Burden of Fluid, Sodium, and Chloride due to Intravenous Fluid Therapy in Patients with Respiratory Support: A Post-hoc Analysis of a Multicenter Cohort Study

Sakuraya M, Yoshihiro S, Onozuka K, Takaba A, Yasuda H, Shime N, et al. A burden of fluid, sodium, and chloride due to intravenous fluid therapy in patients with respiratory support: A post-hoc analysis of a multicenter cohort study.

Ann Intensive Care. 2022;12(1):100.

■ CLINICAL QUESTION

To address the burden due to fluid creep and total sodium and chloride load among patients admitted to critical care unit and receiving mechanical ventilation.

■ WHAT IS ALREADY KNOWN?

- Most if not all critically ill patients are prescribed IV fluids. Even though indispensable in some patients, inappropriate use can lead to fluid overload and increase morbidity as well as mortality. Major indications of fluid therapy are resuscitation and maintenance. Resuscitation fluids are administered early in acute illnesses to correct hypovolemia or to revert shock and maintenance fluids are given later in patients where enteral route is not able to fulfil their daily fluid requirement.[19]
- Of-late, another kind of fluid administered to these group of patients, have been recognized, which is an important source of overall fluid overload. This source of fluid known as "fluid creep" constitutes fluid administered as drug diluent and that is given for maintenance of catheter patency. Though clinicians may consider this paltry in total volume of fluid administered, several recent publications have proved that it comprises a major proportion of total fluid intake, especially in the later part of illness.[20,21]
- Besides fluid, total sodium and chloride load imposed on a critically ill patient may correlate with adverse respiratory and renal outcome.[22,23]
- Though several previous works have reported the contribution of fluid creep, none have studied it specifically in hypoxic and mechanically ventilated patients. These patients may require deep sedation and more vasopressors which may lead to more fluid creep. Fluid creep may also contribute to higher positive fluid balance in such patients with associated worse outcomes.

■ STUDY DESIGN

- The current study is a post-hoc analysis of the "incidence and risk factors for phlebitis and complications due to peripheral venous catheters in critically ill patients (AMOR-VENUS study)".[24]
- The AMOR-VENUS study was a prospective multicenter cohort study of the general ICU population conducted in 23 ICUs in Japan from January 1 to March 31, 2018 and aimed to address the epidemiology of peripheral intravascular catheter (PIVC)-related phlebitis and complications in critically ill patients.

POPULATION STUDIED

- The AMOR-VENUS study included all consecutive adult patients admitted to ICUs of study centers over 3 months of study duration. Excluded were those who refused to participate or had no intravascular catheters during their ICU stay.
- This post-hoc analyses selected only those patients who underwent invasive or noninvasive mechanical ventilation.
- Those discharged within 24 hours of admission, who didn't receive any IV fluids or in whom the ratio of arterial oxygen partial pressure (PaO_2) to fractional inspired oxygen (FiO_2) (P/F ratio) was not recorded were excluded from further analysis.

EXPOSURE AND COMPARATORS

- *Definitions and categorization of fluids*: Fluid therapy was categorized as resuscitation fluid, maintenance fluids, fluids for nutritional therapy (e.g., 25% dextrose solution), or fluid creep.
  - Fluid creep was defined as fluids for drug dilution and fluid administered for maintenance of IV catheters.
  - Fluid given at a rate >166 mL/h was categorized as resuscitation fluid and between 20 and 166 mL/h as maintenance fluid.
  - If administered, at <20 mL/h it was categorized as fluid for catheter patency.
- Besides, fluids could be isotonic or hypotonic crystalloids and fluid creep was further divided based on drugs—antibiotics, sedatives, analgesics, and vasoactive drugs.
- Fluid therapy data was collected till 7 days from admission.
- *Patients' categories*: Patients were divided into three categories based on baseline oxygenation status: (1) patients without hypoxemia (P/F ratio >300), (2) patients with mild hypoxemia (150 <P/F ratio ≤300), and (3) patients with severe hypoxemia (P/F ratio ≤150).

OUTCOMES

- Out of 3,482 patients included in the AMOR-VENUS data, 588 patients who underwent mechanical ventilation were selected for analysis and did not have any exclusion, were included in the analysis.
- 167 without hypoxemia, 297 with mild hypoxemia, and 124 with severe hypoxemia.
- The sample included medical (51%) and surgical (49%) patients. Median SOFA scores were 7, 20% had sepsis or septic shock, and ICU mortality was 7.5%.
- *Total fluid, sodium, and chloride*:
  - A mean total IV fluid volume of 2,662 (range, 1,646–4,059) mL was administered during the first 24 hours after ICU admission.
  - The total amount of IV fluid gradually decreased but remained >1,000 mL/24 h during the entire observation period (7 days).
  - Isotonic crystalloid was the main IV fluid administered within 24 hours, after which hypotonic fluid accounted to major fluid. About 20% of total fluid administered was isotonic even in later part but not in patients with severe hypoxemia.
  - Estimated mean of 300 mEq of both sodium and chloride were administered in first 24 hours that decreased subsequently to 100 mEq/24 h.

- *Fluid creep*:
  - Median fluid creep during first 24 hours was 661 mL (range: 402–984 mL) or 25.2% of total IV volume. Vehicle for antibiotics leads to most administered volume.
  - Total fluid as fluid creep decreased after 24 hours but not in patients with severe hypoxemia.
  - Proportion of fluid creep in total IV fluid increased after 24 hours.
  - Proportion of sodium and chloride load due to fluid creep increased after 24 hours.
  - The most used drug vehicle was normal saline.
- *Multivariate analysis*:
  - Association of septic shock and hypoxemic respiratory failure with total fluids and fluid creep in first 24 hours was tested with a multivariate linear regression model.
  - Overall, septic shock was associated with an increased total fluid volume, sodium, and chloride burdens. However, septic shock was not associated with an increased fluid volume, sodium, and chloride burdens due to fluid creep.
  - In contrast, hypoxemic respiratory failure was associated with a reduction in the total amount of IV fluids, sodium, and chloride. However, hypoxemic respiratory failure was not associated with a reduction in the IV fluids, sodium, and chloride due to fluid creep.

AUTHORS' VIEWPOINT
- This study emphasizes the role of "fluid creep" as a major source of fluid volume, sodium, and chloride burdens.
- Fluid creep tends to decrease throughout ICU days in patients without hypoxemia and in those with mild hypoxemia, but no significant trend was observed in those with severe hypoxemia.
- Sodium and chloride load due to fluid creep was higher in patients with severe hypoxemia and its proportion increased in later part of observation.
- Authors recommend that fluid creep should not be overlooked as a source of IV fluid volume, especially in patients with severe hypoxemia.

STRENGTHS OF THE STUDY
This is the first study to quantify "fluid creep" as well as sodium and chloride load according to oxygenation in adult mechanically ventilated patients, thus providing an important and novel insight in this subgroup of critically ill patients.

DRAWBACKS OF THE STUDY
- Most of the limitations were related to design, being a post-hoc analysis of a prospective observational study conducted for answering another research question, thus limiting the data available.
- No data was available for enteral intake, as the original research focused on use of IV catheters in critically ill patients.
- Data pertaining to urine output which influences the cumulative fluid balance was not available.
- Though authors defined resuscitative fluid as—isotonic crystalloids administered at a certain rate, it was not explicitly labeled in the data set and one cannot be sure as the prescription really meant resuscitative or maintenance fluid.
- No analysis on important outcome data like how mortality and liberation from

mechanical ventilation were associated with fluid creep was provided. Data on oxygenation status was available only for first 24 hours of study enrolment, how subsequent recovery or worsening of hypoxia-influenced fluid therapy, cannot be inferred.
- Lastly, data was exclusively collected from Japanese centers and generalizability to other countries is limited.

■ REVIEWERS' VIEWPOINT
- The study provides fresh knowledge on how hypoxic respiratory failure influences the amount of fluid therapy and fluid creep.
- The study provides important insights to the clinicians caring for the critically ill about the significant contribution of fluid creep to overall fluid overload and importance of actively limiting "fluid creep" to improve patient outcomes.

ARTICLE 5
Restrictive Fluids versus Standard Care in Adults with Sepsis in the Emergency Department (REFACED): A Multicenter, Randomized Feasibility Trial

Jessen MK, Andersen LW, Thomsen MH, Kristensen P, Hayeri W, Hassel RE, et al. Restrictive fluids versus standard care in adults with sepsis in the emergency department (REFACED): A multicenter, randomized feasibility trial.
Acad Emerg Med. 2022;29(10):1172-84.

■ CLINICAL QUESTION
Is it feasible to develop a restrictive IV fluid protocol for ED patients with sepsis without shock and could this protocol decrease volume of IV fluids administered compared to standard care?

■ WHAT IS ALREADY KNOWN?
- Large volume IV fluid is commonly administered in ED especially in the setting of infection, sepsis, and septic shock. In an observational study from three Danish EDs, mean total volume administered over 24 hours in patients with simple infection, sepsis and septic shock were 3,656 mL [standard deviation (SD): 1,675), 3,762 mL (SD: 1,839), and 6,080 mL (SD: 3,978), respectively].[25]
- Fluid boluses are recommended in patients with septic shock aiming at improving cardiac output, which in turn potentially improve tissue perfusion.[2]
- However, role of prophylactic fluid administration in patients with sepsis without shock needs to be studied. Such prophylactic fluid administration had failed to show any beneficial effects in other settings and might even be potentially harmful.[26]
- Several observational studies have also shown an increased mortality and other adverse outcome associated with increasing cumulative fluid balance.[7,8]
- With this background, it is important to see whether it is feasible to restrict fluid volumes in ED patients with sepsis and no shock.

STUDY DESIGN

- This study was an investigator initiated, multicenter, randomized, parallel-group, and open-label feasibility trial.
- The study was conducted in three EDs from Denmark including one University hospital and two regional hospitals and was registered with EU Clinical Trials Register (NCT05076435).

POPULATION STUDIED

- Patients fulfilling all the following criteria were included in the study:
  - Adult patients ≥18 years
  - Unplanned ED admission
  - Sepsis defined as (1) infection suspected by the treating clinician, (2) blood cultures drawn, (3) IV antibiotics administered or planned, and (3) an infection-related increase in the SOFA score ≥2
  - Expected hospital stay >24 hours
- Following patients were excluded from the study:
  - Received ≥500 mL of IV fluids before screening
  - Vasopressors or invasive ventilation started prior to screening
  - Known or suspected severe bleeding judged by the treating clinician
  - Known or suspected pregnancy
  - Not expected to survive the next 24-hours
- All eligible patients were randomly assigned to either restrictive IV fluid administration or standard care groups, in a 1:1 ratio. Randomization was performed using a computer-generated allocation sequence list with varying block sizes stratified by site.
- The assigned treatment protocol was followed in the ED as well as wards or ICUs if the patient was transferred within the 24-hour period.

INTERVENTION GROUP

- A fluid bolus of 250 mL of 350 mL crystalloid could be administered if one or more of the flowing criteria were met. However, it was not a requirement that a fluid bolus was to be administered.
  - Lactate concentration ≥4 mmol/L (arterial or venous)
  - Hypotension [systolic blood pressure (SBP) <90 mm Hg]
  - Mottling beyond edge of kneecap (i.e., Mottling score >2)
  - Severe oliguria defined as urine output <0.1 mL/kg/h in the first 4 hours of admission.
- Treating physician was allowed to violate the protocol and administer additional fluid boluses, if judged to be necessary. However, the physician had to state the reason for violating the protocol.
- IV fluids could be given as carrier for medications (but volume should be reduced if possible) or as replacement for volume lost or as maintenance fluid (if oral/enteral route is contraindicated) or to correct significant electrolyte deficiencies or to ensure a total fluid input of 1 L/24 h (counting all fluids including medications and nutrition).
- Protocol was paused temporarily if a patient underwent surgery during the 24-hour inclusion period. However, clinicians were encouraged to continue restrictive fluid therapy.

CONTROL GROUP

Administration of fluids was at the discretion of clinician.

OUTCOMES

- From November 3, 2021, to December 18, 2021, 2,412 patients were screened, out of whom 383 patients met all inclusion criteria and no exclusion criteria. Finally, 124 patients were randomized—62 patients were assigned to the fluid restriction group and 62 were allocated to the standard care group.
- *Feasibility assessment*: 32% (95% CI 28–37%) of patients meeting all inclusion criteria and no exclusion criteria could be finally included for the study.
  - Baseline characteristics randomized patients and nonrandomized patients were more or less similar at admission.
  - Median (IQR) time from ED admission to randomization was 140 (90–194) minutes.
- Baseline variables were well matched in both intervention groups.
- *Primary outcome*: Mean IV crystalloid volumes at 24-hour were significantly less in the intervention group: 562 (±1,076) mL versus 1,370 (±1,438) mL; mean difference −801 mL (−1257 to −345; $p = 0.001$).
  - This corresponds to a relative decrease in fluid volume by 58%.
  - Median difference was −1,000 mL (95% CI −1,392 to −607).
- 38 of 61 (62%) patients in the restrictive group and 15 of 62 (24%) patients in the standard care group received no IV crystalloid fluids in the first 24 hours.
- *Secondary outcome*: Mean (±SD) of combined oral and IV fluids in the first 24 hours was 2,881 (±1,295) mL in the restrictive group versus 3,720 (±1,623) mL in the standard care group with a mean difference of −840 mL (95% CI −1,364 to −317, $p = 0.002$).
  - There were no significant between group differences in use of mechanical ventilation or initiation of vasopressors or new-onset acute kidney failure at 7 days.
  - There were no differences in-hospital, 30-day, 90-day mortality, or in-hospital length of stay.
- Fluid boluses were administered in 21 of 61 patients despite no criteria fulfilled (protocol violation).

AUTHORS' VIEWPOINT

- The authors concluded that a larger randomized trial is feasible comparing a restrictive fluid protocol with standard care in ED patients with sepsis without shock.
- Despite low randomization to screening ratio, preplanned sample size of 124 patients could be quickly recruited within 6 weeks and the restrictive protocol could significantly reduce 24-hour IV fluid volume.

STRENGTHS OF THE STUDY

- This is the first of its kind study comparing a restrictive fluid strategy with standard care in ED patients with sepsis without shock.
- Inclusion of multiple centers including both teaching and nonteaching hospitals is a big plus for the study.
- Speed at which researchers could recruit their patients in the study is commendable.
- Despite a relatively long delay of 140 minutes between screening to randomization, most patients received no fluid before randomization.

- Inclusion of broad patient populations including older age group, patients with do-not-attempt resuscitation order, or those who are unable to consent, makes the results of the study more generalizable.

DRAWBACKS OF THE STUDY

- Scientific rational behind conducting this study is questionable. Why should a sepsis patient without shock be administered fluid boluses? However, this seems to be a common practice in study EDs, as seen by the observational study published earlier.
- The study was nonblinded. Although considering the nature of the intervention, it is highly improbable to perform blinding in this setting.
- No advanced hemodynamic parameters were used before fluid administration. But this may be okay in the ED setting.
- No differences were observed in mortality or hospital length of stay or adverse effects between groups. The study was not adequately powered to confirm or refute any such differences.

REVIEWERS' VIEWPOINT

Introduction of a fluid restriction protocol can reduce unnecessary fluid administration in ED patients with sepsis and not in shock. In fact, fluid volume administered in the control group of current study is much lower compared to earlier observational study from the same group.

ARTICLE 6

Early Restrictive or Liberal Fluid Management for Sepsis-induced Hypotension

Shapiro NI, Douglas IS, Brower RG, Brown SM, Exline MC, Ginde AA, et al. Early restrictive or liberal fluid management for sepsis-induced hypotension.
N Engl J Med. 2023;388:499-510.

CLINICAL QUESTION

In patients with sepsis-induced hypotension refractory to initial treatment, does a restrictive fluid strategy (with prioritizing vasopressor usage) in first 24 hours of resuscitation, compared to a liberal fluid strategy result in lower all-cause mortality before discharge by day 90?

WHAT IS ALREADY KNOWN?

- Intravenous fluids are widely prescribed in sepsis-induced hypotension with an aim to restore tissue perfusion by potentially increasing cardiac output and MAP. However, fluid therapy is also associated with potential harm including dilutional coagulopathy, fluid overload, and pathological tissue edema.[27]
- Vasopressors are also commonly used in sepsis resuscitation aiming to quickly restore blood pressure, as well as for potentiating improvement in cardiac output by their venopressor effect (and increment in venous return). However, vasopressor therapy comes at a potential cost of tissue ischemia, arrhythmias, and increased cardiac workload.[28]
- Current guidelines suggest administration of large volume IV fluids before initiation

of vasopressors in sepsis-induced hypoperfusion, which is based on low-quality evidence.[2]
- Based on physiological factors, data from observational studies and from small-randomized studies, there is strong rationale in favor of using lesser volume of fluid along with early initiation of vasopressor during sepsis resuscitation.[29] However, a recent large-randomized control study showed no difference in outcomes when comparing restrictive fluid approach compared to standard fluid strategy.
- In the absence of robust data to guide fluids and vasopressor, there is wide practice variability around the appropriate approach to their use especially in the early stage of sepsis resuscitation. Current trial compares the effects of a restrictive fluid strategy (with early use of vasopressors) to a liberal fluid strategy in first 24 hours of sepsis resuscitation.

STUDY DESIGN
- Multicenter, randomized, unblinded superiority trial conducted in 60 US centers, from March 2018 to January 2022.
- The study was funded by NHLBI as a part of Prevention and Early treatment of Acute Lung Injury (PETAL) network.

POPULATION STUDIED
- Adult patients (≥18 years) with suspected or confirmed infection and sepsis-induced hypotension defined as SBP <100 mm Hg after administration of >1,000 mL of IV fluid were included.
- Patients were excluded from the study if the fulfil any of the following criteria:
  - >4 hours since meeting inclusion criteria for sepsis-induced hypotension
  - >24 hours since hospital presentation
  - >3 L IV fluid therapy (including prehospital)
  - Inability to obtain informed consent
  - Pregnancy
  - Evidence of fluid overload
  - Blood pressure is not known or not reported at baseline level
  - Hypotension suspected to be from nonsepsis cause
  - Severe volume depletion from non-sepsis causes
- Patients were randomly assigned using web-based system to either restrictive fluid group or liberal group.

INTERVENTION GROUP
- Restrictive fluid protocol prioritizing vasopressor as the primary treatment for treating hypotension.
- If SBP <100 mm Hg or MAP <65 mm Hg after receipt of 1–3 liters of crystalloid, restrictive fluid strategy is initiated.
  - All bolus and maintenance fluids halted
  - However, up to 2 liters of total fluid boluses were allowed if not already received (including pre-enrolment pretreatment fluid) at discretion of treating team.
- If still mean arterial pressure < 65 mm Hg or SBP <90 mm Hg, titration of vasopressor to achieve MAP >65.
  - Once MAP in target then fluids limited medications and nutrition
- Rescue fluid (500 mL bolus) recommended if:
  - Severe hypotension (SBP <70, MAP <50 mm Hg)
  - Refractory hypotension (SBP <90 or MAP <65 on norepinephrine >20 μg min or equivalent)
  - Rising lactate (value of 4 mmol/L and increasing after 2 hours of therapy)

- Evidence of hypovolemia on echocardiographic evaluation
- Need felt by treating team.

CONTROL GROUP

- Control group received liberal fluid strategy.
- If SBP <100 mm Hg or MAP <65 mm Hg after receiving of 1–3 liters of crystalloid.
  - Halt all maintenance
  - Give 2 liters of additional crystalloid at randomization (to be completed in 180 minutes)
  - Clinical assessment at 1 liter if volume replete forego 2nd liter
- Further 500-mL fluid bolus to be given if:
  - MAP <65 mm Hg
  - Lactate >4 mmol/L and increasing
  - Sinus tachycardia (heart rate >110/min)
  - Requirement of vasopressors to maintain SBP 90 mm Hg or MAP 65 mm Hg
  - Clinical assessment or measured assessment
- Rescue vasopressors allowed if severe hypotension (defined as per restrictive group), lactate >4 mmol/L and increasing after 2 hours, >5 liter total IV fluid given, clinical evidence of fluid overload or treating team felt it to be in best interest of patient.
- All other treatment options were similar in both groups and were at the discretion of treating physician.

OUTCOMES

- 1,563 patients enrolled, out of which 782 assigned to restrictive group and 781 to liberal group.
- Patients in both the groups had similar baseline characteristics and treatment before randomization.
- Both groups received similar volumes of IV fluid before randomization (median 2,050 mL in each group).
- Protocol guided treatments:
  - *At 6 hours after randomization*: Volume of fluid in restrictive versus liberal was median of 500 mL and 2,300 mL, respectively.
  - *At 24 hours after randomization*: Volume of fluid was of median of 1,267 mL in restrictive and 3,400 mL in liberal group.
  - *Vasopressors use in first 24 hours*: 59% patients in restrictive versus 37% patients in liberal group
- *Primary/efficacy outcome*: Death before discharge home by day 90: 14.0% in restrictive group versus 14.9% in liberal group with estimated difference −0.9% (95% CI −4.4–2.6), $p = 0.61$.
- *Safety outcomes*: At 28 days, no significant difference was observed in two groups.
  - Days free from ventilator use
  - Days out of ICU from day 1 to day 28
  - Free from organ support therapy
  - No significant difference in new onset of ARDS was observed between day 1 and day 7.
- *Adverse effects:*
  - Fewer reported adverse events of pulmonary edema in restrictive vs liberal group (0 vs. 3, respectively)
  - Peripheral extravasation of vasopressor in 3 patients among 500 patients who received peripheral vasopressor
- Post-hoc analysis revealed higher rate of ICU admission in restrictive group at 24 hours (67% vs. 59%) and at 7 days (70% vs. 62%)
- No subgroup favored any particular type of fluid strategy.

AUTHORS' VIEWPOINT

- Authors conclude that for the types of patients enrolled in CLOVERS trial, prioritization of either a vasopressor-predominant or fluid-predominant approach resulted in similar patient-centered outcomes.
- They emphasize that since the types of patients included in the trial were representative of patients who present to the hospital with sepsis-induced hypotension, the results of the study is broadly generalizable. However, trial results may not be generalizable patient subgroups such as patients with extremes of volume overload or volume depletion, as they were excluded from the study.
- Authors acknowledge that there may exist some subgroup of patients identifiable with more sophisticated clinical or biologic measurements (e.g., biomarkers to classify subphenotypes) who may still get benefit from preferential use of one approach over other.

STRENGTHS OF THE STUDY

- Biggest strength of the current study is inclusion of large number of patients from multiple centers and randomizing them into two clearly defined groups.
- Protocolized care was provided in both groups.
- Adequately followed both the groups for primary outcome till day 90.
- High adherence to trial protocol was observed in audited patients from both groups—97% in restrictive group and 96% in liberal group.
- There was a clear separation between groups in terms of the amount of fluid given.

DRAWBACKS OF THE STUDY

- The study was limited to a single country (United States).
- Unblinded nature of the study might have introduced some bias to the study. However, given the nature of the study, it may be difficult to achieve blinding.
- Exclusion of certain subgroups of patients might have missed the opportunity to assess whether some specific population might be benefited by a particular approach.
- In the absence of a usual care arm, the study cannot infer about the differences, if any, between both protocolized approach and an unstructured approach.
- Patients enrolled did not seem that sick (baseline mean SBP 93.5 mm Hg and lactate of 2.9 mmol/L).
- Certain interventions suggested by the protocol may not have strong scientific evidence. Example, fluid boluses advised in the liberal group if heart rate is >110 beats/min.
- Advanced hemodynamic assessments like tests for fluid responsiveness or fluid tolerance were not performed routinely in the study population.
- Complete adherence to protocol could not be ensured in the study with some patients in restrictive group receiving vasopressors later than intended and some patients in liberal group receiving lesser fluid volume.

REVIEWERS' VIEWPOINT

- Comparison between two "one-size-fit all" approach in patients with sepsis-induced hypotension failed to show any benefit of one approach over another.

- Sepsis resuscitation should be individualized with thoughtful prescription of fluid and vasopressors (and inotropes) guided by patients' clinical status and hemodynamic parameters including fluid responsiveness and fluid tolerance.
- This study does not change the current practice.

ARTICLE 7

Early Adjunctive Methylene Blue in Patients with Septic Shock: A Randomized Controlled Trial

Ibarra-Estrada M, Kattan E, Aguilera-González P, Sandoval-Plascencia L, Rico-Jauregui U, Gómez-Partida CA, et al. Early adjunctive methylene blue in patients with septic shock: a randomized controlled trial. *Crit Care.* 2023;27(1):110.

■ CLINICAL QUESTION

Could time to vasopressor discontinuation be reduced by early administration of methylene blue as an adjunct, compared to placebo, in patients with septic shock?

■ WHAT IS ALREADY KNOWN?

- Hyperproduction of nitric oxide (NO) by the inducible form of NO synthase (iNOS) plays an important role in the pathogenesis of septic shock by contributing to vasodilation (resulting from vascular hyporeactivity), hypotension, and myocardial depression.[30] Inhibition of NO synthase (NOS) can restore vascular reactivity and potentially reverse hypotension.
- However, a large multicenter randomized study comparing NOS inhibitor N(G)-methyl-L-arginine hydrochloride (546C88) against placebo in patients with septic shock, had to be stopped earlier as the intervention arm showed an increase in mortality. Inhibition of constitutive form of NOS (cNOS) by the nonspecific NOS inhibitor 546C88, might have contributed to this increase in mortality. cNOS is necessary for microcirculatory regulation even in patients with septic shock.[31]
- Methylene blue is a more specific inhibitor of iNOS. Possible potential benefits of this molecule were observed in two randomized studies performed earlier.[32,33] However, both these studies were limited by their small size (20 and 30 patients, respectively), short follow-up (<48 hours), and lack of meaningful patient-centric outcome.

■ STUDY DESIGN

- Investigator initiated, parallel group, double-blind, placebo-controlled, randomized control trial was conducted in a single large medical-surgical ICU of an academic medical center in Mexico.
- The study was approved by institutional review board and registered with clinicaltrials.gov (NCT04446871).

■ POPULATION STUDIED

- Adult patients (≥18 years) with septic shock (sepsis-3 definition—possible or confirmed infection with hypotension

requiring norepinephrine to maintain a MAP ≥65 mm Hg and serum lactate >2 mmol/L after adequate fluid resuscitation) were assessed for inclusion in the study.
- Adequate fluid resuscitation was defined as negative fluid responsiveness by at least two different methods following at least 500 mL bolus of balanced crystalloid.
- Following patients were excluded from the study:
  - 24 hours since initiation of norepinephrine
  - Pregnancy
  - High probability of death within 48 hours
  - Concurrent hemorrhagic, obstructive, or hypovolemic shock
  - Major burn injury
  - Personal or family history of glucose-6-phosphate dehydrogenase deficiency
  - Allergy to MB, phenothiazines, or food dyes
  - Recent intake (<4 weeks) of selective serotonin reuptake inhibitors (SSRIs)
  - Lack of consent
- Patients were randomly assigned to either methylene blue infusion or placebo. Randomization sequence was computer-generated using permuted block with a size of 4 with 1:1 allocation ratio.

■ INTERVENTION

Intravenous infusion of 100 mg of MB diluted in 500 mL of 0.9%. Sodium chloride solution over 6 hours once a day for three doses.

■ COMPARATOR

- 500 mL of 0.9% sodium chloride solution without MB over 6 hours once a day for three doses.
- All infusion bags were prepared at central pharmacy with opaque envelopes to avoid visual identification.
  - Other resuscitation measures including norepinephrine, vasopressin, hydrocortisone, and fluid resuscitation were protocolized with no differences between two groups.

■ OUTCOMES

- 92 patients underwent randomization. One patient in the intervention arm withdrew consent after first-dose of MB and was excluded from the further analysis. Finally, 46 patients were assigned to control group and 45 to intervention group.
- There was no difference in baseline characteristics between two groups. Most common sources of sepsis were pulmonary (49.5%) and intra-abdominal (38.5%). All patients received antibiotics within 3 hours of septic shock diagnosis.
- *Primary outcome*: Time to vasopressor discontinuation was significantly shorter in intervention group compared to control group [69 hours (IQR 59-83) vs. 94 hours (IQR 74-141); $p < 0.001$].
  - Numerically lesser number of patients in the intervention group required reinitiation of norepinephrine infusion within 48 hours of discontinuation (11% vs. 28%; $p = 0.06$).
- *Secondary outcomes*:
  - At 28-day, the number of vasopressor-free days was more in intervention group compared to control group (median difference 1-day; $p = 0.008$).
  - At 28-day, intervention group had lower cumulative fluid balance by 741 mL (95% CI 293-1,188; $p = 0.001$), shorter ICU length of stay (median difference 1.5 days; 95% CI 0.08-2.5,

$p = 0.001$) and shorter hospital length of stay (median difference 2.7 days; 95% CI 0.3–4.6; $p = 0.027$) compared to patients in control group.
- However, there was no significant between group difference in 28-day mortality (33% in intervention group vs. 46% in control group; $p = 0.23$).

■ *Adverse effects*:
- 93% of patients in the intervention group had green–blue discoloration of urine with no clinical consequences.
- Maximum methemoglobin concentration in intervention group was significantly higher [2.9% (IQR 2.2–3.3) vs. 0.5% (IQR 0.4–0.7); $p < 0.001$]. However, it was not clinically relevant.
- There were no differences in other potential adverse effects including change in ejection fraction, PaO_2/FiO_2, serum creatinine, bilirubin, and liver aminotransferases.

■ AUTHORS' VIEWPOINT

- Authors emphasized on the positive effects of early methylene blue infusion, in patients with septic shock, on several clinically important outcomes including reduced vasopressor duration, cumulative fluid balance, ICU, and hospital length of stay.
- The study also does not show any increase in clinically significant adverse effects of methylene blue with the dose used.
- However, authors feel the need for a larger multicenter randomized clinical trial to confirm the findings of the study.

■ STRENGTHS OF THE STUDY

- The biggest strength of the current study is the investigator initiated, double blind randomized study design.
- Other strengths of the study are:
  - Broad inclusion criteria
  - Inclusion of really sick patients in both intervention and control arms (APACHE II score of 22.9 ± 4.4 and 22.4 ± 4.4, respectively)
  - Protocolized care for both groups other than the intervention itself
  - Measures were taken to maintain masking.
  - Adequate follow-up of 28-day.
  - Detail follow-up including all relevant adverse effects

■ DRAWBACKS OF THE STUDY

- Single center study. Certain outcome measures such as ICU or hospital length of stay may not be reproducible in other settings.
- Septic shock diagnosis was mostly made outside the ICU setting with a potential for delay. However, shock diagnosis to intervention time was quite rapid in both intervention and control groups 8.3 ± 1.7 hours and 7.6 ± 2.3 hours, respectively.
- Study was done during COVID-19 pandemic, slowing the recruitment process. However, patients with COVID-19 were excluded from the study and no change was made in the resuscitation protocol.
- Authors could not measure cytokine or nitrate/nitrite serum levels to confirm the mechanism of the effects of methylene blue.
- Despite all measures taken, complete masking could not be made because of the urinary discoloration seen in majority of patients in the intervention arm.

■ REVIEWERS' VIEWPOINT

- Considering the low cost of the drug and absence of any adverse effects of the drug in the dose recommended in this study,

methylene blue should be considered early (with 24 hours of noradrenaline initiation) in patients with septic shock.
- However, a larger multicenter study is desirable before a universal recommendation.

IMPACT ON CURRENT PRACTICE AND TAKE-HOME MESSAGE

- Methylene blue infusion may be considered in patients with septic shock and escalating doses of vasopressors provided there is no contraindication to its use, like personal or family history of glucose-6-phosphate dehydrogenase deficiency, allergy to MB, phenothiazines, or food dyes and recent intake of SSRIs.
- Methylene blue should be used early, i.e., <24 hours of shock onset.
- Dose of methylene blue infusion should be 100 mg to be diluted in 500 mL of 0.9% sodium chloride solution over 6 hours once a day for three doses.

ARTICLE 8

The Increase in Cardiac Output Induced by a Decrease in Positive End-expiratory Pressure Reliably Detects Volume Responsiveness: The PEEP-test Study

Lai C, Shi R, Beurton A, Moretto F, Ayed S, Fage N, et al. The increase in cardiac output induced by a decrease in positive end-expiratory pressure reliably detects volume responsiveness: The PEEP-test study.
Crit Care. 2023;27(1):136.

CLINICAL QUESTION

Could a positive end-expiratory pressure (PEEP) test (transient decrease in PEEP) in critically ill patients who received a low tidal volume (TV) ventilation with a PEEP level ≥10 cmH$_2$O might accurately detect volume responsiveness, defined as positive passive leg raising (PLR test)?

WHAT IS ALREADY KNOWN?

- Predicting volume responsiveness, using various available dynamic tests, is recommended before fluid bolus administration in patients with acute circulatory failure as to avoid unnecessary fluid administration.[2]
- However, validity and reliability of certain dynamic tests of volume responsiveness are questioned in different clinical circumstances, especially in the presence of spontaneous breathing.[34,35] End-expiratory occlusion test is a reliable test to predict volume responsiveness in spontaneously breathing patients who are mechanically ventilated. However, patients with strong respiratory effort may not tolerate rather prolonged (15 seconds) inspiratory hold and may interrupt the test.[36] Hence, there is a requirement for an easy to perform and widely applicable measure to predict volume responsiveness test in mechanically ventilated patients with spontaneous breathing effort.
- One possible way is to take advantage of the effect of positive end expiratory pressure (PEEP) on cardiac output. PEEP

has twofold effect in ventilated patients.[37] First, it may increase the pulmonary vascular resistance and right ventricular afterload by increasing transpulmonary pressure. Second, it may decrease cardiac preload by increasing the right atrial pressure.
- Transient increase in PEEP was proposed as volume responsiveness test in ventilated patients with a low-level PEEP.[38] The reliability of this test may impair in patients with high level of PEEP as increasing PEEP may significantly increase the right ventricular afterload.
- For predicting volume responsiveness, decreasing PEEP in patients who are on high level of PEEP, may closely mimic a preload challenge similar to end-expiratory occlusion or PLR.

STUDY DESIGN

- Investigator initiated, prospective study conducted in the ICUs of two tertiary care hospitals in Paris, France.
- The study was approved by Comité de Protection des Personnes Est-III (2018-A01599-46) and was registered in ClinicalTrials.gov (NCT 04,023,786).

POPULATION STUDIED

- Adult patients (≥18 years), on invasive mechanical ventilation without spontaneous breathing with PEEP ≥10 cmH$_2$O, oxygen saturation (SpO$_2$) ≥90%
  - Ventilated in volume-assist control mode
  - Tidal volume at 6 mL/kg of predicted body weight (PBW)
  - PEEP set by clinicians with plateau pressure goal of ≤30 cmH$_2$O
  - Monitored by transpulmonary thermodilution device

- Following patients were excluded:
  - Patients on extrapulmonary membrane oxygenation (ECMO)
  - Patients having venous compression stockings
  - Contraindication to perform PLR test
  - Decrease in SpO$_2$ <80% during PEEP test
- *Noninclusion*:
  - Refusal to participate
  - Unavailability of the investigators.

INTERVENTION

- *Baseline 1*: After inclusion hemodynamic variables (heart rate, arterial pressure including pulse pressure, PPV, stroke volume variation (SVV), CVP, intra-abdominal pressure (IAP), ventilatory parameters, and cardiac index (CI) measured by transpulmonary thermodilution) were documented.
  - Passive leg raising test was performed to look for volume responsiveness.
  - Patients were deemed to be volume responsive if the pulse contour analysis-derived CI increased by ≥10% after 1-min PLR test.
- *Baseline 2*: After returning to the semirecumbent position and once CI was stabilized, hemodynamic variables were collected again. CI was measured by pulse contour analysis.
  - PEEP-test was performed by reducing PEEP from its baseline level (≥10 cmH$_2$O) to 5 cmH$_2$O for 1 minute.
  - All hemodynamic variables were collected again, including CI measured from pulse contour analysis. The maximal value of CI during the PEEP-test was collected.
- *Baseline 3*: Once the PEEP is increased back to baseline and CI is stabilized, all hemodynamic variables were once again collected.

OUTCOMES

- 64 patients were included, 31 of them were deemed to be volume responsive.
  - 42 patients (66%) had acute respiratory distress syndrome (ARDS) (mild—14, moderate—25, and severe—3).
  - Acute circulatory failure was attributed to septic shock in 28 (44%) patients, vasoplegic nonseptic shock in 33 (52%) patients, and cardiogenic shock in three (5%) patients.
  - In 88% patients' IAP measurements were available. Median IAP was 13 (10–15) mm Hg.
- PEEP test consisted of a median 7 cmH$_2$O (range, 5–10 cmH$_2$O) decrease in PEEP.
  - Desaturation to SpO$_2$ <90% occurred in six (9%) patients (lowest value of 82% in one patient).
  - However, in all these patients SpO$_2$ restabilized to ≥90% after stabilization in baseline 3.
- During PEEP test, CI increased from 2.6 ±0.7 to 2.9 ± 0.8 L/min/m^2. Percentage increase in CI was significantly larger in volume responders compared to volume nonresponders [13% (9–17%) vs. 3% (1–7%), p <0.0001].
  - PEEP test also increased PP to a larger extent in volume responders than in nonresponders [12% (7–21%) vs. 4% (1–11%), p <0.0001].
  - PPV and SVV significantly decreased in volume responders and remained unchanged in volume nonresponders
- PEEP-test induced increase in CI >8.6% predicted a positive PLR test, sensitivity 96.8% (95% CI 83.3–99.9%) and specificity of 84.9% (95% CI 68.1–94.9%). The AUROC was 0.94 (p <0.0001 vs. 0.5).
- Decrease of PPV ≥1% was able to predict volume responsiveness in 57 patients without cardiac arrhythmias. However, AUCROC of 0.81 (95% CI 0.68–0.90) was lower compared to PEEP-induced increase in CI. The sensitivity was 96.6% (95% CI 82.2–99.9%) and a specificity of 50.0% (95% CI 30.6–69.4%).
- An increase in PP ≥4 mm Hg during the PEEP test could also detect volume responsiveness with an AUROC of 0.75 (95% CI 0.62–0.85), sensitivity of 80.7% (62.5–92.5%) and specificity of 69.7% (95% CI 51.3–84.4%).
- *Adverse effects*: 9% of patients had desaturation to a level of SpO$_2$ <90%. However, it did not lead to any adverse outcome.
  - There were no significant cardiac arrhythmias noted during the study.

AUTHORS' VIEWPOINT

- PEEP test was able to reliably detect the volume responsiveness in patients being ventilated with PEEP 10 cmH$_2$O.
- Overall, the test was found to be safe.
- In patients with sinus rhythm, volume responsiveness can also be reliably predicted by a decrease in PPV by ≥1% during PEEP test, albeit with significantly lower specificity.
- An increase in PP by ≥4 mm Hg may also be used as a surrogate for change in CI during PEEP test, but with much lower overall predictability compared to >8.6% increase in CI during test.

STRENGTHS OF THE STUDY

- Clinical question asked in the study is clinically relevant.
- Predictability of volume responsiveness by >8.6% increase in CI by decreasing PEEP to 5 cmH$_2$O from a baseline of 10 cmH$_2$O was comparable to that of PLR-induced change in CI.

- This test could be utilized in predicting volume responsiveness in intubated patients with circulatory shock where PPV/SVV/systolic pulse variation (SPV) is contraindicated and when end-expiratory occlusion maneuver or PLR is not feasible.

- The reliability of the test in patients with very low lung compliance (<20 mL/cmH$_2$O) or with higher IAP (>20 mm Hg) needs to be confirmed.
- The results of the study is applicable only in patients with higher baseline PEEP ≥10 cmH$_2$O.

DRAWBACKS OF THE STUDY

- Study did not include the patients with acute cor pulmonale, in which PEEP test could induce strong decrease in RV afterload thereby increasing CI even in volume responsiveness
- Study neither measured pleural pressure nor mean systemic pressure for effects of PEEP on cardiac preload.

REVIEWERS' VIEWPOINT

- Study was able to establish assessing fluid responsiveness in patients with higher PEEP levels, this may serve as a suitable alternative test in above-mentioned subsets for volume responsiveness.
- However, study was limited to a particular population and demography, and a larger multicenter study is desirable before giving a universal recommendation.

ARTICLE 9

The Vasopressin Loading for Refractory Septic Shock (VALOR) Study: A Prospective Observational Study

Nakamura K, Nakano H, Ikechi D, Mochizuki M, Takahashi Y, Koyama Y, et al. The Vasopressin Loading for Refractory septic shock (VALOR) study: a prospective observational study.
Crit Care. 2023;27(1):294.

CLINICAL QUESTION

Can the hemodynamic response to bolus loading of vasopressin, predict response to subsequent continuous infusion of the drug in patients with septic shock refractory to initial noradrenaline infusion?

WHAT IS ALREADY KNOWN?

- Current guideline recommends vasopressin as the second vasopressor in patients with septic shock on norepinephrine infusion and inadequate MAP.[2] Usual dose of vasopressin is 0.03–0.06 units/min as a fixed-dose infusion.
- Vasopressin has a long half-life of 10–35 minutes (compared to a few minutes for catecholamines) and blood pressure response to vasopressin is slower compared to catecholamines (at a plasma vasopressin concentration of 50 pg/mL and higher).[39] Loading dose of vasopressin followed by a fixed-dose infusion can potentially reach the steady state concentration of the drug earlier and achieve blood pressure target faster.

- Moreover, many patients fail to show meaningful clinical response to vasopressin and continuation of the infusion can only subject patients to unnecessary side effects.[40] Response to initial loading dose of vasopressor can potentially predict subsequent response to infusion.

■ STUDY DESIGN

Prospective observational study. The study was conducted at the Hitachi General Hospital Emergency and Critical Care Center.

■ POPULATION STUDIED

- Patients admitted in the ICU between April 2021 and March 2023 were screened for following inclusion criteria.
  - Age ≥18 years
  - Septic shock (Sepsis-3 criteria)
  - On continuous infusion of norepinephrine ≥0.2 µg/kg/min and requiring vasopressin infusion to achieve target MAP
  - Not on continuous steroid therapy until the administration of vasopressin
  - An arterial line in place
- Patients planned for end-of-life or terminal care were excluded from the study.

■ STUDY PROTCOL

- Vasopressin was administered intravenously as a bolus of 1 U for loading, followed by a continuous infusion at 1 U/h. Before vasopressin bolus, blood sample was collected for endocrinological tests and ProAQT (Getinge, Japan) was connected to the arterial line for arterial pressure waveform analysis.
- Other interventions were not limited by study protocol.
- Patients were classified as responders and nonresponders to vasopressin loading, based on changes in MAP within 3–5 minutes of vasopressin loading (Maximum MAP – Baseline MAP; ΔMAP). Lower tertile of MAP was selected as the cut-off for differentiating responders from nonresponders.
- Epidemiological parameters and hemodynamic variables and any adverse effects of vasopressin infusion were recorded throughout resuscitation. Patients were followed up till hospital discharge.
- Primary outcome of the study was change in "catecholamine index (CAI)" 6-hour (CAI) after vasopressin loading. CAI was calculated as dopamine + dobutamine + (norepinephrine + epinephrine) × 100 µg/kg/min.

■ OUTCOMES

- 92 patients were included in the study. The lower tertile of MAP after vasopressin loading was 22 mm Hg and using this cut-off 62 patients were assigned as responders and remaining 30 as nonresponders.
- Following differences were observed between these two groups:
  - Longer time to administration of vasopressin after initiation of norepinephrine infusion in responders.
  - Lower maximum lactate concentration within 24 hours of study inclusion.
  - There was higher SVV in responders. Other hemodynamic parameters were not significantly different between responders and nonresponders.
  - Lower ACTH concentration in responders with no significant difference in vasopressin or cortisol concentration.
- *Primary outcome*: ΔCAI at 6 hours was significantly lower in responders (median −10 vs. 0; $p < 0.0001$).

- ΔMAP >22 mm Hg (cut-off used to define responders) had sensitivity of 0.92 and specificity of 0.77 for ΔCAI <0 at 6 hours.
- AUROC of ΔMAP following vasopressin loading to predict ΔCAI at 6-hour <0 was 0.843.
- *Secondary outcomes*:
  - Responders had higher urine output and lower cumulative fluid balance at 6-hour.
  - Responders achieve higher stroke volume and dPmax following vasopressor loading.
  - There was no difference in in-hospital mortality, ICU/hospital length of stay or mechanical ventilation days between two groups (study was not adequately powered).
- *Adverse effects*:
  - Ischemia events were recorded in 5 patients, i.e., 5.4% of the cohort.
  - Incidence of digital ischemia was significantly higher in nonresponders (7.1% vs. 0%; $p = 0.030$).
  - Rates of mesenteric or cardiac ischemia were similar in two groups.

AUTHORS' VIEWPOINT

- Increase in MAP following vasopressin loading may be used to predict subsequence responses to its continuous infusion. This strategy may be useful to select appropriate vasopressor strategy in refractory septic shock.
- Vasopressin loading may also achieve a rapid increase in blood pressure without any serious adverse consequences.

STRENGTHS OF THE STUDY

Well-designed prospective study aiming to test a hypothesis with strong physiological basis.

DRAWBACKS OF THE STUDY

- Result of a single center observational study may not be a truly representative one.
- Change in "CAI" at 6-hour was used as primary outcome of the study. However, changes in this parameter depend on how frequently catecholamine infusion rates were changed and the blood pressure target.
- Change in MAP (as absolute value) post-vasopressin loading depends on baseline MAP and vasodilatory status of the patient. Hence, a percentage change in MAP following vasopressin loading may be a more suitable parameter to predict subsequent response to vasopressin infusion.
- Vasopressin dose used in the study (1 U/h) is significantly lower than the usual vasopressin dose suggested by guideline (0.03 U/min or 1.8 U/h for a 60-kg individual). Smaller size and often older age of Japanese patients were quoted by the authors as the reason for this dose reduction.

REVIEWERS' VIEWPOINT

- An important study with a goal to choose appropriate second-line strategy in septic shock refractory to initial noradrenaline infusion. However, findings of this study need to be confirmed in a multicenter and multinational study.
- Instead of absolute increase in MAP, percentage increase in MAP following vasopressin bolus should be considered to define vasopressin responsiveness in future.

IMPACT ON CURRENT PRACTICE AND TAKE-HOME MESSAGE

Widespread implementation of this study results cannot be recommended, till they are confirmed by larger multicenter, multinational study.

REFERENCES

1. Goksel G, Matthias PH, Ince C. Microcirculation: Physiology, pathophysiology and clinical application. Blood Purif. 2020;49:143-50.
2. Evans L, Rhodes A, Alhazzani W, Antonelli M, Coopersmith CM, French C, et al. Surviving sepsis campaign: international guidelines for management of sepsis and septic shock 2021. Intensive Care Med. 2021;47:1181-247.
3. Olcay D, Bulent E, Ince C. Assessment of sublingual microcirculation in critically ill patient: Consensus and debate. Ann Transl Med. 2020;8(12):793.
4. Jung C, Fuernau G, de Waha S, Eitel I, Desch S, Schuler G, et al. Intra-aortic balloon counterpulsation and microcirculation in cardiogenic shock complicating myocardial infarction: An IABP-SHOCK II sub-study. Clin Res Cardiol. 2015;104:679-87.
5. Massey MJ, Hou PC, Filbin M, Wang H, Ngo L, Huang DT, et al. Microcirculatory perfusion disturbances in septic shock: results from the ProCESS trial. Crit Care. 2018;22(1):308.
6. Bruno RR, Schemmelmann M, Wollborn J, Kelm M, Jung C. Evaluation of a shorter algorithm in an automated analysis of sublingual microcirculation. Clin Hemorheol Microcirc. 2020;76:287-97.
7. Boyd JH, Forbes J, Nakada T, Walley KR, Russell JA. Fluid resuscitation in septic shock: a positive fluid balance and elevated central venous pressure are associated with increased mortality. Crit Care Med. 2011;39:259-65.
8. Vaara ST, Korhonen AM, Kaukonen KM, Nisula S, Inkinen O, Hoppu S, et al. Fluid overload is associated with an increased risk for 90-day mortality in critically ill patients with renal replacement therapy: data from the prospective FINNAKI study. Crit Care. 2012;16(5):R197.
9. Maitland K, Kiguli S, Opoka RO, Engoru C, Olupot-Olupot P, Akech SO, et al. Mortality after fluid bolus in African children with severe infection. N Engl J Med. 2011;364(26):2483-95.
10. Malbrain ML, Marik PE, Witters I, Cordemans C, Kirkpatrick AW, Roberts DJ, et al. Fluid overload, de-resuscitation, and outcomes in critically ill or injured patients: a systematic review with suggestions for clinical practice. Anaesthesiol Intensive Ther. 2014;46:361-80.
11. Silversides JA, Major E, Ferguson AJ, Mann EE, McAuley DF, Marshall JC, et al. Conservative fluid management or de-resuscitation for patients with sepsis or acute respiratory distress syndrome following the resuscitation phase of critical illness: a systematic review and meta-analysis. Intensive Care Med. 2017;43:155-70.
12. Hjortrup PB, Haase N, Bundgaard H, Thomsen SL, Winding R, Pettilä V, et al. Restricting volumes of resuscitation fluid in adults with septic shock after initial management: the CLASSIC randomised, parallel-group, multicentre feasibility trial. Intensive Care Med. 2016;42 (11):1695-705.
13. Tenner S, Baillie J, DeWitt J, Vege SS; American College of Gastroenterology. American College of Gastroenterology guideline: Management of acute pancreatitis. Am J Gastroenterol. 2013;108:1400-15;1416.
14. Vege SS, DiMagno MJ, Forsmark CE, Martel M, Barkun AN. Initial medical treatment of acute pancreatitis: American Gastroenterological Association Institute technical review. Gastroenterology. 2018;154:1103-39.
15. Singh VK, Gardner TB, Papachristou GI, Rey-Riveiro M, Faghih M, Koutroumpakis E, et al. An international multicenter study of early intravenous fluid administration and outcome in acute pancreatitis. United European Gastroenterol J. 2017;5:491-8.
16. Mao EQ, Tang YQ, Fei J, Qin S, Wu J, Li L, et al. Fluid therapy for severe acute pancreatitis in acute response stage. Chin Med J (Engl). 2009;122(2):169-73.
17. Mao EQ, Fei J, Peng Y-B, Huang J, Tang Y-Q, Zhang S-D. Rapid hemodilution is associated with increased sepsis and mortality among patients with severe acute pancreatitis. Chin Med J (Engl). 2010;123:1639-44.

18. Di Martino M, Van Laarhoven S, Ielpo B, Ramia JM, Manuel-Vázquez A, Martínez-Pérez A, et al. Systematic review and meta-analysis of fluid therapy protocols in acute pancreatitis: type, rate and route. HPB (Oxford). 2021;23:1629-38.
19. Malbrain MLNG, Langer T, Annane D, Gattinoni L, Elbers P, Hahn RG, et al. Intravenous fluid therapy in the perioperative and critical care setting: executive summary of the international fluid academy (IFA). Ann Intensive Care. 2020;10:64.
20. Van Regenmortel N, Verbrugghe W, Roelant E, Van den Wyngaert T, Jorens PG. Maintenance fluid therapy and fluid creep impose more significant fluid, sodium, and chloride burdens than resuscitation fluids in critically ill patients: a retrospective study in a tertiary mixed ICU population. Intensive Care Med. 2018;44:409-17.
21. Lindén-Søndersø A, Jungner M, Spångfors M, Jan M, Oscarson A, Choi S, et al. Survey of non-resuscitation fluids administered during septic shock: a multicenter prospective observational study. Ann Intensive Care. 2019;9:132.
22. Payen D, de Pont AC, Sakr Y, Spies C, Reinhart K, Vincent JL, et al. A positive fluid balance is associated with a worse outcome in patients with acute renal failure. Crit Care. 2008;12:R74.
23. Zhang Z, Xu X, Fan H, Li D, Deng H. Higher serum chloride concentrations are associated with acute kidney injury in unselected critically ill patients. BMC Nephrol. 2013;14:235.
24. Yasuda H, Yamamoto R, Hayashi Y, Kotani Y, Kishihara Y, Kondo N, et al. Occurrence and incidence rate of peripheral intravascular catheter-related phlebitis and complications in critically ill patients: a prospective cohort study (AMOR-VENUS study). J Intensive Care. 2021;9:3.
25. Jessen MK, Andersen LW, Thomsen MH, Jensen ME, Kirk ME, Kildegaard S, et al. Twenty-four-hour fluid administration in emergency department patients with suspected infection: A multicenter, prospective, observational study. Acta Anaesthesiol Scand. 2021;65:1122-42.
26. de-Madaria E, Buxbaum JL, Maisonneuve P, García García de Paredes A, Zapater P, Guilabert L et al. Aggressive or Moderate Fluid Resuscitation in Acute Pancreatitis. N Engl J Med. 2022; 387:989-1000.
27. Nijssen EC, Rennenberg RJ, Nelemans PJ, Essers BA, Janssen MM, Vermeeren MA, et al. Prophylactic hydration to protect renal function from intravascular iodinated contrast material in patients at high risk of contrast-induced nephropathy (AMACING): a prospective, randomised, phase 3, controlled, open-label, non-inferiority trial. Lancet. 2017;389:1312-22.
28. Self WH, Semler MW, Bellomo R, Brown SM, deBoisblanc BP, Exline MC, et al. Liberal Versus Restrictive Intravenous Fluid Therapy for Early Septic Shock: Rationale for a Randomized Trial. Ann Emerg Med. 2018;72:457-66.
29. Meyhoff TS, Hjortrup PB, Wetterslev J, Sivapalan P, Laake JH, Cronhjort M et al. Restriction of Intravenous Fluid in ICU Patients with Septic Shock. N Engl J Med. 2022;386:2459-70.
30. Hamzaoui O, Georger JF, Monnet X, Ksouri H, Maizel J, Richard C, et al. Early administration of norepinephrine increases cardiac preload and cardiac output in septic patients with life-threatening hypotension. Crit Care. 2010;14(4):R142.
31. Kirkebøen KA, Strand OA. The role of nitric oxide in sepsis—an overview. Acta Anaesthesiol Scand. 1999;43:275-88.
32. López A, Lorente JA, Steingrub J, Bakker J, McLuckie A, Willatts S, et al. Multiple-center, randomized, placebo-controlled, double-blind study of the nitric oxide synthase inhibitor 546C88: Effect on survival in patients with septic shock. Crit Care Med. 2004;32:21-30.
33. Kirov MY, Evgenov OV, Evgenov NV, Egorina EM, Sovershaev MA, Sveinbjørnsson B, et al. Infusion of methylene blue in human septic shock: a pilot, randomized, controlled study. Crit Care Med. 2001;29:1860-7.

34. Memis D, Karamanlioglu B, Yuksel M, Gemlik I, Pamukcu Z. The influence of methylene blue infusion on cytokine levels during severe sepsis. Anaesth Intensive Care. 2002;30:755-62.
35. Michard F, Chemla D, Teboul JL. Applicability of pulse pressure variation: how many shades of grey? Crit Care. 2015;19:144.
36. Teboul JL, Monnet X, Chemla D, Michard F. Arterial pulse pressure variation with mechanical ventilation. Am J Respir Crit Care Med. 2019;199:22-31.
37. Gavelli F, Teboul JL, Monnet X. The end-expiratory occlusion test: Please, let me hold your breath! Crit Care. 2019;23:274.
38. Mahmood SS, Pinsky MR. Heart-lung interactions during mechanical ventilation: The basics. Ann Transl Med. 2018;6:349.
39. Ali A, Aygun E, Abdullah T, Bolsoy-Deveci S, Orhan-Sungur M, Canbaz M, et al. A challenge with 5 cmH$_2$O of positive end-expiratory pressure predicts fluid responsiveness in neurosurgery patients with protective ventilation: an observational study. Minerva Anesthesiol. 2019;85:1184-92.
40. Möhring J, Glänzer K, Maciel JA Jr, Düsing R, Kramer HJ, Arbogast R, et al. Greatly enhanced pressor response to antidiuretic hormone in patients with impaired cardiovascular reflexes due to idiopathic orthostatic hypotension. J Cardiovasc Pharmacol. 1980;2:367-76.
41. Nakamura K, Nakano H, Naraba H, Mochizuki M, Takahashi Y, Sonoo T, et al. Vasopressin Loading for Refractory Septic Shock: A Preliminary Analysis of a Case Series. Front Med (Lausanne). 2021;8:644195.

Section 2

Respiratory/Ventilation/Acute Respiratory Distress Syndrome

Section Editor: Manoj Y Singh

ARTICLE 10

Hydrocortisone in Severe Community-acquired Pneumonia

Dequin PF, Meziani F, Quenot JP, Kamel T, Ricard JD, Badie J, et al. CRICS-TriGGERSep Network. Hydrocortisone in severe community-acquired pneumonia.
N Engl J Med. 2023;388(21):1931-41.

■ CLINICAL QUESTION OR PROBLEM

Does the use of hydrocortisone (with its anti-inflammatory and immunomodulatory effects) compared to a placebo in patients admitted to intensive care unit (ICU) with severe community-acquired pneumonia (CAP) reduce 28-day mortality?[1]

■ WHAT IS ALREADY KNOWN?

Severe CAP is associated with significant mortality and morbidity, especially in patients who need admission to ICU. The use of steroids in this setting has been studied before and has had mixed results. It does find a place in some guidelines, namely the ESICM/SCCM (European Society of Intensive Care Medicine/Society of Critical Care Medicine) guideline but the ATS/ISDA (American Thoracic Society/Infectious Diseases Society of America) have however, recommended against its use.

Last year, Meduri et al. (ESCAPe study group)[2] conducted a double-blind, randomized controlled trial (RCT) in 586 patients (well short of target sample size of 1,420) with severe CAP admitted in ICU. They compared placebo versus use of methylprednisolone over 3 weeks [40-mg intravenous (IV) methylprednisolone for 7 days followed by progressive tapering of the dose over 20-day period]. They reported no significant difference in 60-day mortality [16% vs. 18%, adjusted odds ratio (OR) 0.9 95% confidence interval (CI) 0.57–1.40] and no significant differences in secondary outcomes [shock, acute respiratory distress syndrome (ARDS), multiple organ dysfunction syndrome (MODS)-free days, mechanical ventilation (MV)-free days, ICU and hospital length of stay (LOS)] and complications.

■ STUDY DESIGN

- Multicenter, double-blind, RCT (centralized randomization using web-based

system with 1:1 ration in block sizes of four, which were stratified according to trail site and the use of MV)
- *Power calculation:* 1,146 patients needed to provide 80% power to detect a 25% relative risk reduction in mortality from a baseline of 27%. The study was ended after a planned second interim analysis.

POPULATION STUDIED INCLUDING DEMOGRAPHICS

Inclusion
- Age >18
- Admission to ICU
- CAP diagnosis suggested by ≥2 of cough, purulent sputum, chest pain, and dyspnea
- Focal shadowing on chest X-ray (CXR)/computed tomography (CT) scan
- Severe disease defined by at least one of the following:
  - Pulmonary severity index (PSI) score >130
  - MV
  - High-flow nasal cannula (HFNC) with fraction of inspired oxygen (FiO_2) >0.5 and partial pressure of arterial oxygen (PaO_2)/FiO_2 (P/F) ratio <300
  - Rebreathing mask with P/F ratio-dependent on O_2 flow (e.g., >10 L the P/F <300)
- At least one dose of antibiotics administered.

Exclusion
- Treated by vasopressors for septic shock at time of inclusion
- Clinical history suggesting aspiration
- Treated by invasive MV within last 14 days
- More than 7 days of antibiotics prior
- Polymerase chain reaction (PCR)-positive for influenza
- Use of >15-mg prednisolone (or equivalent)/day for >30 days
- Pregnancy
- Cystic fibrosis (CF), active tuberculosis (TB) or fungal infection and active viral hepatitis or active infection with herpes virus
- Average age was 67 years, 70% male, with chronic obstructive pulmonary disease (COPD) (22%), diabetes (24%), MV (46%), and needing high-flow nasal prong (HFNP) (42%).

INTERVENTION(S) STUDIED
- Assigned patients to receive IV hydrocortisone (200 mg daily for either 4 or 7 days as determined by clinical improvement, followed by tapering for a total of 8 or 14 days)
- Treating tram using predefined criteria to administer for a total of 8 days if the prespecified criteria met on day 4 [P/F >200; breathing spontaneously, day 4 sequential organ failure assessment (SOFA) ≤ day 1 SOFA]
- Median duration was 5 days.

COMPARATOR USED
- Placebo (identically packaged)
- Median duration was 6 days

OUTCOMES EVALUATED
Primary Outcome
Death by day 28: Hydrocortisone 6.2% versus placebo 11.9%
- Absolute risk reduction (ARR): −5.6% (−9.6 to −1.7%), $p = 0.006$
- Number needed to treat (NNT): 17

Secondary Outcomes
- *Comparing hydrocortisone versus placebo group:*

- No significant difference in cumulative incidence of hospital-acquired infection by day 28: 9.8% versus 11.1% and cumulative incidence of gastrointestinal (GI) bleeding by day 28: 2.2% versus 3.3%.
- Median daily dose of insulin by day 7 was significantly greater in intervention group 35.5 versus 20.0 IU/day.
- 90-day mortality was significant lower in intervention group: 9.3% versus 14.7%, with less patients needing intubation and vasopressors on day 28.
- *Selected subgroups:*
  - Comparing hydrocortisone versus placebo, the following subgroups trended to favoring hydrocortisone use:
    * Not mechanically ventilated: 6/222 versus 22/220
      - Risk difference: −7.3 (95% CI −12.6 to −2.0)
    * No culture positivity: 11/189 versus 25/168
      - Risk difference: −9.1 (95% CI −15.0 to −3.1).

■ AUTHORS' VIEWPOINT

Early treatment with hydrocortisone reduced 28-day mortality in those admitted to the ICU with severe CAP.

■ STRENGTH OF THE STUDY

- Multicenter study design, with well-balanced baseline characteristics after randomization and included patients with CAP needing ventilatory support at time of randomization
- Intervention initiated as targeted, within 20 hours of hospital admission
- Minimal loss of follow-up (only two patients).
- Septic shock patients needing steroids were excluded.
- Minimal protocol variation and placebo identical to study drug in packaging.

■ DRAWBACKS OF THE STUDY

- *Single country*: France
- Lower mortality numbers than predicted with only 72 deaths across both arms with a fragility index six patients
- No uniform duration of steroid use (e.g., tapered or not)
- Low microbiological yield (in 45% patients no pathogen identified)
- The subgroup in which no pathogens were isolated trended to favoring steroid use compared to those in whom a pathogen was isolated.

■ REVIEWERS' VIEWPOINT

- Strongly consider the use of steroids in patients admitted with severe CAP, especially in those where the microbiology is negative.
- In a recent systematic review and meta-analysis,[3] Wu et al. included 1,689 patients from seven RCTs, and reported lower 30-day mortality (0.61; 95% CI 0.4400.85, $p < 0.01$, $I^2 = 0\%$), and lower risk of MV requirement, and shorter ICU and hospital LOS with the use of corticosteroids in patients with severe CAP.

■ IMPACT ON CURRENT PRACTICE AND TAKE HOME MESSAGE

Strongly consider the use of steroids in patients admitted with severe CAP, especially in those where the microbiology is negative.

ARTICLE 11

Oxygen-Saturation Targets for Critically Ill Adults Receiving Mechanical Ventilation

Semler MW, Casey JD, Lloyd BD, Hastings PG, Hays MA, Stollings JL, et al; PILOT Investigators and the Pragmatic Critical Care Research Group. Oxygen-Saturation Targets for Critically Ill Adults Receiving Mechanical Ventilation.

N Engl J Med. 2022;387(19):1759-69.

CLINICAL QUESTION OR PROBLEM

We routinely monitor and target oxygen saturation in patients needing invasive MV. Does a target arterial oxygen saturation (SaO_2) of 90%, 94% or 98% impact 28-day mortality and MV-free days?

WHAT IS ALREADY KNOWN?

Oxygen is one of the most common therapies administered in ICU and the optimal oxygenation target remains elusive. Though aiming higher oxygen targets provides a safety net against hypoxemia, but use of high FiO_2 can have potential harms.

A number of trials have compared restrictive and liberal oxygen therapy, with more recent trials showing equipoise between the two groups. While the *OXYGEN-ICU study*[4] demonstrated that lower oxygenation targets [peripheral oxygen saturation (SpO_2) 94–98%/PaO_2 70–100 mm Hg] yield a mortality benefit, the study had a number of methodological issues. *ICU-ROX trial*[5] did not demonstrate any difference in ventilator-free days between conservative and usual oxygen therapy. *$LOCO_2$ trial*[6] demonstrated no difference in 28-day mortality between liberal or conservative oxygenation targets in patients with ARDS. The *HOT-ICU study*,[7] targeting lower oxygenation level of 60 mm Hg did not result in lower 90-day mortality in comparison to targeting higher oxygenation levels of 90 mm Hg in patients with acute hypoxemic respiratory failure.

STUDY DESIGN

- Single center (Nashville USA); patients intubated and mechanically ventilated in emergency department (ED) or ICU were cluster-randomized in this cluster-crossover trial (1 of 3 targets every 2 months, in a randomly generated sequence). This trial could not be blinded.
- Final 7 days of each period were considered as washout period and were not included in analysis.

POPULATION STUDIED INCLUDING DEMOGRAPHICS

Inclusion
- Age >18
- Admission to ICU or ED
- Requiring MV.

Exclusion
- Pregnant, incarcerated, coronavirus disease 2019 (COVID-19)
- Baseline characteristic in the three groups were broadly similar.
- *Age:* 57 versus 59 versus 59 years,

- Commodities like COPD, ischemic heart disease (IHD), myocardial infarction (MI), vasopressor requirements nearly similar.

■ INTERVENTION(S) STUDIED

The mechanically ventilated patients were assigned into one of the two oxygen targets:
1. Lower (SpO_2 90%; range 88–92%)
2. Intermediate (SpO_2 94%; range 92–96%).

The median time from initiation of MV to enrolment was similar. Only changes in the FiO_2 were mandated by the trial protocol. All other aspects of patient care including changes in ventilator settings were left to the discretion of treating team.

■ COMPARATOR USED

Higher oxygen target (SpO_2 98%; range 96–100%).

■ OUTCOMES EVALUATED

Primary Outcome

- Number of alive days and MV-free days at day 28
  - No difference (20 days in lower and 21 days in intermediate and higher group)
    - *Lower versus intermediate:* 0.95 (95% CI 0.79–1.19)
    - *Intermediate versus higher:* 1.0 (95% CI 0.84–01.19)
    - *Lower versus intermediate:* 0.95 (95% CI 0.78–1.14).

Secondary Outcomes

- No significant difference in any pre-specified secondary outcomes
- No difference in 28-day mortality in the three groups (34.8% vs. 34.0% vs. 33.2%).

■ AUTHORS' VIEWPOINT

In mechanically ventilated critically ill patients aiming oxygen saturation to lower, intermediate, and higher oxygenation targets did not impact their outcome.

■ STRENGTH OF THE STUDY

- Good adherence to SaO_2 targets and separation of three study groups
- Large number of patients included in study
- Use of SaO_2 allowed big data set
- Cluster crossover design limited selection bias
- Targeted patient-centered primary outcome.

■ DRAWBACKS OF THE STUDY

- Single-center study
- No surgical patients included in ICU
- FiO_2 target by respiratory therapists, not present in various ICU
- Oxygen saturation for lower group not really met even at FiO_2 of 0.21.

■ REVIEWERS' VIEWPOINT

- Many of us target SaO_2 based on our own biases and interpretation of previous evidence. This trial gives a good insight that targeting intermediate or high SaO_2 is not harmful.
- Until more studies come into light in specific patient population, there is no clinical benefit in targeting a particular SaO_2 level.

■ IMPACT ON CURRENT PRACTICE AND TAKE HOME MESSAGE

Aiming intermediate saturation targets in most patients as good as aiming low SaO_2 targets.

REFERENCES

1. Dequin PF, Meziani F, Le Gouge A. Hydrocortisone in severe community-acquired pneumonia. N Engl J Med. 2023; 389(7):671-2.
2. Meduri GU, Shih MC, Bridges L, Martin TJ, El-Solh A, Seam N, et al; ESCAPe Study Group. Low-dose methylprednisolone treatment in critically ill patients with severe community-acquired pneumonia. Intensive Care Med. 2022;48(8):1009-23.
3. Wu JY, Tsai YW, Hsu WH, Liu TH, Huang PY, Chuang MH, et al. Efficacy and safety of adjunctive corticosteroids in the treatment of severe community-acquired pneumonia: a systematic review and meta-analysis of randomized controlled trials. Crit Care. 2023;27(1):274.
4. Girardis M, Busani S, Damiani E, Donati A, Rinaldi L, Marudi A, et al. Effect of Conservative vs. Conventional Oxygen Therapy on Mortality Among Patients in an Intensive Care Unit: The Oxygen-ICU Randomized Clinical Trial. JAMA. 2016;316(15):1583-9.
5. ICU-ROX Investigators and the Australian and New Zealand Intensive Care Society Clinical Trials Group; Mackle D, Bellomo R, Bailey M, Beasley R, Deane A, Eastwood G, et al; ICU-ROX Investigators the Australian and New Zealand Intensive Care Society Clinical Trials Group. Conservative Oxygen Therapy during Mechanical Ventilation in the ICU. N Engl J Med. 2020;382(11):989-98.
6. Barrot L, Asfar P, Mauny F, Winiszewski H, Montini F, Badie J, et al. $LOCO_2$ Investigators and REVA Research Network. Liberal or Conservative Oxygen Therapy for Acute Respiratory Distress Syndrome. N Engl J Med. 2020;382(11):999-1008.
7. Schjørring OL, Klitgaard TL, Perner A, Wetterslev J, Lange T, Siegemund M, et al; HOT-ICU Investigators. Lower or Higher Oxygenation Targets for Acute Hypoxemic Respiratory Failure. N Engl J Med. 2021; 384(14):1301-11.

Section 3

Neurocritical Care

Section Editor: Ketan Kargirwar
Associate Editor: Sanket Hansora

ARTICLE 12

Treatment for Intracranial Hypertension in Acute Brain Injury: Grading, Timing, and Association with Outcome. Data from the SYNAPSE-ICU Study

Robba C, Graziano F, Guglielmi A, Rebora P, Galimberti S, Taccone FS, et al. On behalf of the SYNAPSE-ICU Investigators. Treatment for intracranial hypertension in acute brain injury: grading, timing, and association with outcome. Data from the SYNAPSE-ICU study.
Intensive Care Med. 2023;49:50-61.

■ CLINICAL QUESTION OR PROBLEM

- To control detrimental increase in intracranial hypertension in acute brain injured patients. When and how it should be done?
- What should be the "therapy intensity level (TIL)"—less aggressive or more aggressive?
- What are the therapeutic approaches for controlling intracranial hypertension in patient with acute brain injury (ABI) during first week since intensive care unit (ICU) admission.
- What are the variabilities in the use of TILs among different pathologies (subarachnoid hemorrhage (SAH), traumatic brain injury (TBI), and intracranial hemorrhage (ICH).
- Is there any association between varying level of TILs and clinical outcomes?

■ WHAT IS ALREADY KNOWN?

- *Blood pressure control:* Uncontrolled blood pressure may associate with higher risk of worsening intracranial bleed and poor neurological outcome.
- *Cerebral perfusion pressure (CPP):* CPP monitoring of severe TBI patients is recommended to decrease 2-week mortality. Maintaining certain cerebral perfusion pressure (60–70 mm Hg) has a favorable outcome.
- *Intracranial hypertension (ICP) thresholds:* Management of severe TBI patients using information from ICP monitoring is recommended to reduce in-hospital and 2-week mortality. Treating ICP >22 mm Hg is recommended because values above this level are associated with increased mortality.
- *Prophylactic hypothermia:* It is not recommended to improve outcome in diffuse injury.

- *Hyperosmolar therapy:* Mannitol effective for control of ICP at doses of 0.25–1 g/kg body weight, however hypotension should be avoided and restrict its use prior to ICP monitoring.
- *Hyperventilation therapy:* Prolonged prophylactic hyperventilation with $PaCO_2$ <25 is not recommended. Hyperventilation should be avoided during first 24 hours after the injury when cerebral blood flow (CBF) is reduced critically.
- *Anesthetics, analgesics and sedatives:* Prophylactic use of barbiturates for burst suppression is not recommended. Although propofol is recommended to control of ICP, it is not recommended for improvement in mortality.
- *Steroids:* Use of steroids is not recommended for reducing ICP.
- *Seizure prophylaxis:* Prophylactic use of valproate or phenytoin is not recommended for late posttraumatic seizure (PTS), however phenytoin is recommended to reduce early PTS.
- *Decompressive craniotomy:* A large frontotemporal craniotomy is recommended for reduced mortality.
- *Cerebrospinal fluid (CSF) drainage:* Initial Glasgow Coma Scale (GCS) <6 during first 12 hours after injury may be considered.

STUDY DESIGN

- It is a multicenter, prospective, international, and observational cohort study.
- Its primary aim was evaluating clinical practice and managing ICP monitoring in AIBs.
- It helped to clarify the current clinical use of ICP monitoring and treatment across the different countries with different resources and its use in various types of AIBs.

POPULATION STUDIED INCLUDING DEMOGRAPHICS

- *Inclusion criteria:*
  - Age: >18 years
  - Diagnosis of ABI following TBI, SAH, ICH
  - Altered level of consciousness: GCS—eye response score of 1, no eye-opening, motor response of 5 or less, not obeying command on admission to ICU
  - Neurological deterioration with no-eye opening and motor score decreased to 5 or less within 48 hours after ICU admission.
- *Exclusion criteria:*
  - Patients not requiring ICU admission and/or being admitted for other form of AIBs.
- A total of 2,395 patients enrolled in Synapse-ICU study
  - 75 without TIL data on day 1 were excluded.
- A total of 2,320 patients were available for this analysis.
  - 1,339 (57.7%) patients were admitted for TBI
  - 409 (17.6%) admitted for SAH
  - 572 (24.7%) admitted for ICH
- Median age was 55 years
- The number of females was 800.
- 1,916 (85.6%) presented with GCS <8 and 744 (34%) had at least one unreactive pupil.
- 409 patients were admitted from low-income countries.

INTERVENTION STUDIED

- Intervention to reduce intracranial hypertension was recorded to the TIL scale on day 1, 3, and 7 of the ICU stay.
- TIL scale: Basic, mild-moderate, and extreme treatment

- Level of TIL during the week was defined as maximum level of treatment over days 1, 3, and 7.
  - eTIL group: Patients receive extreme therapies at least once on days 1, 3, and 7.
  - No-eTIL group: Patients who do not receive extreme therapies.
- Patients primarily decompressed on day 1 were classified according to maximum TIL.
- If a patient received a decompressive craniectomy on day 3, he/she was considered also decompressed on day 7.

■ OUTCOME EVALUATED

- *Primary endpoint:* Prevalence of TIL use in ABI in the first week since ICU admission.
- *Secondary endpoint:* Mortality and Glasgow Outcome Scale Extended (GOSE) collected at 6-month follow-up.
- Unfavorable outcome was defined as a GOSE score of <5.
- Over the first week in ICU, 295 patients received eTIL at least once, while 1,643 patients received mild-moderate at maximum level and remaining 382 patients received no-basic TIL.
- Among 295 eTIL patients, 93 were aggressively treated only on day 1, 35 on day 3, and 50 on day 7. Only 15 subjects were treated with extreme TIL at all time.
- During whole week 305 SAH patients received mild-moderate TIL and 63 received eTIL.
- In TBI group, 932 patients received mild-moderate TIL and 178 eTIL.
- In ICH group, 406 patients treated with mild-moderate TIL and 54 with eTIL.
- Among the patients, who received the eTIL during the week, the most frequent treatments were, in SAH group, decompressive craniectomy, hypocapnia, and metabolic suppression; in TBI metabolic suppression and in ICH hypocapnia.
- There is variability in frequency of use of eTIL was observed.
- Association between TIL and outcomes:
  - At 6 months, 1,331 patients had an unfavorable neurological outcome (GOSE <5) and 934 patients died.
  - Mortality was higher in patients in no-basic TIL group compared to those who received mild-moderate TIL or eTIL.
  - Unfavorable neurological outcome was more frequent in those patients who received eTIL compared to other groups (eTIL 68.5%, mild-moderate 60.5%, no-basic TIL 65.9%).
  - Considering eTIL as reference, the use of no-basic TIL was independently associated with 6 months mortality but use of mild-moderate was not.
  - Analysis according to the type of brain injury, the result was consistent in each pathology.
  - No significant association of TIL group with 6 months neurological outcome was found.
  - Results were consistent when stratifying according to the type of brain injury.
  - Excluding most severe cases, the model showed the statistically significant association between unfavorable neurological outcome and no-basic or mild-moderate TIL comparing with eTIL.

■ AUTHORS' VIEWPOINT

- During the first week of ICU admission, strategies for managing intracranial hypertension, especially mild and moderate treatment, are frequently used in ABI patients.

- There is large variability across centers and countries still exists regarding the use of these therapies.
- The management of intracranial pressure is fundamental in neurocritical care patients to reduce secondary brain damage and improve clinical outcome.
- Considering the lack of definitive randomized controlled trial comparing all aggressive treatment, initiating one of the strategies relies on the balance between risks and benefit, patient clinical condition, and there local practice.
- We found that patients undergoing eTIL were more severe and younger but with better pre-injury condition. This suggests that physicians consider applying these strategies when benefit outweighs the risk.
- Despite the significant variability in ICP practice and treatment, intensive treatments are guided by invasive treatment and there are still significant numbers of patients who receive aggressive treatment without ICP monitoring, thus highlighting the need to provide more universally accepted criteria for its use in ABIs.
- The multivariate analysis on 6 months mortality showed that aggressive treatment could reduce the mortality at 6 months compared to no-basic TIL.
- Even though there might be a potential harm from using high TIL therapies, monitoring and treating these patients can reduce the mortality in selected patients.
- The effect on the neurological outcome remains unclear.

STRENGTH OF THE STUDY

- Data from this large cohort of acute brain injury patients admitted to ICU will provide a detailed description of the patient characteristics, intracranial pressure management strategies, resource use, and their correlation to clinical outcome.
- The results complement other multicenter studies focusing on traumatic brain injury practice and will add information on ICP practice in subarachnoid hemorrhage and intracerebral hemorrhage.
- The presence of centers in low- and middle-income countries will provide robust data about ICP monitoring in these regions.
- The global approach can be considered as the main strength and novelty of the study, since it allows to explore the clinical practice in geographical regions characterized by very different public health issues.

DRAWBACKS OF THE STUDY

- This is observational study therefore it is impossible to draw any causality relationship between the associations found.
- Definition of TIL treatment includes only decompressive craniotomy, hypothermia and metabolic suppression are defined as tier-three therapies.
- Data such as withdrawal of care or escalation of care in the use of TIL, data on duration of metabolic suppression or method of cooling to obtain hypothermia and database at day 1 regarding primary and secondary decompression are lacking.
- There is no universal consensus on definition of neuroworsening.

REVIEWERS' VIEWPOINT

- Treatment of intracranial hypertension is frequently applied in the first week of ICU management of acute brain-injured patients.

- Highly aggressive therapies are still significantly variable across centers and do not follow the staircase approach recommended by most recent guidelines.
- Aggressive strategies benefit 6-month mortality but not 6-month neurological outcome.

IMPACT ON CURRENT PRACTICE AND TAKE HOME MESSAGE

- The findings of the SYNAPSE-ICU study have the potential to influence clinical practice in the management of ICH in acute brain injury. The study may provide valuable insights into the optimal timing of treatment initiation, the selection of appropriate treatment strategies based on ICH severity, and the impact of treatment on patient outcomes.
- Findings from the study indicate that there is considerable variability in the use of ICP monitoring across different centers and countries.
- The study also suggests that ICP monitoring may be associated with a more intensive therapeutic approach and lower 6-month mortality in more severe cases of acute brain injury.
- Additionally, ICP monitoring was found to be associated with better neurological outcomes at 6 month.
- The findings could guide clinicians in making evidence-based decisions and improving patient care in the ICU setting.

ARTICLE 13

Prognostic Factors Associated with Extubation Failure in Acutely Brain-injured Patients: A Systematic Review and Meta-analysis

Taran S, Angeloni N, Pinto R, Lee S, McCredie VA, Schultz MJ, et al. Prognostic Factors Associated with Extubation Failure in Acutely Brain-injured Patients: A Systematic Review and Meta-analysis.
Crit Care Med. 2023;51(3):401-12.

WHAT IS ALREADY KNOWN?

Potential factors associated with extubation failure in acutely brain-injured patients may include:
- *Glasgow Coma Scale score:* The GCS is a neurological scale that assesses a patient's level of consciousness. Lower GCS scores at the time of extubation may indicate a higher risk of extubation failure.
- *Neurological status:* The severity and nature of the brain injury play a crucial role in determining a patient's ability to maintain spontaneous breathing and airway control after extubation.
- *Age:* Older age has been associated with an increased risk of extubation failure in various patient populations, including those with brain injuries.
- *Preexisting medical conditions:* Patients with comorbidities, such as chronic respiratory disorders or cardiovascular diseases, may have a higher likelihood of extubation failure.
- *Duration of mechanical ventilation:* Longer durations of mechanical ventilation may lead to muscle weakness and other complications, increasing the risk of extubation failure.

- *Blood gas parameters:* Abnormal blood gas values, such as low arterial oxygen levels or high carbon dioxide levels, may indicate respiratory insufficiency and predict extubation failure.
- *Rapid shallow breathing index (RSBI):* RSBI is a ratio calculated by dividing the respiratory rate by tidal volume during a spontaneous breathing trial. Higher RSBI values have been associated with an increased risk of extubation failure.

STUDY DESIGN

Cohort studies and randomized trials examining the association of prognostic factors with extubation failure.

This systematic review and meta-analysis were performed following reporting standards for prognostic factor studies, the Cochrane Handbook, and the Preferred Reporting Items for Systematic Reviews and Meta-analysis (PRISMA) guidelines. The review protocol was developed a priori and registered with PROSPERO (CRD42021253310).

POPULATION STUDIED INCLUDING DEMOGRAPHICS

In this systematic review and meta-analysis including 21 studies and 3,274 adult patients with ABI admitted to an ICU. Data were collected on the population, index prognostic factor, comparator prognostic factor, outcome, timing, and setting.

INTERVENTION(S) STUDIED

All meta-analyses were performed using random effects models to account for between-study heterogeneity. Heterogeneity was assessed by visual inspection of forest plots for overlapping point estimates and CIs and formally reported using the I^2 measure.

COMPARATOR USED

Not applicable.

OUTCOMES EVALUATED

- The primary outcome was extubation failure. Additional outcomes included ICU length of stay and mortality at longest follow-up. Where reported they have extracted the reasons for reintubation among patients failing extubation and the proportion of patients receiving a tracheostomy.
- Among patients who failed extubation, the most common reasons for reintubation were excessive secretions [median, 9.7%; interquartile range (IQR), 7.0–50.5%], decreased level of consciousness (median, 16.0%; IQR, 10.2–26.4%), stridor (median, 21.6%; IQR, 16.7–25.6%), and respiratory failure (median, 36.4%; IQR, 17.1–46.7%).
- Between 2.8 and 47.0% of patients received a primary tracheostomy without an extubation attempt.
- Patients failing extubation had a numerically higher mortality at longer follow-up (with the exception of one study) and longer median ICU length of stay compared with patients extubated successfully.

AUTHORS' VIEWPOINT

By synthesizing data from multiple studies, the meta-analysis can identify and quantify the strength of association between various prognostic factors and extubation failure in acutely brain-injured patients.

This information can guide clinical decision-making and inform prognostic discussions with patients and their families.

STRENGTH OF THE STUDY

- Strengths of this systematic review include our use of a preregistered study protocol with few deviations and adherence

to standards for systematic reviews of prognostic factors and updated PRISMA guidelines.
- *Methodological rigor:* Systematic reviews and meta-analyses are considered to be some of the highest levels of evidence in medical research due to their rigorous methodology. This study likely followed strict guidelines for conducting systematic reviews, ensuring that all relevant studies were identified and included, and that the data extraction process was thorough and unbiased.
- *Large sample size:* The strength of a meta-analysis lies in its ability to pool data from multiple studies, creating a larger sample size than any individual study. A substantial sample size increases the statistical power of the analysis, allowing for more reliable and precise estimates of the prognostic factors associated with extubation failure in brain-injured patients.
- *Clinical relevance:* Extubation failure in acutely brain-injured patients is a critical concern for clinicians in intensive care settings. By identifying prognostic factors associated with this outcome, the study provides relevant insights into patient management and may aid in risk stratification and targeted interventions.

■ DRAWBACKS OF THE STUDY

As with all research, potential biases, heterogeneity in study designs, and other confounding factors should be carefully considered when interpreting the results. Researchers should acknowledge these limitations and provide suggestions for future research to further enhance the understanding of this important clinical issue.
- First, although the unadjusted analysis demonstrated that extubation failure was not predicted by specific ABI diagnosis, the credibility of this finding is limited by residual confounding, and subgroup effects by ABI subtype are not excluded.
- Second, although our review suggests the importance of cough and swallow in the decision to extubate, several studies reported these as binary variables (i.e., present or absent). Our analyses, therefore, do not account for the possibility of a dose-response relationship between individual airway factors and extubation failure.
- Third, since our primary meta-analysis included factors that did not adjust for the same set of covariates, readers should apply caution in comparing summary estimates between different prognostic factors or ranking them by their magnitude. However, even where adjustment is performed with similar covariates, direct comparisons between prognostic factors should generally be avoided.
- Fourth, methods to determine eligibility for extubation were highly variable across studies. However, this heterogeneity reflects important real-world differences in policies and practices related to extubation, such that generalizability of our results may be enhanced. Finally, for continuous factors, we were unable to report associations at common thresholds due to differences in prognostic factor reporting across studies, leading to our use of the tertile method.

■ REVIEWERS' VIEWPOINT
- In this case the authors conducted a review of relevant studies investigating extubation failure in acutely brain-injured patients and then performed a meta-analysis to pool the results of these studies for more robust conclusions.

- The meta-analysis may reveal that factors such as the Glasgow Coma Scale (GCS) score, age, presence of intracranial hemorrhage, or certain physiological parameters (e.g., oxygenation, respiratory rate) are significantly associated with a higher risk of extubation failure. These findings can help clinicians identify patients who are at a higher risk of unsuccessful extubation and adjust their management plans accordingly.
- The findings of the meta-analysis can inform prognostic discussions with patients and their families. Clinicians can use this information to better communicate the potential risks and outcomes associated with extubation in acutely brain-injured patients. It can help set realistic expectations and facilitate shared decision-making by providing evidence-based information about the likelihood of successful extubation and potential factors that may impact the outcome.

IMPACT ON CURRENT PRACTICE AND TAKE HOME MESSAGE

Impact on Current Practice

The systematic review and meta-analysis on prognostic factors associated with extubation failure in acutely brain-injured patients can have a significant impact on current medical practice, especially in critical care settings. It provides valuable insights into the factors that may influence the success or failure of extubation in this specific patient population. These findings can help clinicians make more informed decisions when deciding whether and when to extubate brain-injured patients, which is a crucial step in their management.

- *Tailored extubation decisions:* The study's results can guide clinicians in tailoring their extubation decisions based on individual patient characteristics. By identifying specific prognostic factors that may increase the risk of extubation failure, clinicians can take a more personalized approach to extubation, ensuring that patients with a higher likelihood of failure receive appropriate interventions or prolonged mechanical ventilation when necessary.
- *Enhanced patient safety:* Reducing extubation failure rates in brain-injured patients can lead to improved patient safety. Extubation failure can result in adverse outcomes, such as reintubation, prolonged mechanical ventilation, or even complications like ventilator-associated pneumonia. Understanding the factors that contribute to failure can help mitigate risks and prevent potential harm to patients.
- *Resource optimization:* Preventing unnecessary extubation failures can lead to more efficient utilization of healthcare resources. Reintubation and prolonged ventilation are resource-intensive and can strain critical care units. By reducing extubation failure rates, hospitals can potentially allocate resources more effectively, providing better care to other patients in need.

Take Home Message

- The key take home message from this systematic review and meta-analysis is that there are identifiable prognostic factors associated with extubation failure in acutely brain-injured patients. These factors can assist clinicians in making more informed decisions regarding the timing and appropriateness of extubation, ultimately leading to improved patient outcomes.

- Additionally, it highlights the importance of a multidisciplinary approach in managing brain-injured patients. Collaborative efforts between neurologists, intensivists, respiratory therapists, and other healthcare professionals are essential to assess and consider these prognostic factors comprehensively.
- Furthermore, the study underscores the need for ongoing research in critical care medicine to enhance our understanding of extubation management in specific patient populations. Future studies should focus on validating the identified prognostic factors, exploring potential interventions to mitigate extubation failure risks, and refining protocols for extubation decision-making in acutely brain-injured patients.
- Overall, this systematic review and meta-analysis contribute valuable evidence to the field of critical care medicine and provide a basis for more informed and individualized approaches to extubation in brain-injured patients, ultimately striving for better patient outcomes and safety.

ARTICLE 14

Effect of Remote Ischemic Conditioning vs. Usual Care on Neurologic Function in Patients with Acute Moderate Ischemic Stroke: The RICAMIS Randomized Clinical Trial

Chen HS, Cui Y, Li XQ, Wang XH, Ma YT, Zhao Y, et al. Effect of Remote Ischemic Conditioning vs Usual Care on Neurologic Function in Patients with Acute Moderate Ischemic Stroke: The RICAMIS Randomized Clinical Trial.
JAMA. 2022;328(7):627-36.

■ WHAT IS ALREADY KNOWN?

The study aimed to assess the efficacy of remote ischemic conditioning (RIC) as a neuroprotective strategy for acute moderate ischemic stroke. Prior research had indicated the potential neuroprotective effects of RIC in preclinical studies, but robust clinical evidence for its effectiveness in patients with ischemic stroke was lacking.

■ STUDY DESIGN

This was a multicenter, open-label, blinded-endpoint, randomized clinical trial conducted at 55 hospitals in China from December 26, 2018, through January 19, 2021.

■ POPULATION STUDIED INCLUDING DEMOGRAPHICS

The study included 1,893 patients with acute moderate ischemic stroke, with a mean age of 65 years, and 34.1% of participants were women.

■ INTERVENTION(S) STUDIED

Eligible patients were randomly assigned to receive RIC treatment in addition to guideline-based treatment. RIC involved five cycles of cuff inflation for 5 minutes and deflation for 5 minutes to the bilateral upper limbs to 200 mm Hg. This was administered for 10–14 days.

■ COMPARATOR USED

The control group received guideline-based treatment alone.

■ OUTCOMES EVALUATED

The primary endpoint was excellent functional outcome at 90 days, defined as a modified Rankin Scale score of 0–1. Secondary outcomes included favorable functional outcome (mRS scores 0–2), early neurologic deterioration, stroke-associated pneumonia, change in National Institutes of Health Stroke Scale (NIHSS) score, occurrence of stroke or other vascular events, and time to death within 90 days. The authors concluded that RIC significantly increased the likelihood of excellent neurologic function at 90 days for patients with acute moderate ischemic stroke. However, they emphasized the need for further trials to replicate these findings.

■ AUTHORS' VIEWPOINT

- Remote ischemic conditioning is a noninvasive and well-tolerated neuroprotective therapy that has shown promise in patients with acute moderate ischemic stroke.
- *Neuroprotection:* RIC activates endogenous tissue repair mechanisms, which can help protect the brain from further damage and promote neurological recovery.
- *Cardiovascular protection:* RIC has been shown to have cardiovascular benefits, including improving blood flow and reducing the risk of cardiovascular events.
- *Feasibility and safety:* RIC is a noninvasive and well-tolerated therapy that can be applied within 24 hours after stroke, including in patients receiving standard stroke treatments such as thrombolysis or mechanical thrombectomy.

■ STRENGTH OF THE STUDY

- *Rigorous methodology:* The Remote Ischemic Conditioning in Acute Moderate Ischemic Stroke (RICAMIS) study is designed with careful consideration of various factors, including appropriate inclusion criteria, random allocation of participants, standardized intervention protocols, and robust outcome measures. This rigorous methodology enhances the validity and reliability of the study's findings.
- *Targeted patient population:* The RICAMIS study focuses specifically on patients with acute moderate ischemic stroke. This targeted approach allows for a more precise evaluation of the potential benefits of RIC in this specific subgroup of stroke patients.
- *Functional outcome assessment:* The primary outcome measure of the RICAMIS study is functional outcome, assessed using validated stroke scales such as the modified Rankin Scale (mRS) or the NIHSS. By utilizing these standardized measures, the study aims to provide meaningful and clinically relevant data on the impact of RIC on patients' functional recovery.
- *Potential clinical relevance:* If the RICAMIS study demonstrates positive results, it has the potential to influence clinical practice and stroke management guidelines. The findings may support the adoption of RIC as an adjunctive therapy in the acute management of moderate ischemic stroke, potentially improving patient outcomes and enhancing the standard of care.
- *Ethical considerations:* The RICAMIS study adheres to rigorous ethical guidelines, ensuring informed consent, patient confidentiality, and protection of participants' rights. This commitment to

ethical conduct demonstrates the study's integrity and further strengthens the credibility of its findings.

DRAWBACKS OF THE STUDY

- First, the open-label design did not allow blinding of the assigned treatment to participants and physicians. Blinded end-point assessments were performed to reduce observer bias, but assessment of the success of outcome blinding was not performed.
- Second, a structured interview was used to assess the mRS disability score, which may have affected the accuracy of assessors in distinguishing how much of an individual's disability was due to stroke versus nonstroke.
- Third, there may have been outcome measurement bias in the full analysis set and selection bias in the exclusions after randomization.
- The relatively large amount of dropout after randomization may have introduced attrition bias, although there was a similar proportion of dropout in the RIC versus control group.
- Fourth, data regarding physiotherapy and speech language therapy were not collected and could not be assessed for possible confounding.
- Fifth, confirmation of these findings is required, including in non-Chinese populations, given potential differences compared with other populations in body mass, comorbid factors, and patterns of cerebrovascular disease of patients with AIS.

REVIEWERS' VIEWPOINT

- The RICAMIS study has the potential to bring about practice-changing implications in the management of acute moderate ischemic stroke if its findings demonstrate positive results.
- The target condition of acute ischemic stroke has a massive disease burden but limited treatment options currently beyond IV thrombolysis (which is only applicable to a small subset). Even minor benefits could impact many lives.
- Clinically relevant outcomes are being assessed—functional independence and disability at 90 days. Positive results on such patient-centered outcomes could strongly support implementation.
- An international, multi-center trial design will help minimize bias and ensure inclusion of a diverse population, supporting broader applicability of findings.

IMPACT ON CURRENT PRACTICE AND TAKE HOME MESSAGE

- *Integration of RIC in stroke management guidelines:* If the RICAMIS study shows that RIC improves functional outcomes in patients with acute moderate ischemic stroke, it may lead to the inclusion of RIC as a recommended neuroprotective strategy in stroke management guidelines. Healthcare professionals may be encouraged to consider RIC as part of the overall treatment plan for this patient population.
- *Adoption of RIC as an adjunctive therapy:* Positive results from the RICAMIS study could lead to the adoption of RIC as an adjunctive therapy alongside standard care for acute moderate ischemic stroke. Healthcare providers may consider incorporating RIC protocols into the acute stroke management pathway to potentially enhance neuroprotection and improve patient outcomes.
- *Development of RIC protocols:* The RICAMIS study may provide insights into

the optimal protocols for applying remote ischemic conditioning in acute moderate ischemic stroke. The study's findings, along with further research, could guide the development of standardized RIC protocols, including the duration, frequency, and intensity of RIC cycles, to maximize its neuroprotective effects.
- *Consideration of RIC in prehospital settings:* If RIC is shown to be beneficial in the RICAMIS study, there may be considerations for implementing RIC protocols in prehospital settings, such as during ambulance transport or in emergency medical services. This could provide an opportunity for early initiation of RIC and potentially extend the therapeutic window for neuroprotection.
- *Further research and refinement:* The RICAMIS study's findings, whether positive or negative, may stimulate further research and refinement of RIC protocols in acute moderate ischemic stroke. Subsequent studies could explore the optimal timing of RIC initiation, the potential benefits in different stroke subtypes, and the long-term effects of RIC on functional recovery and quality of life.

ARTICLE 15

Transfusion Guidelines in Traumatic Brain Injury: A Systematic Review and Meta-analysis of the Currently Available Evidence

Montgomery EY, Barrie U, Kenfack YJ, Edukugho D, Caruso JP, Rail B, et al. Transfusion Guidelines in Traumatic Brain Injury: A Systematic Review and Meta-analysis of the Currently Available Evidence.
Neurotrauma Rep. 2022;3(1):554-68.

■ WHAT IS ALREADY KNOWN?

- *Timing of transfusion:* Timing is an important consideration in transfusion management for TBI patients. Early initiation of transfusion, particularly in cases of severe hemorrhage, may help improve outcomes by maintaining adequate tissue oxygenation.
- *Transfusion thresholds:* The optimal transfusion threshold for TBI patients is still a matter of debate. The TRICC trial, which included ICU patients but not specifically TBI patients, found no difference in 90-day mortality between a restrictive transfusion threshold (hemoglobin level of 7 g/dL) and a liberal threshold (hemoglobin level of 10 g/dL).[1-3] However, more recent studies have not provided definitive superiority of one strategy over the other.
- *Outcomes:* Several studies have assessed the association of blood transfusion thresholds with clinical outcomes in TBI patients. On study found that transfusion when the initial hemoglobin level was >10 g/dL was associated with decreased survival. Another study suggested that transfusion was associated with worse outcomes with a hemoglobin threshold <9 or 10 g/dL, but improved outcomes in patients with a hemoglobin level <7 and 8 g/dL.
- *Risk factors:* Several risk factors have been identified for the need for blood transfusion in TBI patients. These include

older age, lower GCS score, higher Injury Severity Score (ISS), and higher head Abbreviated Injury Scale (AIS) score.
- *Complications:* Blood transfusions in TBI patients can lead to various complications. These include acute respiratory distress syndrome (ARDS), infections, and adverse reactions to blood products.
- *Coagulopathy management:* Traumatic brain injury patients often experience coagulopathy, which increases the risk of bleeding and complications. The use of antifibrinolytic agents, such as tranexamic acid, has shown promise in reducing mortality and improving outcomes in TBI patients with coagulopathy.

STUDY DESIGN

A systematic review and meta-analysis was conducted using PubMed, Google Scholar, and Web of Science electronic database.

POPULATION STUDIED INCLUDING DEMOGRAPHICS

Traumatic brain injury patients who require blood transfusion and those did not require it. The transfusion triggers in traumatic brain injury. Studied population age, sex, Glasgow Coma Scale (GCS), ISS, and head AIS.

INTERVENTION(S) STUDIED

Traumatic brain injury patients who were not transfused blood, number of patients who were transfused blood, transfusion hemoglobin (Hgb) threshold, age, GCS on presentation, ISS on presentation, mean number of packed RBC (pRBC) transfusions, complication rate, and mortality rate.

COMPARATOR USED

Traumatic brain injury patients who did not require RBC transfusion.

OUTCOMES EVALUATED

Follow-up outcomes of interest included mortality, length of stay (LOS), and Glasgow Outcome Scale [GOS; or Glasgow Outcome Scale-Extended (GOSE)].

AUTHORS' VIEWPOINT

- Traumatic brain injury is a complex condition that can lead to significant morbidity and mortality. The management of TBI includes various aspects such as surgical intervention, prevention of secondary brain injury, and optimization of systemic factors.
- Transfusion of blood products, such as packed red blood cells (PRBCs), platelets, and fresh frozen plasma (FFP), is often considered in the management of TBI to maintain adequate oxygen delivery to the brain and prevent coagulopathy. However, the optimal transfusion thresholds and ratios in TBI remain a topic of debate.
- Several systematic reviews and meta-analyses have been conducted to evaluate the available evidence on transfusion guidelines in TBI, but the results have been somewhat conflicting. Some studies have suggested that a more liberal transfusion strategy with higher hemoglobin thresholds may improve outcomes in TBI patients, while others have not found a significant benefit or have even suggested potential harm with liberal transfusion practices.
- Standardized criteria regarding the definition of TBI severity, inclusion of anemic patients, Hgb monitoring, indications for transfusion, and consideration of the unique oxygenation requirements of cerebral tissue are important foundations on which to build future studies to more definitively answer this important question.

■ STRENGTH OF THE STUDY

- *Comprehensive literature search:* The systematic review and meta-analysis will involve a comprehensive search of multiple electronic databases, ensuring a thorough identification of relevant studies. This approach minimizes the risk of missing important evidence.
- Transfusion status and GCS on admission were independent predictors for long-term functional outcome is important to consider these associations in the context of transfusion threshold analyses, given that outcomes between groups may simply be the result of transfused patients being sicker and more likely to receive transfusion.
- The meta-analysis determined that transfused patients have higher rates of mortality, which likely suggests that patients who require a transfusion have an inherently worse prognosis at baseline, but further clarification is warranted given the heterogeneity of included studies.
- *Inclusion of different study designs:* The article plans to include both randomized controlled trials (RCTs) and observational studies, allowing for a broader assessment of the available evidence. This inclusion of different study designs increases the robustness and generalizability of the findings.
- *Quality assessment:* The article mentions the use of appropriate tools to assess the quality of included studies, such as the Cochrane Risk of Bias Tool for RCTs and the Newcastle-Ottawa Scale for observational studies. This quality assessment helps ensure that the included studies are methodologically sound and minimizes the risk of bias.
- *Data extraction and analysis:* The article describes a standardized data extraction process, which involves two independent reviewers extracting data from the selected studies. This approach enhances the reliability and accuracy of the data. Additionally, the planned meta-analysis using appropriate statistical methods allows for the estimation of pooled effect sizes, providing a quantitative summary of the findings.
- *Potential impact on clinical practice:* The article highlights the potential impact of the study findings on clinical practice. By synthesizing the currently available evidence, the study aims to inform transfusion guidelines in traumatic brain injury and ultimately improve patient outcomes. This practical relevance enhances the significance of the research.

■ DRAWBACKS OF THE STUDY

Weaknesses of the article may include:
- Inclusion criteria are inconsistent regarding the definition of TBI, whether anemic versus non-anemic patients are eligible for inclusion, follow-up time, and the specific definitions "restrictive" and "liberal" transfusion thresholds.
- *Variability in definitions:* Definitions of transfusion triggers/thresholds, anemia levels, and outcomes were not standardized between studies, introducing some uncertainty.
- *Potential publication bias:* Additionally, only two included studies were RCTs that sought to directly compare outcomes in TBI patients between transfusion thresholds. The remaining studies were post hoc analyses of RCTs or unmatched retrospective analyses, which are more subject to selection and confounding bias. The inclusion of both RCTs and post hoc analysis may introduce heterogeneity in terms of study design, patient populations, and interventions.

- *Variability in transfusion strategies:* Transfusion strategies may vary across studies, including thresholds for transfusion, type of blood products used, and timing of transfusions. This heterogeneity could limit the ability to draw firm conclusions and make specific recommendations for clinical practice.
- *Quality of included studies:* Although the article mentions the use of quality assessment tools, the overall quality of the included studies may vary. The inclusion of studies with high risk of bias or low methodological quality could introduce potential sources of bias and impact the reliability of the findings.
- *Potential confounding factors:* The observational studies included in the analysis may be prone to confounding, as they rely on existing data and may not have controlled for all potential confounders. This could introduce biases and affect the accuracy of the estimated treatment effects.

REVIEWERS' VIEWPOINT

- It is important to note that the management of TBI is highly individualized and depends on various factors, including the severity of the injury, the patient's clinical condition, and the presence of associated injuries. The decision to transfuse blood products in TBI should be based on a careful assessment of the patient's hemodynamic status, coagulation profile, and the presence of active bleeding.
- There is still a need for a systematic review and meta-analysis to comprehensively evaluate the currently available evidence and address the remaining uncertainties in transfusion guidelines for traumatic brain injury.

IMPACT ON CURRENT PRACTICE AND TAKE HOME MESSAGE

- Current literature appears to support restrictive transfusion protocols (Hgb <7 g/dL) compared to liberal thresholds (Hgb <10 g/dL), but the quality and consistency of evidence is mixed.
- The management of TBI is highly individualized, and the decision to transfuse RBCs should be based on the patient's specific needs. Factors such as the severity of the injury, presence of active bleeding, and hemodynamic stability should be taken into account.

REFERENCES

1. Gobatto ALN, Link MA, Solla DJ, Bassi E, Tierno PF, Paiva W, et al. Transfusion requirements after head trauma: a randomized feasibility-controlled trial. Crit Care. 2019;23(1):89.
2. Warner MA, O'Keeffe T, Bhavsar P, Shringer R, Moore C, Harper C, et al. Transfusions and long-term functional outcomes in traumatic brain injury. J Neurosurg. 2010;113(3):539-46.
3. McIntyre LA, Fergusson DA, Hutchison JS, Pagliarello G, Marshall JC, Yetisir E, et al. Effect of a liberal versus restrictive transfusion strategy on mortality in patients with moderate to severe head injury. Neurocrit Care. 2006;5(1):4-9.

Section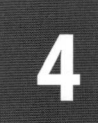

Gastroenterology/Hepatobiliary

Section Editor: Lalita Gouri Mitra
Associate Editors: Jagdeep Sharma, Harsimran Singh Walia

ARTICLE 16

A Randomized Trial of Albumin Infusions in Hospitalized Patients with Cirrhosis

China L, Freemantle N, Forrest E, Kallis Y, Ryder SD, Wright G, et al. ATTIRE Trial Investigators. A randomized trial of albumin infusions in hospitalized patients with cirrhosis.
N Engl J Med. 2021;384:808-17.

CLINICAL QUESTION OR PROBLEM

Cirrhosis is a global problem, with an estimated 1 million deaths occurring annually, and is the third leading cause of death in adults aged 45–64 years.[1] In the UK, over 3% of all critically ill patients admitted to the intensive care unit (ICU) have cirrhosis.[2,3] These patients are immunosuppressed and more than one-fourth suffer a bacterial infection, causing a fourfold increase in mortality.[4] Patients with acute-on-chronic liver failure (ACLF) who develop a bacterial infection have a higher mortality than those without bacterial infection.

WHAT IS ALREADY KNOWN?

Albumin, which is solely produced in the liver at a rate of 12–25 g/day, is the most abundant plasma protein in the human body, with a total body pool of 250–300 g for a 70-kg adult.[5] Poor synthetic liver function in cirrhosis and ACLF, leads to lower plasma albumin levels than in healthy people. Approximately two-thirds of the body's albumin is stored in the extravascular space and one-third in the intravascular space. This ratio can change dramatically during critical illness, with up to a 300% increase of transcapillary movement during septic shock, resulting in increased losses due to transfer to lumen of the gastrointestinal tract, pleural and intra-alveolar space, and wounds which are nonexchangeable regions.

Apart from its oncotic effect, albumin also functions to bind and transport endogenous and exogenous compounds, maintains acid–base balance, has anticoagulant properties, and supports microvascular function and the immune system.

The excess of the eicosanoid prostaglandin E2 (PGE2) in cirrhotic patients attributes to immunosuppression as it inhibits the secretion of cytokines from macrophages, hence the ability to destroy the bacteria decreases and this effect is not seen in patients without cirrhosis.[6] Albumin binds and inactivates PGE2, potentially reversing this PGE2-mediated immunosuppression, increasing the possibility that exogenously administered albumin may prevent some of the excess infections, and deaths, as seen in cirrhotics.

STUDY DESIGN, POPULATION STUDIED INCLUDING DEMOGRAPHICS, INTERVENTION(S) STUDIED, COMPARATOR USED, OUTCOMES EVALUATED

The ATTIRE (Albumin to Prevent Infection in Chronic Liver Failure) trial (2016–2019) was a parallel group, open-label, multicenter (35 UK centers), stratified, randomized controlled trial (RCT) evaluating a strategy of maintaining a serum albumin above 30 g/dL in hospitalized patients with decompensated cirrhosis. Inclusion criteria were: patients aged over 18 years, enrolment within 72 hours of being hospitalized for an acute decompensation of cirrhotic liver disease and those with a serum albumin level of <30 g/dL, and an expected duration of hospitalization of at least 5 days. The exclusion criteria were advanced hepatocellular carcinoma with a life expectancy of <8 weeks, those receiving palliative care and severe cardiac dysfunction.

Recruited patients were randomly allocated to either the intervention or control group in a 1:1 ratio, via an online service incorporating a minimization algorithm. Patients were stratified by center, MELD (Model for End-Stage Liver Disease) score, number of organ dysfunctions, serum albumin level, and the use of antibiotics. The intervention group received daily infusions of 20% human albumin solution (HAS), targeting a serum albumin level >35 g/L, with the aim of achieving a level >30 g/L. A tiered daily-dosing regimen for albumin administration was suggested—patients with a serum albumin level of 30–34 g/L received 100 mL 20% HAS; 26–29 g/L, 200 mL 20% HAS; 20–25 g/L, 300 mL 20% HAS; and <20 g/L, 400 mL 20% HAS. Albumin was administered for up to 14 days or discharge from hospital. The control group received standard care. Albumin administration was permissible for standard indications, such as large-volume paracentesis, spontaneous bacterial peritonitis (SBP), and hepatorenal syndrome (HRS).

The primary outcome was a composite of infection, renal dysfunction, and death between days 3 and 15 post-randomization. The presence of an infection was confirmed by the treating clinicians and supporting information sought for blinded validation by a panel of physicians. Renal dysfunction was defined as a 50% increase in serum creatinine from baseline or an absolute increase of 0.3 mg/dL (26.5 µmol/L), or the introduction of renal replacement therapy.

With an expected incidence of the composite primary outcome of 30% in the control group, and a 10% attrition rate, 433 patients per group were required to identify a 30% reduction, from 30% to 21%, with 80% power at the 5% significance level. Analyses were performed on an intention-to-treat basis. The primary outcome was also assessed by stratum.

Secondary outcomes included the individual components of the primary outcome, plus time to outcome, transplantation within 6 months, and safety and tolerability of HAS as well as several more and additional exploratory outcomes. 9,273 patients were screened, 1,563 were eligible, and 829 were randomized. One patient withdrew and 51 had more than one randomization, leaving

777 patients for analysis, with 380 allocated to the albumin group and 397 to the control group.

Groups were largely similar at baseline, although there were slightly more females in the albumin group (123 vs. 104; 32% vs. 26%) The mean patient age was 54 years, 97% were managed in a general ward, approximately 90% had cirrhosis due to alcohol, approximately 65% had worsening ascites as the reason for admission to hospital, albumin levels were similar between groups, as were measures of function the major organ systems. Patients were typically recruited on the day after hospital admission, with a mean (±SD) albumin level of 23.2 ± 3.7 g /L. Both groups were treated for similar durations of time: albumin group, median 8 days [interquartile range (IQR) 6-15] and control group, median 9 days (6-15). Exposure to albumin differed significantly between the two groups. Patients in the albumin group received more albumin [median 200 vs. 20 g; adjusted mean difference 143; 95% confidence interval (CI) 127-158 g]. 49% of the control group received no albumin. The mean serum albumin level in the intervention group was 30 g/L for the intervention period.

The composite primary endpoint occurred in 29.7% of the albumin group and 30.2% of the control group [adjusted odds ratio (aOR) 0.98; 95% CI 0.71-1.33; $p = 0.87$]. The primary outcome did not differ when assessed according to strata. For the components of the primary endpoint, new infections occurred in 20.8% of the albumin group and 17.9% of the control group (aOR 1.22; 95% CI 0.85-1.75); renal dysfunction in 10.5% and 14.4%, respectively (aOR 0.68; 95% CI 0.44-1.11); and death in 7.9% and 8.3%, respectively (OR 0.95; 95% CI 0.56-1.59).

Secondary outcomes occurred at similar rates in the two groups. At 6 months, 34.7% of the albumin group and 30.0% of the control group had died (aOR 1.27; 95% CI 0.93-1.73). There were 87 serious adverse events in the albumin group and 72 in the control group, including more respiratory complications, with an excess of episodes of lung infection (15 vs. 8) and pulmonary edema (15 vs. 4). However, there were less episodes of multiorgan failure in the albumin group (23 vs. 31).

■ REVIEWERS' VIEWPOINT

The ATTIRE trial was an extensive program to evaluate the effectiveness of albumin supplementation in hospitalized patients with cirrhosis. It started with an initial phase 2 feasibility study involving 400 patients. This confirmed both safety and the incrementation of serum albumin with exogenous administration. This initial component included a stop/go assessment for progression to the phase 3 trial.

The ATTIRE trial raises fundamental questions about the efficacy of albumin in the management of patients with cirrhosis. The interventional group received ten times the dose of albumin as the control group. There was a clear separation between groups in terms of exposure to the interventional agent. To maximize the likelihood of a beneficial effect, albumin was administered at an early time point. The trial also appears adequately powered to identify a potential effect, should it have occurred. However, no beneficial effects were seen, but there were signs of harm from albumin administration, particularly to the respiratory system.

This trial addressed the same issue of the SAFE trial,[7] published 20 years ago which demonstrated no benefit from the addition of albumin to critically ill patients, regardless of their serum albumin level. Although there was a possible sign of improvement in those with severe sepsis in the SAFE trial [relative risk (RR) 0.87; 95% CI 0.74–1.02; p = 0.09], the subsequent Albumin Italian Outcome Sepsis (ALBIOS) trial,[8] which directly investigated this subgroup, did not find superior outcomes with this strategy. Interestingly, in the ALBIOS trial, the subgroup with septic shock had better outcomes with albumin administration, but this requires further prospective study, being a subgroup effect found in a post hoc analysis. The recently published small FRISC trial[9] examined the administration of albumin in patients with cirrhosis and infection-induced hypotension and found no short-term benefits.

While the premise of the trial was to restore immune function with albumin in a group uniquely immunocompromised, the intervention also brings undesirable physiological stresses. The SAFE trial demonstrated that albumin has a superior volume expanding effect to saline, by a magnitude of 1.3:1. Portal hypertension is a significant complication of decompensated cirrhosis, often culminating in life-threatening upper gastrointestinal bleeding. In a Spanish multicenter RCT,[10] a liberal transfusion threshold was inferior to a more conservative threshold, possibly due to an increased portal pressure from a higher volume of transfusion.

In ATTIRE, 24 patients suffered an adverse gastrointestinal bleed who had an initial variceal bleed, (7/11 albumin group vs. 3/13 control group). 60% of patients with cirrhosis have cirrhotic cardiomyopathy,[11] which impedes systolic and diastolic dysfunction as well as electrophysiological function, due to which the heart may be the most vulnerable organ to suffer from a relative state of volume overload. Both the ATTIRE and CONFIRM trials reported an excess of pulmonary edema or respiratory failure in those receiving albumin, but no difference in the other main mediators of decompensation, namely, hepatic encephalopathy (HE), acute kidney injury (AKI)/HRS, and SBP. Deaths occurring within 2 days of entry into the study were excluded from the analysis, which reduces the possibility of immediate harm from albumin being recognized. Benefit from the intervention would carry over into the trial period from days 3 to 15 (no infection or renal impairment and ongoing survival), while harm arising from the trial intervention resulting in death, such as volume overload presenting as pulmonary edema, heart failure, venous congestion-induced AKI, would potentially be unmeasured in the death component of the composite primary outcome.

EVIDENCE FROM PREVIOUS STUDIES

In the Italian ANSWER trial,[12] 440 patients with cirrhosis and uncomplicated ascites were randomized to receive either 40 g of HAS twice weekly for 2 weeks, and then 40 g weekly, for up to 18 months, or standard care. It was an investigator-initiated, multicenter, randomized, parallel, open-label, pragmatic trial examining the long-term administration of albumin in patients with decompensated cirrhosis. The serum albumin level rose from 31 to 40 g/L in the albumin group and remained unchanged in the control group. Amongst the 431 analyzed patients, 18-month survival was significantly higher in the group receiving albumin, 77% versus 66% [hazard ratio (HR) 0.62; 95% CI 0.40–0.95]. Non-liver-related adverse events occurred at similar rates of 22% each.

The ALB-CIRINF[13] was a French open-label, multicenter, RCT in 193 consecutive patients admitted to hospital with cirrhosis and sepsis. Participants were blindly allocated to receive antibiotics with 20% HAS, at a dose of 1.5 g/kg on day 1 and 1 g/kg on day 3, or antibiotics alone. The primary outcome was the rate of renal failure at 3 months and occurred in 14.3% of the albumin group and 13.5% of the control group ($p = 0.88$). The albumin group were slower to develop renal failure (mean 29.0 ± 21.8 vs. 11.7 ± 9.1 days, $p = 0.018$). Mortality at 3 months was similar (albumin group, 70.2% vs. control, 78.3%; $p = 0.16$). More patients developed pulmonary edema in the albumin group, prompting the early termination of the trial.

Guevara[14] and colleagues also undertook a parallel group RCT comparing antibiotics with or without albumin in 110 patients with cirrhosis and infections other than SBP. HAS was administered at a dose of 1.5 g/kg on day 1 and 1 g/kg on day 3. The use of antibiotics was protocolized. Albumin was only administered to the control group for the management of type 1 HRS. Groups were similar at baseline, except for a lower mean serum sodium in the albumin group (129 vs. 132 mmol/L). Infection resolved in the majority of patients (94%) and was equal between the two groups. There was no difference in the unadjusted primary outcome of survival at 3 months (albumin group, 82.6% vs. control group, 80.4%). In a per-protocol adjusted analysis, those receiving albumin had a superior 3-month survival (HR 0.294; 95% CI 0.091–0.954; $p = 0.04$).

In 1999, Sort and colleagues compared the administration of cefotaxime with or without the addition of HAS in 126 patients with cirrhosis and SBP.[15] HAS was given at a dose of 1.5 g/kg on day 1 and 1 g/kg on day 3. The dose of cefotaxime was adjusted according to renal function. Groups were similar at baseline. 61 of the 63 patients in the cefotaxime plus albumin group received their assigned albumin. Both groups had similar rates of resolution of sepsis (>90%). The primary outcomes were the development of renal impairment and mortality. Renal impairment occurred in 33% of the cefotaxime only group and 10% of the cefotaxime and albumin group ($p = 0.01$). Three-month mortality was 41% and 22%, respectively ($p = 0.03$).

The ALBIOS,[8] a large Italian trial in 100 ICUs was published in 2014, followed on from the SAFE trial, and investigated the subgroup effect of improved mortality in patients with severe sepsis seen in this trial from the ANZICS (Australian and New Zealand Intensive Care Society) group. It evaluated maintaining a serum albumin level >30 g/L in critically ill adult patients in the ICU. 1,810 patients were randomized and analyzed, 903 in the albumin group and 907 in the control group. Groups were similar at baseline, with median Sequential Organ Failure Assessment (SOFA) scores of 8, approximately 80% receiving mechanical ventilation and 62% being in a state of shock. The albumin group received significantly more albumin and had a higher serum albumin level. There was no difference in the primary outcome of 28-day mortality; albumin group, 31.8% versus control, 32.0% (RR 1.00; 95% CI 0.87–1.14; $p = 0.94$).

The recent single-center, open-label randomized FRISC trial[9] compared saline with albumin for resuscitation in 308 cirrhotic patients with sepsis-induced hypotension. Participants received either a 250 mL bolus of 5% HAS over 15–30 minutes, followed by 50 mL/h over the next 3 hours, or a 30 mL/kg bolus of 0.9% saline over 15–30 minutes, followed by 100 mL/h of saline over the next 3 hours. The primary outcome was the reversal of hypotension, defined as an increase in mean arterial blood pressure above 65 mm Hg at 3 hours. Groups were similar at baseline, with patients having an average mean arterial pressure of 53 mm Hg. More patients in the albumin group had a reversal of their hypotension at 3 hours, 11% vs. 3.2% (OR 3.9; 95% CI 1.42–10.9; p = 0.008). Mortality was also lower in the albumin group at 1 week; 43.5% versus 38.3%; p = 0.03.

The American College of Gastroenterology issued updated guidelines[16] in February, 2022 on the management of patients with ACLF. A strong recommendation, based on moderate quality evidence, was issued recommending not to use albumin infusions to maintain a serum albumin level >30 g/L with the aim of preventing renal dysfunction, infections, or death.

IMPACT ON CURRENT PRACTICE AND TAKE HOME MESSAGE

One should not target a serum albumin level >30 g/L in hospitalized patients with cirrhosis since the ATTIRE trial identified an increase in adverse events with no improvement in outcomes with this strategy.

ARTICLE 17

Terlipressin plus Albumin for the Treatment of Type 1 Hepatorenal Syndrome

Wong F, Pappas SC, Curry MP, Reddy KR, Rubin RA, Porayko MK, et al. CONFIRM Study Investigators. Terlipressin plus albumin for the treatment of type 1 hepatorenal syndrome.
N Engl J Med 2021;384:818-28.

CLINICAL QUESTION OR PROBLEM

Acute-on-chronic liver failure is the sudden decompensation of cirrhosis with associated organ failures.[17] The global prevalence amongst patients admitted to hospital with decompensated cirrhosis is 35%, and 90-day mortality rate is 58%.[18] Worldwide, alcohol is the most common underlying cause of cirrhosis (45%), with infection being the most frequent precipitant of ACLF (35%) and AKI being the most prevalent organ failure (49%).[18] For patients with HRS-AKI (previously termed type 1 HRS),[19] 90 day survival without transplantation is approximately 45%.[20]

International Club of Ascites-AKI defines HRS-AKI as AKI in the presence of cirrhosis and ascites, with a lack of response to 2 consecutive days of diuretic withdrawal and plasma volume expansion with 1 g/kg of albumin, having ruled out shock, nephrotoxic drugs, and structural kidney disease.[19] HRS-AKI is a functional disorder, with splanchnic and systemic vasodilation reducing the effective circulating blood volume, triggering sodium and water retention, and leading to ascites formation in the presence of portal hypertension. Intense renal vasoconstriction occurs due to activation of the renin–angiotensin–aldosterone, vasopressin, and sympathetic systems, causing renal ischemia.[21] Treatment with a vasopressor which specifically acts on the splanchnic circulation to reduce the splanchnic/systemic vasodilation may reverse this.

Most trials undertaken to date have shown improvements in renal function, but no clear effect has been seen on mortality.[18] Since the trials to date were small, a larger RCT may fill the lacuna in the knowledge.

STUDY DESIGN, POPULATION STUDIED INCLUDING DEMOGRAPHICS, INTERVENTION(S) STUDIED, COMPARATOR USED, OUTCOMES EVALUATED

The CONFIRM trial was a binational (60 centers in the USA and Canada; 2016-2019), multicenter, stratified, parallel group, double-blind, RCT comparing terlipressin and albumin with placebo and albumin in patients with type 1 HRS.

Inclusion Criteria

Patients were adults with cirrhosis, ascites, and a diagnosis of type 1 HRS based on the 2007 and 2015 International Ascites Club diagnostic criteria.[22,23] Patients were required to have rapidly progressive deteriorating renal function with a serum creatinine ≥2.25 mg/dL (199 µmol/L) and no sustained improvement in renal function at least 48 hours after diuretic withdrawal and the beginning of plasma volume expansion with albumin, defined as a sustained serum creatinine decrease of 20% or a decrease <2.25 mg/dL.

Exclusion Criteria

A serum creatinine level greater than 7 mg/dL (619 µmol/dL), one or more large volume paracentesis of ≥4 L within 2 days of randomization, sepsis, or other uncontrolled bacterial infection and have received <2 days of antimicrobial therapy for infection, were in shock, had received nephrotoxic agents within the previous 4 weeks, had an estimated life expectancy of <3 days, a superimposed acute liver injury other than acute alcoholic hepatitis, intrinsic renal disease, severe cardiovascular disease, renal replacement therapy within 4 weeks, ongoing use of vasopressors, or transjugular intrahepatic portosystemic shunt (TIPS) within 30 days.

Patients were centrally randomized in a 2:1 ratio to the terlipressin group, stratified by a serum creatinine above or below 3.4 mg/dL (301 µmol/L), and large-volume paracentesis within the previous 3-14 days. The intervention group received 1 mg of terlipressin intravenously every 6 hours up to a maximum of 14 days which was administered as a bolus injection over 2 minutes. The dose of terlipressin could be increased to 2 mg every 6 hours if the serum creatinine decreased by <30% by day 4 and after a minimum of 10 doses had been administered. Terlipressin was continued until 24 hours after the creatinine value was ≤1.5 mg/dL (133 µmol/L) or up to a maximum of 14 days. It was to be discontinued if the serum creatinine was maintained at or above the baseline value on day 4 and after a minimum of 10 doses have been administered. In addition, terlipressin was discontinued if the patient underwent renal replacement therapy, liver transplantation, TIPS, renal replacement therapy, or suffered cardiac or mesenteric ischemia. The control group received a visually identical placebo which was also reconstituted in 5 mL of saline and administered in the same fashion. Patients in both groups were recommended to receive albumin infusions at a dose of 1 g/kg to a maximum of 100 g on day 1, and 20-40 g from day 2 onward. Patients with a partial response to the study intervention (0.3 mg/dL (26 µmol/L) from baseline.

The design, and results, are consistent with the other evidence in the field. Had the therapy been started at an earlier timepoint it may have proven more efficacious. Following points are to be noted:

- The premise of the trial is based on the vasodilatory hypothesis of HRS-AKI, as described in the introduction.[24] However, HRS-AKI can be due to other mechanisms other than splanchnic vasodilation, ineffective circulating blood volume, and intrinsic renal ischemia.
- Numerous other processes not affected by terlipressin have been suggested to contribute to HRS-AKI, including cirrhotic cardiomyopathy, systemic inflammation, hepato-adrenal syndrome, bile cast nephropathy, intra-abdominal hypertension, and a complex neural hepatorenal reflex dependent on liver osmoreceptors, chemoreceptors, and baroreceptors.[25] The rationale of expanding the circulatory volume with albumin and reversing the vasodilatory state with terlipressin appearing sound may be successful in treating HRS-AKI (which was the primary outcome), as terlipressin is a vasopressin analog with a specific vasopressor effect on the splanchnic circulation.
- However, it is less clear if this course of management improves the outcome of a patient with ACLF.

■ WHAT IS ALREADY KNOWN?

The results of the three major trials in this field (CONFIRM, OT-0401,[26] and REVERSE[20]) show that advance liver failure, with a mortality rate of >15% at 28 days, ultimately overwhelms any organ-specific improvements seen in the kidney. Although the intervention group demonstrated improved renal function without improved survival, five subgroups were examined post hoc, with three demonstrating benefits. Patients with alcoholic hepatitis (31% vs. 8%), patients with a baseline serum creatinine between 3 and 5 mg/dL (28% vs. 6%), and patients with systemic inflammatory response syndrome (26% vs. 4%), all had higher incidences of reversal of HRS with terlipressin therapy, in contrast to placebo. Patients whose serum creatinine values were either >5 mg/dL or <3 mg/dL had little benefit. Patients with a baseline mean arterial pressure <70 mm Hg also appeared to benefit (26% vs. 4%) but the 95% confidence limits overlapped between the terlipressin and placebo groups.

This probably reflects that patients who are sick with a serum creatinine >3 mg/dL may benefit, but if they are too sick with a serum creatinine <5 mg/dL may not benefit. Some patients showed improvement due to higher inflammatory measures due to the anti-inflammatory effect of albumin in addition to vasopressor support, while hypotensive patients were supported by the addition of a vasopressor alone.

The 20 additional cases of death due to respiratory failure were seen in the terlipressin and albumin group ($n = 22$) in comparison with the placebo group ($n = 2$). In the REVERSE trial, there was a slightly higher incidence of pulmonary edema in the group receiving terlipressin (10.8% vs. 7.4%). This phenomenon was also seen in the ATTIRE trial, investigating the maintenance of a serum albumin level >30 g/L in hospitalized patients with cirrhosis (15 vs. 4 patients). It may be that the combination of additional afterload on the left ventricle from vasopressin, combined with volume expansion from albumin, in a population with both ischemic heart disease and cirrhotic cardiomyopathy, leads to pulmonary edema, cardiopulmonary dysfunction, and death. The placebo group received a greater volume of albumin, and it is possible that it is the combination of terlipressin and albumin, rather than albumin alone, which may be harmful in this trial. The administration of terlipressin to patients with cirrhosis is known to increase left ventricular afterload and end-diastolic volume, with resultant reduction in cardiac output and ejection fraction.[27]

The small open-label TAHRS trial[28] compared terlipressin plus albumin (n = 23) with albumin alone (n = 23) in 46 patients with cirrhosis and HRS. Terlipressin was administered at a dose of 1–2 mg intravenously every 4 hours. In both groups, albumin was administered at a dose initially of 1 g/kg, followed by 20–40 g/day. The primary outcomes were improvement of renal function and survival at 3 months. Improvement of renal function was defined as complete (reduction in serum creatinine below 133 µmol/L) or partial (reduction in serum creatinine >50% but with an end-of-treatment value ≥133 µmol/L). Renal function improved in 43% of patients in the terlipressin plus albumin group and 8.7% of patients in the albumin group. The median time to improvement of renal function in the terlipressin and albumin group was 11 days. Survival at 3 months did not differ significantly between the two groups, 27% (terlipressin and albumin group) versus 19% (albumin group); p = 0.7. Amongst those in the terlipressin and albumin group, patients with type 2 HRS were more likely to achieve improvement in renal function than patients with type 1 HRS (67% vs. 35%). Rates of adverse events were similar between the two groups.

The OT-0401 trial by Sanyal and colleagues (2004–2006) was a randomized, double-blind, placebo-controlled, multicenter clinical trial conducted in the USA, Germany, and Russia. It compared terlipressin plus albumin (n = 56) with placebo plus albumin (n = 56) in 112 patients with acute or chronic liver disease and type 1 HRS.[26] Terlipressin was administered at a dose of 1 mg every 6 hours. This could be doubled after 4 days if the serum creatinine had not decreased by at least 30%. In both groups, albumin was administered at a dose of 100 g on day 1, and 25 g daily thereafter, up to a maximum of 14 days. The primary outcome was treatment success at day 14, defined as a serum creatinine level ≤1.5 mg/dL on two occasions at least 48 hours apart, without dialysis, death, or recurrence of type 1 HRS by day 14. Patients in the terlipressin plus albumin group (6.3 days) and placebo plus albumin group (5.8 days) received the study drugs for similar lengths of time. The primary outcome occurred in more patients in the terlipressin plus albumin group (25% vs. 12.5%, p = 0.093). More patients in the terlipressin plus albumin group also had reversal of their HRS, defined as a decrease in serum creatinine ≤1.5 mg/dL (34% vs. 13%, p = 0.008). Overall survival (42.9% vs. 37.5%, respectively; p = 0.839) and transplant-free survival to day 180 were similar between the two groups.

The REVERSE study[20] was published in 2016. It compared terlipressin plus albumin (n = 97) with placebo plus albumin (n = 99) in 196 patients with cirrhosis, ascites, and type 1 HRS. This multicenter, double-blind, parallel group, RCT took place in 50 centers in the USA and two in Canada. Similar to the other trials, terlipressin was administered at a dose of 1 mg every 6 hours and could be doubled to 2 mg on day 4 if the serum creatinine value had decreased by <30% of the baseline value. Albumin was administered to both groups at a dose of between 20 and 40 g/day. Study drugs could be discontinued after 4 days if the serum creatinine remained at baseline or higher. The study period was for up to 16 days. The primary endpoint was confirmed reversal of HRS, defined as 2 serum creatinine values of 1.5 mg/dL, at least 40 hours apart, while receiving treatment without renal replacement therapy or liver transplantation.

Patients were similar at baseline. The primary outcome occurred in 19.6% of the terlipressin and albumin group and 13.1% of the placebo and albumin group ($p = 0.22$). HRS reversal, defined as at least 1 serum creatinine value ≤ 1.5 mg/dL while on treatment was achieved in 23.7% of patients receiving terlipressin and albumin and 15.2% of those receiving placebo and albumin ($p = 0.13$). Overall survival and transplant-free survival were similar between groups. There were more ischemic events in the terlipressin and albumin group.

Mohamed and colleagues performed a systematic review and meta-analysis, incorporating 8 RCTs totaling 974 patients, comparing terlipressin plus albumin with albumin alone in patients with either type 1 or 2 HRS.[29] Of the included population, 61% of patients were male, their mean age was 55 ± 10 years, 56% had alcoholic liver disease, mean Child–Pugh score was 10.4 ± 1.8, mean arterial pressure was 76 ± 11 mm Hg, mean serum sodium 132 ± 6 mmol/L, mean serum creatinine 3.6 ± 1.2 mg/dL, mean serum albumin 3.4 ± 1 g/dL, and mean total bilirubin 13 ± 13 mg/dL. Compared with the placebo and albumin group, patients treated with terlipressin and albumin had a higher incidence of reversal of HRS (RR 2.08; 95% CI 1.51–2.86; $p < 0.001$) but no 90-day survival benefit (RR 1.09; 95% CI 0.84–1.43; $p = 0.52$).

IMPACT ON CURRENT PRACTICE AND TAKE HOME MESSAGE

The results of the CONFIRM trial, in addition to previous trials in the field, show that the routine use of the combination of terlipressin with albumin in patients with HRS-AKI is effective in improving renal function, but not mortality and further work is required to clarify their role.

ARTICLE 18

The Comparative Effectiveness of Vasoactive Treatments for Hepatorenal Syndrome: A Systematic Review and Network Meta-Analysis

Pitre T, Kiflen M, Helmeczi W, Dionne JC, Rewa O, Bagshaw SM, et al. The comparative effectiveness of vasoactive treatments for hepatorenal syndrome: a systematic review and network meta-analysis.
Crit Care Med. 2022;50(10):1419-29.

CLINICAL QUESTION OR PROBLEM

Comparative vasoactive therapies' efficacy in treating HRS.

WHAT IS ALREADY KNOWN?

Cirrhosis can result in complications such as HRS.[30] Depending on increases in serum creatinine, HRS is categorized as type 1 or type 2.[19,30] Type 1 HRS is frequently fatal with a median duration of survival of weeks to months, however type 2 HRS has a more insidious onset with the highest risk of death in the weeks after diagnosis. HRS causes refractory renal failure and indicates a dismal prognosis in cirrhotic individuals. Following a diagnosis of HRS, conventional therapies include stopping the use of nephrotoxic medications and diuretics, increasing intravascular volume with albumin, and using vasoconstrictor medications like terlipressin or norepinephrine.[19,30,31] In individuals with HRS-1, vasopressor pharmacotherapy may correct the hemodynamic abnormalities linked to advanced cirrhosis and enhance renal perfusion and function.[32]

Terlipressin is a synthetic vasopressin analog with vasoconstrictor activity in both splanchnic as well as systemic vasculature.[33] This activity results in reduced portal hypertension and decreased portal blood flow which is the main culprit of hemodynamic abnormalities associated with advanced cirrhosis. Systemic hemodynamics is improved, and renal perfusion pressure is raised as a result of the redistribution of circulatory volume from the splanchnic to the systemic circulation.[34,35] These patients' renal hemodynamics are further improved by the increased effective arterial volume, which significantly lowers compensatory renal and systemic vasoconstrictor activities.[36]

Terlipressin has been identified as one of the most promising medicines after the effectiveness of some of these therapies was evaluated by RCTs. Terlipressin is used for HRS-1 in many parts of the world and is part of the Clinical Practice Guidelines in Europe. Terlipressin administration increased rates of HRS reversal in a recent open-label RCT when compared to norepinephrine.[31] However, prior systematic studies only identified evidence with low to extremely low certainty.[37-40]

New trials that have been published since previous evaluations may offer more accurate estimates that would increase the certainty of the evidence. Considering the relative efficacy of pharmacological therapies for HRS, this article is a comprehensive review and network meta-analysis (NMA).

POPULATION STUDIED INCLUDING DEMOGRAPHICS

Eligibility Criteria

Published and abstract reports of RCTs were included that randomized hospitalized adults (≥18 years old) with HRS type 1 or 2 to any pharmacologic agent used for the treatment of HRS.

Route of medication administration or language of publication was not the eligibility criteria. Information was gathered from MEDLINE, Embase, Cochrane Central Register of Controlled Trials, Medline In-process and other non-indexed citations, Scopus, and Web of Science from inception until October 13, 2021. Data was collected from following outcomes: reversal of HRS (as defined by individual study investigators), mortality, transplant-free survival, and severe adverse outcomes (as defined by the study authors). For mortality, the longest follow-up time provided was included.

Statistical Method

Drugs were classified into nodes, based on molecule and mechanism of action and constructed network plots using STATA Version 17.0 (Stata Corp LLC, College Station, TX).[41] For all outcomes, a frequentist random-effects NMA using the "net meta package in R 2.0" was performed.[42] Network estimates were produced by NMA based on direct and indirect estimates.

INTERVENTION(S) STUDIED, AND OUTCOMES EVALUATED

A frequentist random-effects NMA was run using the "net meta package in R 2.0" for all outcomes.[42] Based on the direct and indirect estimates, a NMA yields network estimate. For comparisons with head-to-head data, direct estimates are computed based on conventional pairwise meta-analyses.[43,44] Through indirect loops, contributions from common comparators are used to produce indirect estimates. Using the NMA analytical framework, this facilitates the computation of network estimates, which are pooled estimates of direct and indirect evidence. This gives us several benefits, such as increasing the estimates' accuracy and enabling direct comparisons between medication treatments that have not been the subject of clinical trials.

Pairwise inverse variance random-effects meta-analysis was performed using restricted maximal likelihood estimator. Utilizing a chi-square test, interpretation of the I^2 statistic, and visual inspection of CIs, study heterogeneity was evaluated. We display I^2 for each network separately. I^2 values between 0 and 39% were regarded as minor, 40–60% as moderate, 60–75% as substantial, and over 75% as significant heterogeneity. Examining funnel plots allowed us to determine publication bias when estimates contained 10 or more research. An incoherence test was conducted using node splitting. Meta-regression was used to examine the impact of predetermined subgroups. Risk of bias (RoB) (high or probably high vs. low or probably low), type 1 versus type 2 HRS, cirrhosis etiology (alcoholic vs. viral vs. metabolic), and severity of liver disease (MELD and Child–Pugh as continuous variables) were the subgroups that were analyzed.

When statistical evidence of a subgroup effect was found, instrument was used for assessing the Credibility of Effect Modification Analyses tool to assess credibility in the subgroup effect (ICEMAN).[45] The effect of interventions was summarized using absolute risk reduction and corresponding 95% CIs. The median risk in the placebo arm across all eligible trials was used to compute the baseline risk. Additionally, absolute risk per 1,000 people was calculated using RR, with a positive sign suggesting more incidents per 1,000 people and a negative sign indicating fewer events per 1,000 people.

■ NEW ISSUES ADDRESSED

An updated summary of the research comparing the efficacy of various therapies for type 1 HRS is provided in this review. It includes freshly released, sizable, randomized trials that were not covered in earlier evaluations.[31,32] High certainty evidence was found to support the reversal of type 1 HRS with terlipressin, but very low certainty evidence was found to support the reversal of type 1 HRS with octreotide and midodrine. This is especially interesting because terlipressin is not readily available, whereas octreotide and midodrine are often used in hospitals across North America for patients with HRS. Norepinephrine, however less effective than terlipressin but more certain than Octreotide + Midodrine, may reverse type 1 HRS. There is low certainty evidence that terlipressin may reduce mortality in patients with HRS, however an uncertain impact was found of the other drugs under investigation on the outcome of mortality.

■ AUTHORS' VIEWPOINT

Terlipressin aids in HRS reversal and norepinephrine might make it better. Terlipressin could lower mortality. Even though octreotide + midodrine therapy can be provided in the ward, first triage to ICU or high dependency units for norepinephrine may be more suitable until terlipressin is accessible in North American hospitals.

STRENGTH OF THE STUDY

The strengths of our review are increased low RoB trial data, careful data collection, and review process, and use of updated GRADE (Grading of Recommendations Assessment, Development and Evaluation) methods.

DRAWBACKS OF THE STUDY

Limitations include inconsistent definitions of some outcomes, such as HRS reversal, and evidence of low or very low certainty for other comparisons and outcomes, such as adverse events. Furthermore, the eligibility for and reception of a liver transplant may have a negative impact on our estimate of mortality. Furthermore, information on transplant-free survival was not collected. Even while not all of these RCTs looked at ICU patients, there are differences in how high-dependency units and ICUs are used around the world. In many jurisdictions, administration of several of the researched therapies (including norepinephrine) necessitates ICU stay. Terlipressin can also be administered as a bolus, although an RCT evaluating the relative efficacy of bolus versus infusion discovered that infusion resulted in fewer side effects.[46] Terlipressin infusion typically necessitates admission to a high-dependency facility. Due to this, the findings of this report are relevant to ICU practitioners.

REVIEWERS' VIEWPOINT

Terlipressin should be used in patients with type 1 HRS with renal failure and it has high certainty of evidence supporting its use now. Terlipressin increases HRS reversal as was proven in CONFIRM trial also, but it was associated with serious adverse events including respiratory failure. The use of Midodrine and Octreotide as a treatment option is now debatable after this meta-analysis. If access to terlipressin is an issue, then norepinephrine can be used in patients with HRS and is proven to be better than combination of octreotide and midodrine.

IMPACT ON CURRENT PRACTICE AND TAKE HOME MESSAGE

This is the first study to report high-certainty evidence for the use of terlipressin in type 1 HRS patients as well as low-certainty evidence for the use of norepinephrine. This systemic review and NMA has raised questions on the effectiveness of midodrine and octreotide as a treatment option, which is possibly even more significant. These findings should cause medical facilities all across North America to reevaluate the usefulness, cost-effectiveness, and function of terlipressin in the treatment of patients with confirmed HRS.

Compared to the more popular combination of octreotide and midodrine, greater norepinephrine use for HRS may be advantageous in the absence of access to terlipressin. This would include changing the proper initial care setting from a medical ward to ICUs or high-dependency units that can deliver norepinephrine.

ARTICLE 19

Thromboelastography-guided Therapy Enhances Patient Blood Management in Cirrhotic Patients: A Meta-analysis Based on Randomized Controlled Trials

Hartmann J, Dias JD, Pivalizza EG, Garcia-Tsao G. Thromboelastography-guided therapy enhances patient blood management in cirrhotic patients: a meta-analysis based on randomized controlled trials. *Semin Thromb Hemost.* 2023;49(2):162-72.

INTRODUCTION

The patients with decompensated cirrhosis have both bleeding and thrombotic tendencies. Effective blood management and optimizing coagulation of these patients need precise identification of the issues involved.[47-50] Emphasis on patient blood management is also important as liberal transfusion of blood and blood products in cirrhotic patients is associated with increased mortality.[51-53] Standard tests of coagulation such as prothrombin time/international normalized ratio (INR) and activated partial thromboplastin time do not provide accurate prediction of the risk of bleeding in cirrhotic patients.

CLINICAL PROBLEM AND PAST RESEARCH

Thromboelastography (TEG) can rapidly assess and predict the risk of thrombosis and bleeding tendency. Various organizations have recommended transfusion algorithms based on use of TEG. American Gastroenterological Society update states that use of TEG in their setting is yet to be established.[54] There is lack of robust evidence for the use of TEG-guided therapy in the perioperative period. This meta-analysis was undertaken to determine, if TEG-guided therapy can optimize patient blood management, improve outcomes and reduce mortality compared with standard coagulation testing.

Wang et al. in 2010 studied TEG-guided blood transfusion in patients undergoing orthotopic liver transplantation. The patients monitored with TEG required less transfusion of fresh frozen plasma (FFP) and reduced blood loss. Though the differences in total fluid administration and 3-year survival rates were similar in both the groups.[55]

De Pietri et al. in 2016 studied TEG-guided transfusion of blood and blood products in patients of cirrhosis with severe coagulopathy undergoing invasive procedures. Patients included had an INR >1.8 and/or platelet count <50,000. The FFPs will be transfused if reaction time® was >40 minutes and platelets will be transfused if maximum amplitude <30 mm. They observed reduced transfusion of blood products with TEG-guided transfusion protocol.[56]

Kumar et al. in 2020 evaluated the use of TEG in patients of cirrhosis with significant coagulopathy presenting with non-variceal bleeding.[57] The bleed was diagnosed on upper GI endoscopy. Only 26.7% of patients managed with TEG-guided transfusion required transfusion of all three components (viz., FFPs, platelets, and cryoprecipitates) against 87.2% in the standard care group. Seven patients in TEG group required no blood transfusion. But there were no significant differences in failure to control bleeds, failure to prevent rebleeds, and mortality rates between the intervention and comparator groups.[57]

Rout et al. in 2020 studied the patients of cirrhosis presenting with acute variceal bleed. The primary outcome was to assess the difference in transfusion requirements of FFP and platelets with TEG-monitored therapy. Rebleeding at 5 days and 42 days, with 6-week mortality were the secondary outcomes of the study.[58]

Vuyyuru et al. in 2020 studied the cirrhotic patients with coagulopathy undergoing liver-related procedures. A total of 58 patients were recruited in both the groups (TEG vs. standard coagulation testing). Most common procedure performed was percutaneous liver biopsy, followed by transjugular intrahepatic portosystemic shunt, percutaneous acetic acid injection, and transarterial chemo-embolization. Only nine patients in TEG group received transfusions compared to all patients in standard of care (SOC) (p <0.001). In TEG group, six received FFP (p = 0.753 vs. SOC), two received platelets (p <0.001 vs. SOC), and one (3.4%) patient received both FFP and platelet (p ≥0.999 vs. SOC) transfusion. None of the patients in either group developed procedure-related bleeding complications until 5 days post-procedure.[59]

■ STUDY DESIGN

This study was conducted according to PRISMA guidelines and registered in the PROSPERO database. The literature review research was conducted in MEDLINE, Cochrane, and EMBASE database. The RCTs of adult patients >18 years of age with cirrhosis comparing TEG-based transfusion protocols with standard practices were identified. The analysis was performed using the DerSimonian–Laird random effects method, which is the most commonly used standard for meta-analysis with random effects and assumes that treatment effects vary between studies according to a random distribution, regardless of heterogeneity between studies. Using I^2 statistics, substantial heterogeneity was assumed if I^2 value was >50%. The outcomes being binary in nature were expressed as RR. Three of the five studies reported Kaplan–Meier survival curves, with focus on assessing the mortality rates at 7 days.

It included the RCTs comparing management with TEG (TEG 5,000 analyzer or MonoTem-A) to standard coagulation testing. Majority of studies used standard coagulation testing algorithm, 50×10^9/L levels for platelet transfusion and INR >1.8 for transfusion of FFP.

■ RESULTS

The primary outcomes were the number of units of platelets and FFP transfused. Secondary outcomes included adverse events, mortality, hospital/ICU stay, utilization of individual blood products, blood loss/excessive bleeding events, and intervention outcomes.

The meta-analysis of pooled data showed reduced platelet transfusion in TEG-monitored group. Five times lower platelet transfusion was recorded which was statistically significant [RR (95% CI) = 0.17 (0.03–0.90); p = 0.04]. The data also showed reduced FFP transfusion in TEG-monitored group, though the reduction in rates of transfusion were not statistically significant. [RR (95% CI) = 0.34 (0.10–1.16); p = 0.09].

The detailed secondary outcomes of this meta-analysis are listed as follows:
- *Mortality:* Various studies analyzed this at different time points (from 5 days to 3 years). In patients of cirrhosis TEG-monitored therapy helped reduce mortality at 7 days as compared to control group. No difference in mortality was reported at any later time points between the groups.
- *Utilization of individual blood products:* The use of thromboelastogram suggested

a statistically significant reduction in the use of any blood product [RR (95% CI) = 0.24 (0.15–0.38); p <0.001], FFP and platelets combined [RR (95% CI) = 0.48 (0.34–0.68); p <0.001], and cryoprecipitate [RR (95% CI) = 0.64 (0.51–0.79); p <0.001]. There was no significant difference regarding transfusion of packed red blood cells in both the groups.

- *Adverse events:* The use of TEG helped in significant reduction of serious transfusion-related acute lung injury in patients of cirrhosis with non-variceal bleed. Other than this, there were no significant differences of adverse events between the groups. Two studies[57,58] found that the chances of bleeding within 5 days and rebleeding after 5 days were comparable in both the groups.

■ REVIEWERS' VIEWPOINT

Effective patient blood management can help reduce transfusion requirements, as transfusion in itself is associated with adverse outcomes. But it is important that these patient blood management strategies be confirmed with high quality randomized trials. The TEG-guided therapy enhances the patient blood management by significantly reducing the transfusions of platelets, all blood products, and combined FFP and platelets in patients with cirrhosis who are bleeding or undergoing surgical interventions/liver transplant compared to patients managed with standard coagulation testing. The use of TEG also helped in reducing the 7-day mortality, bleeding, and also reducing the incidence of serious transfusion-related reactions in patients with advanced cirrhosis.

The American Gastroenterology. Association (AGA) 2019 clinical practice update on coagulation in cirrhosis states that TEG may eventually have a role in evaluation of clotting in patients of cirrhosis, but currently lacks validated target levels. The Society of Critical Care Medicine (SCCM) guidelines 2020 for the management of adults with acute and ACLF who are undergoing procedures provide conditional guidance for the use of TEG in preference to measuring INR, platelet, and fibrinogen.[60] These guidelines are based on evidence from old RCTs. The recent trials are included in this meta-analysis.

This study by Hartmann et al. includes recent high-quality RCTs comparing TEG-guided therapy versus standard coagulation testing in patients of cirrhosis. They have used a thoroughly investigated and strategic approach for identification, study design, and statistical methods. Few studies included in this meta-analysis can be a steppingstone data for future guidelines as they were not included in the 2020 SCCM guidelines or 2019 AGA update. The results of this analysis are very clear and precise. They are in synchronization with results from other published meta-analysis by Tangcheewinsirikul et al.[61] and Kovalic et al.[62] Though the studies using rotational thromboelastometry (ROTEM) are scarce, this study by Hartmann et al. corroborated by other meta-analysis of RCTs and/or nonrandomized observational studies that included the limited data on ROTEM suggested these results may be applicable across comparable viscoelastic testing platforms.

This study restricted to RCTs utilizing TEG, and reporting data on the use of devices TEG 5000 and MonoTEM-A. Due to this, the results cannot be assumed to be directly transferrable to other devices. As TEG came into use much earlier, its data is overrepresented with very scarce literature regarding ROTEM using ROTEM device.

SUMMARY

It was abundantly clear that the use of TEG-guided therapy in patients with cirrhosis enhances patient blood management effectively. It may turn out to be a cornerstone in reducing the use of blood products, particularly platelets, without increasing the risk of bleeding while reducing early 7-day mortality. However, more studies in particular RCTs are needed, and evidence-based diagnostic and monitoring protocols and algorithms would help to support implementation in specific clinical settings where patients with cirrhosis are at risk of bleeding complications.

ARTICLE 20

Use of Albumin Infusion for Cirrhosis-related Complications: An International Position Statement

Bai Z, Méndez-Sánchez N, Romeiro FG, Mancuso A, Philips CA, Tacke F, et al. Liver Cirrhosis-related Complications (LCC)—International Special Interest Group. Use of albumin infusion for cirrhosis-related complications: an international position statement.
JHEP Rep. 2023;5(8):100785.

INTRODUCTION

Liver cirrhosis and its associated complications impose a significant economic burden on various countries.[63,64] Human albumin is most commonly used to treat decompensated cirrhosis.[65] The role of albumin is well established in treating HRS, SBP, and large-volume paracentesis (>5 L). It has also been proposed as a disease-modifying agent in decompensated cirrhosis.[66] Its use can help decrease mortality in patients with cirrhosis. Various published RCTs aimed at expanding the therapeutic use of human albumin have provided conflicting conclusions.

PAST RESEARCH AND CLINICAL PROBLEM

The previous surveys conducted by the European Foundation for the Study of Chronic Liver Failure and American Association for the Study of Liver Diseases showed the use of human albumin in the treatment of HRS, SBP, ascites, large-volume paracentesis, non-SBP infections, hyponatremia, HE, muscle cramps, hypoalbuminemia, peripheral edema, and gastrointestinal bleeding.[67,68]

Caraceni et al. published an ANSWER trial in 2018.[12] The patients with cirrhosis and uncomplicated ascites who were being treated with anti-aldosteronic drugs >200 mg/day and frusemide >25 mg/day were administered human albumin 40 g twice weekly for 2 weeks and then 40 g weekly for 18 months. The overall 18-month survival was significantly higher in patients treated with human albumin as compared to patients given standard treatment (Kaplan–Meier estimates 77% vs. 66%; $p = 0.028$), resulting in a 38% reduction in the mortality HR (0.62) (95% CI 0·40–0·95).

In the MACHT trial, 2018, midodrine and intravenous albumin were administered to patients with decompensated cirrhosis on the waiting list for liver transplantation. Midodrine, an alpha-adrenergic vasoconstrictor, helped improve these patients' circulatory dysfunction. The patients received midodrine 15–30 mg/day and albumin 40 mg every 15 days. It did not reduce the incidence of complications, viz., renal failure, hyponatremia, infections, HE, gastrointestinal bleeding, or mortality at 1 year.[69]

In the ATTIRE trial, in 2021, 20% albumin was infused daily in hospitalized patients with decompensated cirrhosis with serum albumin levels of <3 g/dL. The target was to attain >3 g/dL serum albumin levels. The incidence of new infections, renal dysfunction, or death between days 3 and 15 after initiation of treatment was noted. There was no significant difference in outcomes in the targeted albumin group compared to the standard group. They also reported an increased incidence of life-threatening severe events in patients receiving daily albumin infusions.

The current recommendations regarding the use of human albumin in patients with cirrhosis remain inconsistent, so they organized an expert panel of investigators to formulate an international position statement regarding the use of human albumin infusion by comprehensively reviewing the best available evidence.

METHODS AND STUDY DESIGN

Considering the global scope of this position statement, investigators were selected from worldwide. 31 out of 84 invited investigators from 19 countries responded and accepted the invitation. The Delphi consensus process was performed for this international statement following three rounds.

In the first round of Delphi, two members did a high-quality literature search from the PubMed database using Albumin and Cirrhosis as keywords. These were emailed to 13 members from multiple countries to discuss the significance of these topics and revision to the main document.

In the second Delphi round, 33 members were sent a five-point Likert scale questionnaire, with an additional option of "do you know" response option. They also provided free-text comments to explain their choice. The values were percentages and median values as indicators of agreement on the 5-point scales and variances and IQR as consensus indicators. The level of understanding with an item was rated either as "very high" (median of 5, ≥80% agreement, IQR = 0), "high" (median of 4 or 5, ≥80% agreement, IQR = 1), "moderate" (median of 1), or "low" (median of 2).

In the final advisory meeting, a pre-voting link to an online questionnaire was sent to 33 group members to reassess the level of agreement with these statements. This was followed by an online meeting and a questionnaire to all 33 members for final approval of the position statements.

WHAT REVIEWERS, THINK, WITH THE RESULTS OF THIS POSITION STATEMENT

After the three Delphi round consensus process, all the members finally agreed on the following 12 position statements without other comments.

1. Human albumin infusion must be used to differentiate HRS-associated AKI from prerenal AKI. Human albumin has a more substantial and prolonged duration effect on plasma expansion. International Club of Ascites recommends a 1 g/kg dose of up to 100 g daily for at least 2 days and diuretic withdrawal.
2. The infusion of human albumin should be used to manage HRS. Renal failure in HRS is caused due to severe reduction

in the adequate circulatory volume and cardiovascular dysfunction leading to renal hypoperfusion and intrarenal vasoconstriction. So, the recommended treatment is to use a vasoconstrictor and a plasma expander. So, the position statement suggests the use of human albumin for treating HRS at the dose of 20–40 g daily and the infusion of human albumin should be maintained until a serum creatinine level <1.5 mg/dL is achieved.

3. Post-paracentesis circulatory dysfunction (PPCD) is a common complication of large-volume paracentesis. It can accelerate the re-accumulation of ascites and induce complications, such as hyponatremia, renal dysfunction, HE, and reduced mortality. It recommends using human albumin to prevent circulatory dysfunction after large-volume paracentesis at a dose of 8 g/L of removed ascitic fluid. Albumin infusion at the same amount can be considered in cirrhotic patients with ACLF or AKI and ascites undergoing paracentesis of <5 L, though more quality evidence is required. If the economic issues can be resolved long-term, regular human albumin infusion can be used to improve ascites, prevent other complications of liver cirrhosis, and prolong survival in patients with uncomplicated ascites requiring diuretics.

4. SBP, the most common type of bacterial infection in cirrhosis, is defined as an infection of the ascitic fluid without any surgically treatable intra-abdominal source of infection. Sort et al. did an RCT on the effect of intravenous albumin on renal impairment and mortality in patients with cirrhosis and SBP. 126 patients were randomized to receive cefotaxime alone ($n = 63$) or in combination with human albumin ($n = 63$). The dose of human albumin was 1.5 g/kg at diagnosis and 1 g/kg on day 3. The rate of improvement of SBP was not significantly different between the two groups (98% vs. 94%, $p = 0.36$). However, the cefotaxime plus human albumin administered group had a significantly lower incidence of AKI (10% vs. 33%, $p = 0.002$), mortality at 1 month (10% vs. 29%, $p = 0.01$), and mortality at 3 months (22% vs. 41%, $p = 0.03$) than the cefotaxime alone group.[15] Human albumin infusion should prevent and improve survival in cirrhotic patients with SBP, particularly those with a baseline serum bilirubin of >4 mg/dL or a serum creatinine of >1 mg/dL.

Bai et al.[70] recommend the use of human albumin infusion to prevent AKI and improve survival in cirrhotic patients with SBP, particularly those with a baseline serum bilirubin of >4 mg/dL or a serum creatinine of >1 mg/dL. Non-SBP infections, including urinary tract infections, pneumonia, skin infections, bacteremia, and septic shock, account for a significant part of all bacterial infections in patients with decompensated cirrhosis.[71,72] The infusion of human albumin does not prevent renal impairment or improve survival in patients with cirrhosis affected by non-SBP infections other than septic shock.

5. HE is a serious complication of cirrhosis, which adversely affects the quality of life. A significantly higher incidence of HE is seen in patients of cirrhosis and hypoalbuminemia. Simón-Talero et al. published effects of intravenous albumin in patients with cirrhosis and episodic HE in 2013.[73] The administered dose of human albumin was 1.5 g/kg on day 1 and 1 g/kg on day 3, in addition to the standard

treatment with laxatives and rifixamin. There were no significant differences in the resolution of HE at day 4 in both the groups. But the survival rates at 90 days was significantly higher in patients treated with albumin.

The HEAL study explored the role of human albumin infusion in patients with prior HE who had already used standard treatment. Forty-eight patients were randomly assigned to the albumin ($n = 24$) and saline ($n = 24$) groups with albumin dose of 1.5 g/kg weekly over 5 weeks. The human albumin group had significantly higher rates of reversal and improvement of HE. Alongside, there was a significant reduction of interleukin 1b (IL-1b) and endothelial dysfunction markers after treatment with albumin.[74] The current evidence indicates that human albumin given at a dose of 20-40 g daily can be considered to treat overt encephalopathy, especially in cirrhotic patients with hypoalbuminemia.

6. Patients with cirrhosis and ascites usually suffer from hyponatremia. Ninety percent of these cases are of hypervolemic hyponatremia. It is associated with worse outcomes in cirrhotic patients. The ANSWER and ATTIRE trial significantly improved hyponatremia in patients treated with human albumin. A meta-analysis included thirty studies, including 25 RCTs and five cohort studies.[70] Among cirrhotic patients without hyponatremia, the albumin group had a significantly lower incidence of hyponatremia and a higher serum sodium level than the control. Among cirrhotic patients with hyponatremia, the albumin group had a significantly higher rate of resolution of hyponatremia than the control group. The position statement recommends that human albumin be used to manage hyponatremia in selected patients with cirrhosis, but the optimal dosage and schedule need to be defined better with more randomized trials.

7. In the FRISC trial, 154 patients were treated with 5% human albumin intravenous bolus, 250 mL over 15-30 minutes, followed by a maintenance infusion of 50 mL/h for 3 hours (20 g total). It led to better reversal of hypotension and decreased mortality at 1 week than patients treated with saline.[9] In the ALPS trial, 50 cirrhotic patients with sepsis-induced hypotension were treated with a dose of 0.5-1.0 g/kg human albumin over 3 hours. The proportion of patients with mean arterial pressure above 65 mm Hg at 3 hours was significantly higher in the albumin group than in the plasmalyte group.[75] Human albumin can be considered for the management of cirrhotic patients with septic shock, with a transfusion strategy of 5% HAS is intravenously infused at a dosage of 250 mL over 15-30 min, followed by a maintenance infusion of 50 mL/h until hemodynamically stable.

8. Human albumin-associated adverse events: In the ATTIRE trial, the median dose of 20% albumin solution was 200 g during a median hospitalization stay of 8 days but only 20 g during a median hospitalization stay of 9 days in the control group. The albumin group had a higher incidence of pulmonary edema than the control group (6% vs. 2%). In the ALPS trial, the 20% albumin was given at a dose of 0.5-1.0 g/kg over 3 hours and six patients developed pulmonary edema. No patient in the plasmalyte group developed pulmonary edema. In ANSWER and MACHT trials, none of

the patients developed pulmonary edema. The dose of 20% albumin in both trials was 40 g weekly and 40 g every 15 days. In the FRISC trial, none of the patients developed pulmonary edema. High-dose albumin over a short duration must be used cautiously except in SBP; a restrictive strategy can help avoid pulmonary complications. Anaphylactic reactions are rare and no clear evidence supports the association of albumin infusion with an increased risk of portal hypertension-related bleeding.

SUMMARY AND FUTURE RESEARCH

The dosage of human albumin in various studies is based on the agreement of expert opinions and clinical experience. Large-scale RCTs are warranted to confirm the optimal dosage and duration of human albumin infusion and its role in HE, hyponatremia, and various other complications associated with cirrhosis to maximize its efficacy and minimizing the risk of associated adverse effects. Human albumin improves circulatory dysfunction and may counteract systemic inflammation and oxidative stress. It can be used as a therapeutic approach to manage various complications associated with cirrhosis.

REFERENCES

1. Ginès P, Krag A, Abraldes JG, Solà E, Fabrellas N, Kamath PS. Liver cirrhosis. Lancet. 2021;398(10308):1359-76.
2. Blachier M, Leleu H, Peck-Radosavljevic M, Valla DC, Roudot-Thoraval F. The burden of liver disease in Europe: a review of available epidemiological data. J Hepatol. 2013;58(3):593-608.
3. McPhail MJ, Parrott F, Wendon JA, Harrison DA, Rowan KA, Bernal W. Incidence and outcomes for patients with cirrhosis admitted to the United Kingdom critical care units. Crit Care Med. 2018;46(5):705-12.
4. Acevedo J, Fernández J. New determinants of prognosis in bacterial infections in cirrhosis. World J Gastroenterol. World J Gastroenterol. 2014;20(23):7252-9.
5. Nicholson JP, Wolmarans MR, Park GR. The role of albumin in critical illness. Br J Anaesth. 2000;85(4):599-610.
6. O'Brien AJ, Fullerton JN, Massey KA, Auld G, Sewell G, James S, et al. Immunosuppression in acutely decompensated cirrhosis is mediated by prostaglandin E2. Nat Med. 2014;20(5):518-23.
7. Finfer S, Bellomo R, Boyce N, French J, Myburgh J, Norton R; Safe Study Investigators. A comparison of albumin and saline for fluid resuscitation in the intensive care unit. N Engl J Med. 2004;350(22):2247-56.
8. Caironi P, Tognoni G, Masson S, Fumagalli R, Pesenti A, Romero M, et al. ALBIOS Study Investigators. Albumin replacement in patients with severe sepsis or septic shock. N Engl J Med. 2014;370(15):1412-21.
9. Philips CA, Maiwall R, Sharma MK, Jindal A, Choudhury AK, Kumar G, et al. Comparison of 5% human albumin and normal saline for fluid resuscitation in sepsis induced hypotension among patients with cirrhosis (FRISC study): a randomized controlled trial. Hepatol Int. 2021;15(4):983-94.
10. Villanueva C, Colomo A, Bosch A, Concepción M, Hernandez-Gea V, Aracil C, et al. Transfusion strategies for acute upper gastrointestinal bleeding. N Engl J Med. 2013;368(1):11-21.
11. Razpotnik M, Bota S, Wimmer P, Hackl M, Lesnik G, Alber H, et al. The prevalence of cirrhotic cardiomyopathy according to different diagnostic criteria. Liver Int. 2021;41(5):1058-69.
12. Caraceni P, Riggio O, Angeli P, Alessandria C, Neri S, Foschi FG, et al. ANSWER Study Investigators. Long-term albumin administration in decompensated cirrhosis (ANSWER): an open-label randomised trial. Lancet. 2018;391(10138):2417-29.

13. Thévenot T, Bureau C, Oberti F, Anty R, Louvet A, Plessier A, et al. Effect of albumin in cirrhotic patients with infection other than spontaneous bacterial peritonitis. A randomized trial. J Hepatol. 2015;62(4):822-30.
14. Guevara M, Terra C, Nazar A, Solà E, Fernández J, Pavesi M, et al. Albumin for bacterial infections other than spontaneous bacterial peritonitis in cirrhosis. A randomized, controlled study. J Hepatol. 2012;57(4):759-65.
15. Sort P, Navasa M, Arroyo V, Aldeguer X, Planas R, Ruiz-del-Arbol L, et al. Effect of intravenous albumin on renal impairment and mortality in patients with cirrhosis and spontaneous bacterial peritonitis. N Engl J Med. 1999;341:403-9.
16. Bajaj JS, O'Leary JG, Lai JC, Wong F, Long MD, Wong RJ, et al. Acute-on-Chronic Liver Failure Clinical Guidelines. Am J Gastroenterol. 2022;117(2):225-52.
17. Arroyo V, Moreau R, Jalan R. Acute-on-chronic liver failure. N Engl J Med. 2020;382(22):2137-45.
18. Mezzano G, Juanola A, Cardenas A, Mezey E, Hamilton JP, Pose E, et al. Global burden of disease: acute-on-chronic liver failure, a systematic review and meta-analysis. Gut. 2022;71(1):148-55.
19. Angeli P, Ginès P, Wong F, Bernardi M, Boyer TD, Gerbes A, et al. Diagnosis and management of acute kidney injury in patients with cirrhosis: Revised consensus recommendations of the International Club of Ascites. J Hepatol. 2015;62(4):968-74.
20. Boyer TD, Sanyal AJ, Wong F, Frederick RT, Lake JR, O'Leary JG, et al. REVERSE Study Investigators. Terlipressin plus albumin is more effective than albumin alone in improving renal function in patients with cirrhosis and hepatorenal syndrome type 1. Gastroenterology. 2016;150(7):1579-89.e2.
21. Biggins SW, Angeli P, Garcia-Tsao G, Ginès P, Ling SC, Nadim MK, et al. Diagnosis, Evaluation, and Management of Ascites, Spontaneous Bacterial Peritonitis and Hepatorenal Syndrome: 2021 Practice Guidance by the American Association for the Study of Liver Diseases. Hepatology. 2021;74(2):1014-48.
22. Garcia-Tsao G. Terlipressin and Intravenous Albumin in Advanced Cirrhosis—Friend and Foe. N Engl J Med. 2021;384(9):869-71.
23. Angeli P, Bernardi M, Villanueva C, Francoz C, Mookerjee R, Trebicka J, et al. EASL Clinical Practice Guidelines for the management of patients with decompensated cirrhosis. J Hepatol. 2018;69(2):406-60.
24. Schrier RW, Arroyo V, Bernardi M, Epstein M, Henriksen JH, Rodés J. Peripheral arterial vasodilation hypothesis: a proposal for the initiation of renal sodium and water retention in cirrhosis. Hepatology. 1988;8(5):1151-7.
25. Simonetto DA, Gines P, Kamath PS. Hepatorenal syndrome: pathophysiology, diagnosis, and management. BMJ. 2020;370:m2687.
26. Sanyal AJ, Boyer T, Garcia-Tsao G, Regenstein F, Rossaro L, Appenrodt B, et al. Terlipressin Study Group. A randomized, prospective, double-blind, placebo-controlled trial of terlipressin for type 1 hepatorenal syndrome. Gastroenterology. 2008;134(5):1360-8.
27. Krag A, Bendtsen F, Mortensen C, Henriksen JH, Møller S. Effects of a single terlipressin administration on cardiac function and perfusion in cirrhosis. Eur J Gastroenterol Hepatol. 2010;22(9):1085-92.
28. Martín-Llahí M, Pépin MN, Guevara M, Díaz F, Torre A, Monescillo A, et al. TAHRS Investigators. Terlipressin and albumin vs. albumin in patients with cirrhosis and hepatorenal syndrome: a randomized study. Gastroenterology. 2008;134(5):1352-9.
29. Mohamed MMG, Rauf A, Adam A, Kheiri B, Lacasse A, El-Halawany H. Terlipressin effect on hepatorenal syndrome: updated meta-analysis of randomized controlled trials. JGH Open. 2021;5(8):896-901.
30. Francoz C, Durand F, Kahn JA, Genyk YS, Nadim MK. Hepatorenal syndrome. Clin J Am Soc Nephrol. 2019; 14:774-81.
31. Arora V, Maiwall R, Rajan V, Jindal A, Muralikrishna Shasthry S, Kumar G, et al. Terlipressin is superior to noradrenaline in

the management of acute kidney injury in acute on chronic liver failure. Hepatology. 2020;71:600-10.
32. Zheng JN, Han YJ, Zou TT, Zhou YJ, Sun DQ, Zhong JH, et al. Comparative efficacy of vasoconstrictor therapies for type 1 hepatorenal syndrome: a network meta-analysis. Expert Rev Gastroenterol Hepatol. 2017;11:1009-18.
33. Jamil K, Pappas SC, Devarakonda KR. In vitro binding and receptor-mediated activity of terlipressin at vasopressin receptors V1 and V2. J Exp Pharmacol. 2017;10:1-7.
34. Kiszka-Kanowitz M, Henriksen JH, Hansen EF, Møller S, Bendtsen F. Effect of terlipressin on blood volume distribution in patients with cirrhosis. Scand J Gastroenterol. 2004;39:486-92.
35. Mukhtar A, Salah M, Aboulfetouh F, Obayah G, Samy M, Hassanien A, et al. The use of terlipressin during living donor liver transplantation: effects on systemic and splanchnic hemodynamics. Crit Care Med. 2011;39(6):1329-34.
36. Ginès P, Solà E, Angeli P, Wong F, Nadim MK, Kamath PS. Hepatorenal syndrome. Nat Rev Dis Primers. 2018;4:23.
37. Facciorusso A, Chandar AK, Murad MH, Prokop LJ, Muscatiello N, Kamath PS, et al. Comparative efficacy of pharmacological strategies for management of type 1 hepatorenal syndrome: a systematic review and network meta-analysis. Lancet Gastroenterol Hepatol. 2017;2:94-102.
38. Wang H, Liu A, Bo W, Feng X, Hu Y. Terlipressin in the treatment of hepatorenal syndrome: a systematic review and meta-analysis. Medicine (Baltimore). 2018;97:e0431.
39. Allegretti AS, Israelsen M, Krag A, Jovani M, Goldin AH, Schulman AR, et al. Terlipressin versus placebo or no intervention for people with cirrhosis and hepatorenal syndrome. Cochrane Database Syst Rev. 2017;6:CD005162.
40. Best LM, Freeman SC, Sutton AJ, Cooper NJ, Tng EL, Csenar M, et al. Treatment for hepatorenal syndrome in people with decompensated liver cirrhosis: a network meta-analysis. Cochrane Database Syst Rev. 2019; 9:CD013103.
41. Chaimani A, Higgins JP, Mavridis D, Spyridonos P, Salanti G. Graphical tools for network meta-analysis in STATA. PLoS One. 2013;8:e76654.
42. Rücker G, Krahn U, König J, Efthimiou O, Davies A, Papakonstantinou T. (2023). Package Netmeta. [online] Available from https://cran.r-project.org/web/packages/netmeta/netmeta.pdf [Last accessed November, 2023].
43. Higgins JPT, Thomas J, Chandler J, Cumpston M, Li T, Page MJ, et al. Cochrane Handbook for Systematic Reviews of Interventions, 2nd edition. Chichester: John Wiley & Sons; 2019.
44. Rouse B, Chaimani A, Li T. Network meta-analysis: An introduction for clinicians. Intern Emerg Med. 2017;12:103-11.
45. Ghosh S, Choudhary NS, Sharma AK, Singh B, Kumar P, Agarwal R, et al. Noradrenaline vs terlipressin in the treatment of type 2 hepatorenal syndrome: a randomized pilot study. Liver Int. 2013;33:1187-93.
46. Cavallin M, Piano S, Romano A, Fasolato S, Frigo AC, Benetti G, et al. Terlipressin given by continuous intravenous infusion versus intravenous boluses in the treatment of hepatorenal syndrome: a randomized controlled study. Hepatology. 2016;63: 983-99.
47. Tripodi A. Hemostasis abnormalities in cirrhosis. Curr Opin Hematol. 2015;22(05): 406-12.
48. Tripodi A, Primignani M, Chantarangkul V, Dell'Era A, Clerici M, de Franchis R, et al. An imbalance of pro- vs anti-coagulation factors in plasma from patients with cirrhosis. Gastroenterology. 2009;137(06):2105-11.
49. Blasi A, Cardenas A. Invasive procedures in patients with cirrhosis: a clinical approach based on current evidence. Clin Liver Dis. 2021;25(02):461-70.
50. Lisman T, Hernandez-Gea V, Magnusson M, Roberts L, Stanworth S, Thachil J, et al. The concept of rebalanced hemostasis in patients with liver disease: communication from the ISTH SSC working group on hemostatic management of patients with liver disease. J Thromb Haemost. 2021;19(04): 1116-22.

51. Odutayo A, Desborough MJ, Trivella M, Stanley AJ, Dorée C, Collins GS, et al. Restrictive versus liberal blood transfusion for gastrointestinal bleeding: a systematic review and meta-analysis of randomised controlled trials. Lancet Gastroenterol Hepatol. 2017;2(5):354-60.
52. Mohanty A, Kapuria D, Canakis A, Lin H, Amat MJ, Rangel Paniz G, et al. Fresh frozen plasma transfusion in acute variceal haemorrhage: results from a multicentre cohort study. Liver Int. 2021;41(08): 1901-8.
53. Zheng W, Zhao KM, Luo LH, Yu Y, Zhu SM. Perioperative single-donor platelet apheresis and red blood cell transfusion impact on 90-day and overall survival in living donor liver transplantation. Chin Med J (Engl). 2018;131(04):426-34.
54. O'Leary JG, Greenberg CS, Patton HM, Caldwell SH. AGA clinical practice update: coagulation in cirrhosis. Gastroenterology. 2019;157(01):34-43.e1.
55. Wang SC, Shieh JF, Chang KY, Chu YC, Liu CS, Loong CC, et al. Thromboelastography-guided transfusion decreases intraoperative blood transfusion during orthotopic liver transplantation: randomized clinical trial. Transplant Proc. 2010;42(7):2590-3.
56. De Pietri L, Bianchini M, Montalti R, De Maria N, Di Maira T, Begliomini B, et al. Thromboelastography-guided blood product use before invasive procedures in cirrhosis with severe coagulopathy: a randomized, controlled trial. Hepatology. 2016;63(02):566-73.
57. Kumar M, Ahmad J, Maiwall R, Choudhury A, Bajpai M, Mitra LG, et al. Thromboelastography-guided blood component use in patients with cirrhosis with nonvariceal bleeding: a randomized controlled trial. Hepatology. 2020;71(1):235-46.
58. Rout G, Shalimar, Gunjan D, Mahapatra SJ, Kedia S, Garg PK, et al. Thromboelastography-guided blood product transfusion in cirrhosis patients with variceal bleeding: a randomized controlled trial. J Clin Gastroenterol. 2020;54(03):255-62.
59. Vuyyuru SK, Singh AD, Gamanagatti SR, Rout G, Gunjan D, Shalimar. A randomized control trial of thromboelastography guided transfusion in cirrhosis for high-risk invasive liver-related procedures. Dig Dis Sci. 2020;65(07):2104-11.
60. Nanchal R, Subramanian R, Karvellas CJ, Hollenberg SM, Peppard WJ, Singbartl K, et al. Guidelines for the management of adult acute and acute-on-chronic liver failure in the ICU: cardiovascular, endocrine, hematologic, pulmonary, and renal considerations. Crit Care Med. 2020;48(03):e173-e191.
61. Tangcheewinsirikul N, Moonla C, Uaprasert N, Pittayanon R, Rojnuckarin P. Viscoelastometric versus standard coagulation tests to guide periprocedural transfusion in adults with cirrhosis: a meta-analysis of randomized controlled trials. Vox Sang. 2022;117(04):553-61.
62. Kovalic AJ, Khan MA, Malaver D, Whitson MJ, Teperman LW, Bernstein DE, et al. Thromboelastography versus standard coagulation testing in the assessment and reversal of coagulopathy among cirrhotics: a systematic review and meta-analysis. Eur J Gastroenterol Hepatol. 2020;32(03): 291-302.
63. Asrani SK, Devarbhavi H, Eaton J, Kamath PS. Burden of liver diseases in the world. J Hepatol. 2019;70(1):151-71.
64. GBD 2017 Cirrhosis Collaborators. The global, regional, and national burden of cirrhosis by cause in 195 countries and territories, 1990-2017: a systematic analysis for the Global Burden of Disease Study 2017. Lancet Gastroenterol Hepatol. 2020;5: 245-66.
65. Arroyo V, García-Martinez R, Salvatella X. Human serum albumin, systemic inflammation, and cirrhosis. J Hepatol. 2014;61(2): 396-407.
66. Caraceni P, Abraldes JG, Ginès P, Newsome PN, Sarin SK. The search for disease-modifying agents in decompensated cirrhosis: from drug repurposing to drug discovery. J Hepatol. 2021;75:S118-S134.

67. Bajaj JS, O'Leary JG, Wong F, Kamath PS. Variations in albumin use in patients with cirrhosis: an AASLD members survey. Hepatology. 2015;62:1923-4.
68. Caraceni P, Pavesi M, Baldassarre M, Bernardi M, Arroyo V. The use of human albumin in patients with cirrhosis: a European survey. Expert Rev Gastroenterol Hepatol. 2018;12:625-32.
69. Solà E, Solé C, Simón-Talero M, Martín-Llahí M, Castellote J, GarciaMartínez R, et al. Midodrine and albumin for prevention of complications in patients with cirrhosis awaiting liver transplantation. A randomized placebo-controlled trial. J Hepatol. 2018;69:1250-9.
70. Bai Z, Wang L, Lin H, Tacke F, Cheng G, Qi X. Use of human albumin administration for the prevention and treatment of hyponatremia in patients with liver cirrhosis: a systematic review and meta-analysis. J Clin Med. 2022;11:5928.
71. Fernández J, Navasa M, Gómez J, Colmenero J, Vila J, Arroyo V, et al. Bacterial infections in cirrhosis: epidemiological changes with invasive procedures and norfloxacin prophylaxis. Hepatology. 2002;35:140-8.
72. Arvaniti V, D'Amico G, Fede G, Manousou P, Tsochatzis E, Pleguezuelo M, et al. Infections in patients with cirrhosis increase mortality four-fold and should be used in determining prognosis. Gastroenterology. 2010;139:1246-56.
73. Simón-Talero M, García-Martínez R, Torrens M, Augustin S, Gómez S, Pereira G, et al. Effects of intravenous albumin in patients with cirrhosis and episodic hepatic encephalopathy: a randomized double-blind study. J Hepatol. 2013;59:1184-92.
74. Fagan A, Gavis EA, Gallagher ML, Mousel T, Davis B, Puri P, et al. A doubleblind randomized placebo-controlled trial of albumin in patients with hepatic encephalopathy: HEAL study. J Hepatol. 2023;78:312-21.
75. Maiwall R, Kumar A, Pasupuleti SSR, Hidam AK, Tevethia H, Kumar G, et al. A randomized-controlled trial comparing 20% albumin to plasmalyte in patients with cirrhosis and sepsis-induced hypotension [ALPS trial]. J Hepatol. 2022;77:670-82.

Section 5

Nephrology

Section Editor: Kanwalpreet Sodhi
Associate Editors: Manu Gupta, Atul Phillips, Basjinder Kaur

ARTICLE 21

Customized Citrate Anticoagulation versus No Anticoagulant in Continuous Venovenous Hemofiltration in Critically Ill Patients with Acute Kidney Injury: A Prospective Randomized Controlled Trial

Ratanarat R, Phairatwet P, Khansompop S, Naorungroj T. Customized citrate anticoagulation versus no anticoagulant in continuous venovenous hemofiltration in critically Ill patients with acute kidney injury: a prospective randomized controlled trial.
Blood Purif. 2023;52(5):455-63.

CLINICAL QUESTION OR PROBLEM

Compared to anticoagulant-free therapy, does the use of a customized citrate-based regional anticoagulant increase the life of the filter or reduce bleeding in critically ill patients with acute kidney injury (AKI) on continuous renal replacement therapy (CRRT)?

WHAT IS ALREADY KNOWN?

Continuous renal replacement therapy (CRRT) mandates continuous anticoagulation to maintain the patency and functionality of the extracorporeal circuit. Several recent trials have established the efficacy of regional citrate anticoagulation (RCA) in CRRT and have reported that citrate treatment is associated with longer circuit life, lesser bleeding, and fewer transfusions in critically ill patients.[1] However, commercial citrate solutions are costly and may not be available in some countries, leading to limited usage of RCA in low- to middle-income countries.

Intensive care unit (ICU) nurses or pharmacists can make a customized RCA solution by combining hypertonic trisodium citrate solution with a hypotonic replacement solution, which is less expensive than commercial citrate solution. However, the efficacy and safety of customized RCA are yet unestablished. The Indian guidelines on renal replacement therapy (RRT) suggest against the use of custom-made fluids for replacement but have made no recommendation for customized anticoagulant solutions.[2]

STUDY DESIGN

- Single-center randomized controlled trial registered retrospectively with the

Thai Clinical Trials Registry (TCTR) on September 24th, 2021.
- Duration: March 2018 to November 2020.
- Randomization: Patients were randomly assigned in a 1:1 ratio to receive no anticoagulation or customized RCA for continuous venovenous hemofiltration (CVVH) in a block of four randomizations. The random allocation sequence was generated by using sequentially numbered opaque envelopes and computer randomization. Sealed opaque envelopes were used to allocate eligible patients by a statistician who did not take part in the study.

POPULATION STUDIED INCLUDING DEMOGRAPHICS

A total of 37 patients in each group were needed to provide 80% power (type II error of 0.20) and 5% significance (type I error of 0.05) to detect a 20% increase in circuit life span in the customized RCA group as compared to the no-anticoagulation group, considering the average estimated circuit life span of 20.4 ± 3.1 hours.

Inclusion criteria: All patients admitted to ICU with AKI aged ≥18 years, with or without contraindication for systemic anticoagulation fulfilling at least one of the following criteria for initiating CVVH were enrolled:
- Refractory volume overload
- Refractory hyperkalemia
- Uremic symptom
- Refractory metabolic acidosis

Exclusion criteria:
- Need for systemic anticoagulation
- Chronic renal replacement therapy
- Pregnancy
- Breastfeeding
- Severe acute liver failure or waiting list for liver transplantation
- Serum Na >160 mEq/L, HCO_3 >40 mEq/L or pH >7.5
- Uncontrolled bleeding
- Persistent symptomatic hypocalcemia or total calcium (tCa): Ionized calcium (iCa) ratio >2.5
- No informed and signed consent
- Previous allergic reaction to citrate.

Demographics and Baseline Characteristics

A total of 259 patients were screened, 78 were randomized and two were excluded after randomization.
- 38 in customized RCA group.
- 38 in the no-anticoagulant group.
- The intervention and control groups had similar baseline characteristics, including the severity of illness and organ failure were assessed using the Acute Physiology and Chronic Health Evaluation II (APACHE II) and the Sequential Organ Failure Assessment (SOFA) on the day of CVVH recruitment (day 0); and the proportion of patients on mechanical ventilation in each group.

INTERVENTION STUDIED

No-anticoagulant group: In the group receiving no anticoagulation, a custom-made 2-bag formula of bicarbonate-based replacement fluid or commercial replacement fluid (Accusol-35®, Nikkiso) was used.

Customized regional citrate anticoagulation group:
- The custom-made calcium-free trisodium citrate replacement fluid was supplied by the hospital pharmacy and mixed by ICU nurses.
- Potassium chloride and 50% magnesium sulfate ($MgSO_4$) were added as needed in replacement fluid.
- If the systemic iCa level before CVVH initiation was <4.01 mg/dL (1 mmol/L), 20 mL of 10% calcium gluconate was

administered intravenously, and a calcium infusion protocol was started targeting systemic iCa levels of 4.01–4.81 mg/dL (1.0–1.2 mmol/L).
- The circuit iCa was not measured.
- The first measurement of iCa was done after initiation of CVVH for 1 hour and followed up every 2–6 hours.
- In case of citrate accumulation, CVVH was continued with no anticoagulation.

OUTCOME EVALUATED

Primary outcomes:
- Survival time of the first filter (1st circuit life span) in hours—the customized RCA group ($p < 0.001$) had a significantly longer life span as compared to anticoagulation free group [median 44.9 hours (IQR, 20.0, 72.0 hours) vs. 14.3 hours (IQR, 7.0, 22.0)].
- Number of filters used within the first 72 hours of therapy—less filter changes were required in the RCA group as compared to anticoagulation-free group [median 2.0 (IQR, 1.0, 2.0) vs. 2.5 (IQR, 1.0, 3.0); $p < 0.015$].

Secondary outcomes: No significant difference between the two groups were found in: 14-day mortality (23.7% vs. 34.2%, $p = 0.312$); 28-day mortality (34.2% vs. 31.6%, $p = 0.807$); length of ICU stay [14.0 days (IQR, 6.0, 28.0) vs. 11.0 days (IQR, 7.0, 15.0 days) $p = 0.242$]; or renal recovery, i.e. urine output (UO) >30 mL/hour and successful discontinuation RRT (36.8% vs. 34.2%, $p = 0.811$). Bleeding was similar; 2.6% in both groups while citrate accumulation occurred in 13.2% of the customized RCA group.

AUTHORS' VIEWPOINT

Regional anticoagulation with a customized citrate-based replacement solution improved circuit and filter survival and decreased costs in CVVH compared to an anticoagulant-free strategy. This regimen is safe, feasible, and suitable for low- to middle-income countries.

STRENGTH OF THE STUDY

- Balanced baseline characteristics, especially APACHE II, SOFA, and proportion of mechanically ventilated patients, were comparable in both groups.
- Citrate fluid was used as both buffer solution and an anticoagulant, making the protocol less complex, less costly, and easier to implement.
- Higher illness severity scores as compared to other similar studies.
- Low selection bias—computerized random sequence generation and allocation concealment done by using opaque sealed envelopes.
- Low attrition bias—outcome data from each primary and secondary outcome has been comprehensively reported for all randomized patients.
- Low reporting bias—all outcomes mentioned in the clinical trial registry (TCTR ID: TCTR20210924001) have been reported by the authors.

DRAWBACKS OF THE STUDY

- Single center study
- Small sample size
- Performance bias—whether the participants or researchers were blind to the study group allocated, has not been clearly described, and assuming a high risk of performance bias.
- Detection bias—measures used, if any, to blind outcome assessment from knowledge of which intervention a participant received have not been described. Thus, a high risk of detection bias could be assumed.

- Because the RCA system requires high measurement accuracy for measuring iCa, it should not be used in hospitals where iCa measurement is not available.
- Only CVVH modality was evaluated for CRRT, however the reason for this has not been duly explained.
- The reason for mortality has not been described or compared.

■ REVIEWERS' VIEWPOINT

Although previous literature has reported use of customized dialysis fluids but this is one of the pilot studies reporting outcomes with customized regional citrate solution for anticoagulation during CVVH. Among critically ill patients with AKI receiving CRRT, anticoagulation with affordable customized regional citrate, compared with no-anticoagulation, increased filter life span, with no difference in mortality, ICU stay and bleeding complications. However, this being a single-center non-blinded randomized controlled trial (RCT) with small sample size, conclusive evidence from multicenter large-scale trials or systematic reviews with meta-analysis is required for formulating guidelines and recommendations.

The study reports citrate accumulation in 13.2% of patients receiving customized RCA, whereas several research done in the past employing relatively expensive commercially available citrate solutions have reported variable rates of citrate accumulation, from 0.7 to 9.2%. Although citrate accumulation may lead to discontinuation of RCA, no significant increase in mortality has been reported in patients developing citrate accumulation.

■ TAKE HOME MESSAGE

Customized RCA solutions might be an economically viable option for CRRT when compared to commercially available RCA solutions, especially in resource-limited settings and thereby have a potential in the Indian perspective. This study showed that customized RCA can also be used in severely critically ill patients with caution as associated risk of citrate accumulation is present with no higher risk of mortality. Validation with large RCT can further aid in standardizing use of customized RCA.

ARTICLE 22

Regional Citrate Anticoagulation (RCA) in Critically Ill Patients Undergoing Renal Replacement Therapy (RRT): Expert Opinion from the SIAARTI-SIN Joint Commission

Pistolesi V, Morabito S, Pota V, Valente F, Di Mario F, Fiaccadori E, et al. Regional citrate anticoagulation in critically ill patients undergoing renal replacement therapy: expert opinion from the SIAARTI-SIN joint commission.

J Anesth Analg Crit Care. 2023;3(1):7.

■ CLINICAL QUESTION OR PROBLEM

Regional citrate anticoagulation is being recommended as the first-line anticoagulation strategy during CRRT in patients with AKI,[3] but still there are many gray areas for the routine clinical RCA use which need clarity for practical day-to-day clinical application.

WHAT IS ALREADY KNOWN?

Renal Replacement Therapy is considered as a support therapy for critically ill patients with severe AKI, providing control of solutes, fluid balance and acid–base status. An effective anticoagulation strategy is routinely required during RRT to maintain the patency of the extracorporeal circuit, to minimize the downtime period, and decrease blood loss due to filter clotting. RCA introduced into clinical practice for CRRT since early 1990s, has gained a wider acceptance with the development of simplified and safe protocols. Various guidelines on RRT support the use of RCA as the first-line anticoagulation strategy during CRRT in patients without contraindications to citrate, regardless of the patient's bleeding risk. But still there are many controversies and gray areas for the routine RCA use. The position statement by the experts from the "SIN—Società Italiana di Nefrologia", and "SIAARTI–Società Italiana di Anestesia, Analgesia, Rianimazione e Terapia Intensiva" (SIAARTI-SIN) joint commission discusses the use of RCA in different RRT modalities and in combination with other extracorporeal organ support systems.

Position Statements

The clinical aspects of RCA use in RRT have been divided into five sections. The panel has defined certain questions in each section and formulated the position statements as answers to these questions, based on the latest evidence.

Section 1: Should RCA be Considered as First Choice of Anticoagulation Modality for RRT?

Position statement: *If allowed by local resources (e.g., RCA not approved for CRRT use in the USA), RCA be considered as the first choice of anticoagulation modality for RRT, provided the use of citrate has been carefully evaluated.*

Issues related to the costs of CRRT solutions dedicated to RCA could be a potential concern for its extensive use which is nullified by the lower bleeding rates and the longer filter lifespan, potentially leading to global cost saving.

Section 2: RRT Modalities and the use of Regional Citrate Anticoagulation

1. Can RCA protocols be applied to all modalities of RRT?

    Position statement: W*ith properly defined protocols, RCA can be safely applied to all modalities of RRT, including prolonged intermittent renal replacement therapy (PIRRT).*

2. Can low or high concentration citrate solutions be indifferently selected for all RRT modalities?

    Position statement: *High concentration solutions can be potentially used in all RRT modalities including* convective, diffusive, and mixed RRT modalities, but are preferentially used in diffusive ones.

    Low citrate concentration solutions represent part of dialysis dose (as predilution replacement fluid) and are compatible only with convective or mixed RRT modalities.

    Based on their citrate content, commercially available RCA solutions can be classified into high citrate (hypertonic in sodium), generally adopted for diffusive modalities (CVVHD and SLED), versus low citrate concentration (isotonic in sodium), widely used in convective or mixed modalities (CVVH, CVVHDF) and in some SLED variants (e.g. SLED-f). To avoid the risk of hypernatremia and metabolic alkalosis, the hypertonic citrate solutions can be combined with customized dialysis solutions characterized by low sodium and low bicarbonate concentration aimed at optimizing electrolyte and buffer balance in CRRT. The physiologic sodium content of isotonic solutions allows the use of standard sodium concentration replacement fluid and/or dialysate.

Section 3: RCA in Specific Extracorporeal Organ Support Systems Combined with RRT

Several extracorporeal organ support systems, such as extracorporeal membrane oxygenation (ECMO), extracorporeal CO_2 removal ($ECCO_2R$), left ventricular assist device (LVAD), liver support systems, and therapeutic apheresis could be used alone or in combination with RRT in specific clinical settings in the ICU. The Extracorporeal Life Support Organization (ELSO) guidelines do not recommend a specific anticoagulant for ECMO, although systemic unfractionated heparin (UFH) is the most commonly used. RCA could not be conceptually used as an anticoagulation strategy for the ECMO circuit since the citrate flow rates required for the extremely high blood flow of ECMO (50–80 mL/kg/minute) are much higher than the conventional range of 150–200 mL/minute used in CRRT/PIRRT, which would lead to systemic hypocalcemia and a very high citrate load, largely overcoming physiological citrate metabolic rate. Although systemic anticoagulation represents the standard anticoagulation strategy during ECMO, RCA has been successfully used for anticoagulation to prevent repeated CRRT circuit clotting.

1. Is RCA applicable in specific extracorporeal organ support systems combined with RRT?
   Position statement: *The use of RCA for anticoagulation of integrated systems such as $ECCO_2R$ and CRRT requires further studies aimed at defining specific protocols. The citrate load related to the high blood flow rate that characterizes $ECCO_2R$ appears to be the main limit for its application in this setting.*
   Position statement: *The use of RCA for anticoagulation of albumin dialysis circuit has been successfully reported in patients with liver failure. However, the risk of citrate accumulation needs careful monitoring.*
2. Is RCA applicable during ECMO?
   Position statement: *The use of RCA for anticoagulation of CRRT circuit in the setting of ECMO (integrated or in a parallel system) is feasible and allows a prolonged lifespan.*

Section 4: Potential Limitations to RCA and Monitoring in High-risk Patients

1. Do relative or absolute contraindications to RCA exist?
   Position statement: *RCA should be avoided in worsening lactic acidosis regardless of the cause (tissue hypoxia, mitochondrial dysfunction, and impaired liver clearance).*
2. During RCA, which parameters should be monitored to identify citrate accumulation/toxicity?
   Position statement: *Systemic ionized calcium (iCa) and acid-base parameters must be routinely measured to assess the trend toward hypocalcemia and worsening metabolic acidosis.*

The total calcium/ionized calcium (Total Ca/iCa) ratio should be calculated to confirm citrate accumulation (threshold >2.5).

3. How can the condition of citrate net overload and insufficient citrate load be distinguished from citrate accumulation/toxicity?

Position statement: *Citrate accumulation/toxicity is characterized by a triad of systemic ionized hypocalcemia, increased need for calcium supplementation, and worsening metabolic acidosis. Citrate net overload and insufficient citrate load represent easily manageable conditions related to acid-base imbalances due to suboptimal RCA-CRRT parameters setting.*

While following RCA strategy for anticoagulation, it is imperative to look for citrate toxicity and distinguish it from other acid-base disturbances like citrate net overload and insufficient citrate delivery **(Table 1)**.

If citrate level exceeds the body's capacity (liver, skeletal muscle, and kidney cortex) to metabolize citrate through Krebs' cycle, eventually progressive accumulation occurs. Important signs of citrate accumulation include an increased effort aimed at maintaining physiologic levels of serum iCa concentration (i.e., increase in calcium substitution needs), worsening of metabolic acidosis, and a rising trend of total/ionized calcium (Ca/iCa) ratio to >2.5 value. Citrate accumulation requires stringent monitoring for hypocalcemia that must be prevented and treated. But net citrate overload is a benign condition that requires only adjustments of machine settings. Citrate overload occurs due to excessive citrate load and/or low clearance in the hemofilter, and is characterized by an integrity in the capacity to metabolize citrate resulting in metabolic alkalosis due to an increased production of bicarbonate from citrate anion metabolism in the Krebs' cycle.

TABLE 1: Differentiation between citrate accumulation and other benign conditions.

	Citrate accumulation	**Citrate net overload**	**Insufficient citrate load**
Cause	Reduced capacity to metabolize citrate	Excessive citrate administration or buffer needs	Insufficient citrate administration or buffer needs
Total Ca/iCa ratio	>2.5	Normal (<2.5)	Normal (<2.5)
Acid-base disturbance	Metabolic acidosis	Metabolic alkalosis	Metabolic acidosis
Severity	High	Low	Low
Possible interventions	• ↓blood flow rate (QB) • ↑dialysate flow rate (QD) • ↑post-dilution replacement fluid rate (QRpost) • ↓ target citrate dose • Stop RCA; switch to alternative anticoagulation strategies	• ↓blood flow rate (QB) • ↑dialysate flow rate (QD) • ↑post-dilution replacement fluid rate (QRpost) • ↓ target citrate dose	• ↑blood flow rate (QB) • ↓dialysate flow rate (QD) • ↓post-dilution replacement fluid rate (QRpost) • ↑ target citrate dose

Section 5: Optimization of RRT Solutions to Prevent Electrolyte Derangements during RCA

Electrolyte disturbances are potentially modifiable complications associated with CRRT. Calcium supplementation needed during RCA-RRT can be significantly reduced by using calcium-containing dialysate and/or replacement fluid. RCA-RRT is characterized by a negative magnesium mass balance, especially with the use of low concentration citrate solutions. Phosphate depletion is common in critically ill patients, especially during prolonged or continuous RRT modalities. The use of phosphate-containing dialysate and/or replacement fluids, as a variable proportion of dialysis dose, allows to minimize the need for phosphate supplementation. The questions addressed by the expert panel included:

- Can calcium containing solutions be used in specifically designed RCA protocols?

    Position statement: *Specifically designed RCA protocols, including calcium containing dialysate fluids and/or replacement fluids, allow to minimize the need for calcium supplementation and appear to ensure a longer filter life span.*

- Can phosphate-containing solutions be used in the setting of RCA-CRRT?

    Position statement: *The adoption of phosphate containing solutions as a quote of dialysis dose has been reported as safe and effective in preventing CRRT-induced hypophosphatemia, also in the setting of RCA.*

- Could an even magnesium balance be obtained with available CRRT solutions when properly designed RCA-CRRT protocols are applied?

    Position statement: *The loss of magnesium during RCA is only partially balanced by the standard commercially available CRRT solutions; further refinements of magnesium concentration in RCA-dedicated CRRT fluids are needed to approach an even magnesium balance, especially in protocols adopting low magnesium levels.*

■ REVIEWERS' VIEWPOINT

Regional citrate anticoagulation should be the first choice of anticoagulation during RRT with evidence-based advantages of longer filter life span and minimal bleeding risks, with vigilant monitoring for potential citrate toxicity, especially in patients with deranged citrate metabolism. Common dyselectrolytemias associated with CRRT can be corrected with RCA protocols using modified solutions. The article unfolds many myths associated with the use of RCA for anticoagulation during CRRT. The position statement highlights in an elaborate manner the usefulness, safety, and cost effectiveness of using RCA in various RRT modalities when utilized with careful monitoring of electrolytes to avoid potential electrolyte complications associated with it.

■ TAKE HOME MESSAGE

Regional citrate anticoagulation can be safely used for anticoagulation during different RRT modalities, keeping a strict watch on citrate toxicity!!

ARTICLE 23

Higher Blood Pressure versus Normotension Targets to Prevent Acute Kidney Injury: A Systematic Review and Meta-regression of Randomized Controlled Trials

Tran PNT, Kusirisin P, Kaewdoungtien P, Phannajit J, Srisawat N. Higher blood pressure versus normotension targets to prevent acute kidney injury: a systematic review and meta-regression of randomized controlled trials.
Critical Care. 2022;26:364.

CLINICAL QUESTION OR PROBLEM

What is the effect of high versus normal mean arterial pressure (MAP) on AKI incidence or progression across common clinical settings like shock, cardiac or non-cardiac surgery?

WHAT IS ALREADY KNOWN?

Acute kidney injury is a multi-causal disease and remains a global health burden with approximately 1.7 million deaths per year worldwide. AKI pathophysiology is complex with renal hypoperfusion due to shock being one of the important causes. While long standing hypertension causes constriction of renal arterioles leading to impaired filtration, decreased blood flow in shock states causes renal damage within a short span. Till date, no effective pharmacology therapy has been developed to either prevent or treat AKI, hence managing the hemodynamics becomes imperative, aiming at maintaining a physiological MAP to ensure sufficient renal perfusion pressure and microcirculatory blood flow. Fluid resuscitation and administration of vasopressors are the mainstay of hypoperfusion treatment but the target MAP is not specified. The literature on higher blood pressure (BP) targets is controversial.[4] This study is a comprehensive review with meta-analysis based on RCTs that examined the effect of high versus normal MAP on AKI incidence or progression across common settings of shock, cardiac or noncardiac surgery.

STUDY DESIGN

- Systematic review and meta-analysis with meta-regression as per PRISMA guidelines.
- Studies searched between November 2021 and May 2022 on MEDLINE, EMBASE, the Cochrane Library, and SCOPUS for RCTs comparing higher and lower BP targets in shock or perioperative period. The search questions were based on three concepts:
  - Shock, postcardiac arrest, and perioperative patients
  - Blood pressure target, and
  - Randomized controlled trial.

Inclusion criteria
All studies that met all of the following criteria were included:
- Randomized controlled trial with two or more arms targeting higher BP as compared to lower BP targets, which served as normotension level;
- Studies reporting renal outcomes such as incidence or rates of any stage of AKI (as per KDIGO (Kidney Disease Improving Global Outcome), RIFLE, AKIN criteria, or other equivalent definitions) or rates of RRT receipt.

Exclusion criteria
Studies on animal research, studies in the pediatric population (<15 years of age) or obstetrics were excluded.

■ STUDIES INCLUDED IN REVIEW

A total of 8,285 citations were retrieved, of which 2,417 duplicates were removed. After full-text and result seeking, 15 studies were classified as "ongoing" and five as "awaiting classification". In the full-text assessment 12 (six multicenter and six single center) studies were reviewed including three on shock, four in noncardiac surgery and five studies in cardiac surgery.

■ OUTCOME EVALUATED

- Renal outcome was the primary endpoint in six out of 12 studies.
- Of the 5,759 total patients, 3,282 (57.0%) were in shock, 1,687 (29.3%) were non-cardiac and 790 (13.7%) patients have had a cardiac surgery.
- Baseline characteristics varied across studies and studies recruited mostly elderly male patients.
- Effect of higher MAP on AKI in shock patients:
  - Targeting MAP higher than normotension did not significantly prevent AKI progression or reduce RRT receipt rate, with risk ratios and 95% CIs of 1.10 (0.93, 1.29) and 1.03 (0.92, 1.16), respectively.
  - Subgroup analysis on 1,466 shock patients with premorbid hypertension revealed significantly lower risk of RRT receipt in higher MAP arm, with RR of 1.20; $p <0.05$; while 1,767 shock patients without premorbid hypertension showed no significant difference.
- Effect of higher MAP on AKI in cardiac surgery patients.
  - In cardiac surgery patients, targeting MAP above 60 mm Hg or different levels of high MAP (60–70 mm Hg, 70–80 mm Hg, and above 80 mm Hg) versus normotension did not have significant difference in rate of AKI or RRT receipt, all with $p <0.05$.
- Effect of higher MAP on AKI in noncardiac surgery patients
  - In noncardiac surgery patients, targeting a higher MAP compared to normotension or subgroup analysis on different levels of high MAP (75–95 mm Hg and 95–110 mm Hg) versus normotension did not result in significantly lower AKI or RRT receipt rates, with $p >0.05$.

■ AUTHORS' VIEWPOINT

- In shock and perioperative patients (both cardiac and noncardiac surgery), targeting higher MAP generally was not superior to normotension in terms of preventing AKI occurrence or progression, 28-day mortality, or persistent organ dysfunction.
- Targeting a physiological MAP of 65 mm Hg is necessary to safeguard key organs by ensuring peripheral perfusion and microcirculatory blood flow.
- Meta-regression models show no significant link between MAP and AKI after adjusting for patient group, hypertension, mean age, and risk of bias (RoB).
- Shock patients with hypertension revealed a renoprotective effect of higher MAP (>70 mm Hg) on reducing the RRT receipt rate as chronic hypertension shifts the renal autoregulation to the right and therefore a higher MAP is required to maintain adequate perfusion pressure.

Nephrology

■ STRENGTH OF THE STUDY

- Robust methodology for data extraction and risk of bias assessment was used. The authors used a preregistered protocol with a comprehensive literature search and independently using Cochrane RoB updated version (RoB-2).
- Majority of the studies included were RCTs comparing different MAP targets on renal outcome.
- Usage of meta-regression using comprehensive meta-analysis version 3 to examine the relationship between predefined potential moderators strengthens the statistical analysis.
- Funnel plots were performed for primary outcome synthesis and inspected for any asymmetry, so as to detect publication bias.

■ DRAWBACKS OF THE STUDY

- Limited number of studies in each patient group (septic shock, cardiac surgery, noncardiac surgery), which may result in underpowered statistical findings and make multivariable analysis in the meta-regression models difficult.
- Prespecified subgroup analysis could not be performed due to lack of available results.
- Varied AKI definitions were used and most studies used mortality at different time intervals as an outcome measure hence, the sample size was inadequately powered to detect difference in kidney outcomes.
- The baseline characteristics of patients varied across studies in terms of age and sex.
- Varied BP targets of intervention across the studies could also be a cause of bias.
- Hypertension percentage was not reported in the original publications and a close approximation was imputed by use if antihypertensive medications were used.
- Sequential analysis was not attempted due to the anticipated heterogeneity of the included populations.

■ REVIEWERS' VIEWPOINT

One of the most common causes of AKI especially in shock and surgery-related AKI is renal hypoperfusion. MAP is the fundamental driver of organ perfusion and therefore optimizing hemodynamics is the priority for the prevention and treatment of AKI in these settings. Maintaining a physiological MAP is necessary to ensure sufficient kidney perfusion pressure and microcirculatory blood flow but literature still has conflicting results with regard to the benefit of high MAP and good renal outcomes. This systematic review is methodologically sound addressing a clearly focused question whether a higher MAP prevents AKI and the authors conducted a comprehensive literature search using relevant research databases. The characteristics of the studies including the study participants and description of the intervention were well outlined.

But to achieve a higher MAP, fluids and vasopressors were used. It is known that norepinephrine, in an attempt to increase BP, can aggravate renal medullary hypoxia and thereby cause AKI which can be a confounding factor. The studies that analyzed the effect of hypertension in cardiac and noncardiac surgical patients were heterogeneous in their definition of AKI, primary outcomes and different target MAP which could have led the studies to be underpowered. Also these studies had a high risk of bias, wide confidence intervals with an inconsistent effect in their random-effect meta-analyses despite large sample sizes. Publication bias was noted due to asymmetric funnel plot in studies for cardiac and noncardiac surgeries.

Targeting a higher MAP in shock or perioperative patients may not reduce the onset or progression of AKI, but in shock patients with premorbid hypertension, targeting MAP over 70 mm Hg might have a renoprotective impact.

TAKE HOME MESSAGE

There is no role of targeting higher MAP in preventing AKI in normotensive shock or perioperative scenario. For septic shock patients having chronic hypertension, maintaining a higher MAP may reduce the RRT administration rate, suggesting a renoprotective impact of higher MAP, possibly more beneficial in elderly population.

ARTICLE 24

Decreased Renal Perfusion during Acute Kidney Injury in critical COVID-19 assessed by Magnetic Resonance Imaging: A Prospective Case Control Study

Luther T, Eckerbom P, Cox E, Lipcsey M, Bülow S, Hultström M, et al. Decreased renal perfusion during acute kidney injury in critical COVID-19 assessed by magnetic resonance imaging: a prospective case control study.
Crit Care. 2022;26(1):262.

CLINICAL QUESTION OR PROBLEM

Is AKI in critically ill patients with coronavirus disease of 2019 (COVID-19) associated with decreased renal perfusion, reduced renal oxygenation, and increased water retention in the kidneys, and can these differences in perfusion, oxygenation and water diffusion be identified using magnetic resonance imaging (MRI) in critically ill COVID-19 patients with or without AKI?

WHAT IS ALREADY KNOWN?

Acute kidney injury is a common accompaniment in hospitalized patients with COVID-19, with a reported incidence of 40–50%, with around 20% receiving RRT and is independently associated with increased mortality. Several hypotheses have been put forth regarding the pathogenesis of AKI in COVID-19 including decreased renal perfusion, increased renovascular resistance, altered renal hemodynamics brought on by high PEEP and sedative medications in patients receiving mechanical ventilation and an inability to decrease kidney oxygen consumption, which, when combined with reduced perfusion and oxygen delivery, results in renal hypoxia. It is yet uncertain whether these mechanisms cause AKI or are merely a manifestation of it. Modern noninvasive multiparametric magnetic resonance imaging (mpMRI) techniques provide unique opportunities to investigate renal tissue characteristics in AKI, including perfusion, oxygenation, and water diffusion.

■ STUDY DESIGN

A prospective case control sub-study of the MR-Evaluation of Renal Function in Septic Patients (MERSEP) study conducted at a tertiary care University Hospital in Sweden (Clinical Trials ID: NCT02765191).

■ POPULATION STUDIED

Adult patients admitted to the ICU with polymerase chain reaction (PCR)-confirmed COVID-19 and AKI or at risk of developing AKI were screened for inclusion.

The exclusion criteria were:
- Pregnancy
- Preexisting renal failure
- Contraindications for MRI (e.g., pacemaker or certain metal implants)
- Deterioration or instability in vital parameters to a degree where MRI is not feasible (e.g., dependence on prone positioning).

Using data from healthy volunteers the researchers claim that group sizes of $n = 10$ would have statistical power $(1-\beta)$ of ≥ 0.8 and alpha coefficient ≤ 0.05 for a 20% difference in total renal blood flow and 10% difference in oxygenation.

All patients recruited to the study were allocated to AKI or NO AKI groups.

Acute kidney injury (AKI) group: Fulfillment of the KDIGO creatinine criteria at the day of the MRI examination, or within 12 hours after the MRI examination. The UO criteria were disregarded as the authors claimed that oliguria without a reduction in glomerular filtration (GFR) was commonplace.

All other patients were assigned to the NO AKI group (controls).

Nineteen patients being treated in ICU for COVID-19 fulfilling the inclusion criteria were recruited to this study.

- Ten in the AKI group
- Nine in the NO AKI group.

All recruited patients completed at least one MRI scan session.

The baseline clinical and demographic characteristics of both groups were equitable.

■ INTERVENTION STUDIED

Patients were mechanically ventilated using a Maquet Servo-i MR-Conditional ventilator and transferred to the MRI scanner by specialist ICU-staff. Throughout the test, the sedation and vasoactive therapy were maintained, and saturation was measured using pulse oximetry and invasive arterial pressure. Patients were scanned on a 3T MR scanner in a supine position for 35–40 minutes. Healthy volunteers' data was collected from formerly published research carried out on the same field strength and MR scanner and was added post hoc for secondary comparison of measurements of renal perfusion and oxygenation to facilitate interpretation. The radiologist interpreting the MRI was blind to the AKI status.

The major *multiparametric renal MRI measures* studied were:

Magnetic resonance imaging phase contrast: The measurement of blood flow in renal arteries and veins was done using bipolar gradients and ECG gating. Global renal perfusion was measured by dividing the total blood flow to the kidney by the total kidney volume (TKV). Renal resistive index (RI) was also calculated on phase contrast.

Arterial spin labeling (ASL): ASL is a subtraction technique where arterial blood water is labelled prior to imaging. Differences in signals were determined by subtracting imaging data with and without labeling. The resulting ASL images depend on tissue perfusion, and a kinetic model is used to calculate regional perfusion in the cortex and medulla. This technique was used to estimate the regional perfusion of the cortex and medulla.

Blood oxygen level dependent—a relative measure of oxygenation (BOLD): Deoxyhemoglobin, which is paramagnetic, shortens the transverse relaxation constant of T2 intensity, which is the inverse of the relaxation rate, and is influenced by changes in hematocrit and tissue water content.

T2 relaxation under spin tagging (TRUST): Renal TRUST is a novel technique used to measure renal venous saturation. Spin tagging of blood was used to separate signals from venous blood from surrounding tissues, and data was collected across a range of T2-weighted echo times. Validation studies are mainly from the central nervous system to study the sagittal sinus.

Diffusion weighted imaging (DWI): DWI determines signals from the Brownian motion of water in tissue by acquiring data at a range of b-values, which is increased in the presence of edema. Intravoxel incoherent motion (IVIM) bi-exponential model was used to calculate measures of renal water diffusion such as pure diffusion (D) separated from pseudo-diffusion (D*) and perfusion fraction (fp).

T2-weighted imaging and T1 and T2 mapping: T2-weighted sequences were used to measure TKV by manipulating signal intensity and contrast between tissues. T1 mapping was performed using a respiratory triggering inversion recovery technique with a curve fitting function, while T2 mapping was performed using a respiratory triggered gradient- and spin-echo (GRASE) scheme.

But all these parameters could not be obtained in all subjects due to technical issues related to the scanner or significant artifacts within the data.

■ OUTCOME EVALUATED

- *Global perfusion (mL/100 g/minute):* The AKI group had lower total renal blood flow (RBF) than the NO AKI group (645 mL/minute vs. 859 mL/minute, $p = 0.037$), which was similar to that of healthy controls (825 mL/minute). However, adjusting RBF by total kidney volume attenuated the differences between groups and made it non-significant.
- *Renal resistive index:* RI was higher in the AKI group compared to the NO AKI group (0.90 vs. 0.79, $p = 0.046$).
- *Regional renal tissue perfusion measured by ASL:* Cortical perfusion computed by ASL showed significant differences between groups ($p < 0.001$). The AKI group had the lowest cortical perfusion at 76 mL/100 g/minute, while the NO AKI group had cortical perfusion of 146 mL/100 g/minute ($p = 0.015$). Cortical perfusion was lower in the NO AKI group compared to healthy volunteers (197 mL/100 g/minute; $p = 0.009$). The AKI group had lower medullary perfusion than the NO AKI group (28 mL/100 g/minute, 47 mL/100 g/minute; $p = 0.03$).
- *Regional and global oxygenation estimated by BOLD R2* and TRUST:* No differences in cortical or medullary oxygenation between the groups were observed. Cortical R2* was 17/s in both the AKI and NO AKI groups. R2* in the renal medulla was 29/s in AKI patients versus 27/s in NO AKI patients.
- *Regional tissue composition and water diffusion:* The AKI and NO AKI groups did not differ in terms of cortical and medullary apparent diffusion coefficient (ADC), D, D*, or fp, or tissue composition (cortical T1 and T2 and medullary T1).

Nephrology

■ AUTHORS' VIEWPOINT

In this study, novel state-of-the-art techniques (mpMRI) were utilized to demonstrate that critically ill COVID-19 patients with AKI have decreased total, cortical, and medullary renal blood flow without any significant difference in renal oxygenation or water retention, when compared to patients who did not have AKI.

■ STRENGTH OF THE STUDY

- Utilization of a novel multiparametric MRI technology to understand the pathophysiology of AKI in COVID-19 infection.
- This being a preliminary research as well as a control group comprising of COVID-19 patients who were treated in the ICU but did not have AKI, added substance to the observations that were presented.
- Healthy volunteer data from an existing cohort with identical mpMRI sequences were added post hoc for secondary comparison of measured parameters. This validated the findings of the control group despite a low sample size. Higher illness severity scores as compared to other similar studies.
- *Low reporting bias:* All outcomes mentioned in the clinical trial registry (Clinical Trials ID: NCT02765191) have been reported by the authors.
- *Low detection bias:* Researchers interpreting the results of mpMRI were blind toward the AKI status of the patient.
- The use of ASL MRI in this study demonstrated reduced regional perfusion in both renal cortex and medulla, overcoming the major limitation with phase contrast MRI used in previous studies which could not investigate regional hypoperfusion.
- No conflict of interests as reported by the authors.
- The design of the study, the collection of data, the interpretation of the results, as well as the writing of the manuscript were all completely independent of the funding bodies.

■ DRAWBACKS OF THE STUDY

- Single center study, with a small sample size.
- *Selection bias:* To include patients in the AKI group, only the creatinine arm of the KDIGO criteria was used. The authors' explanation for this variation was a high incidence of oliguria in COVID-19 patients with no decrease in GFR. But this exclusion would have produced a bias.
- *Performance bias:* Whether the participants or researchers were not blind to the study group allocated, however as the groups were decided based on AKI status of the patient, blinding does not seem to be feasible.
- Because of the novelty of mpMRI technique, reproducing the findings of this study at a large scale involving multiple centers could be challenging.
- Only CVVH modality was evaluated for renal replacement therapy, however the reason for this has not been duly explained.
- The reason for mortality has not been described or compared.

■ REVIEWERS' VIEWPOINT

Noninvasive mpMRI techniques offer novel possibilities to investigate perfusion, oxygenation, and tissue characteristics in any type of kidney disease. With the use of this noninvasive modality, the investigators found that patients with COVID-19-related AKI had significantly lower regional perfusion of the renal cortex and medulla when compared to patients with COVID-19 without AKI and a cohort of healthy volunteers. However, this reduced perfusion was only observed on ASL, with no difference in global perfusion of kidneys observed on phase contrast studies, and no statistical difference seen between global and regional renal oxygenation on evaluation by various techniques during mpMRI. Kidneys maintained renal oxygenation in spite of hypoperfusion and no plausible reason for the same could be postulated. The study does not support hypoperfusion-induced renal hypoxia as a specific feature of early AKI in COVID-19. So, changes in hemodynamics leading to decreased renal perfusion cannot yet be conclusively proven as a major pathogenic mechanism responsible for AKI in COVID-19 infection.

■ TAKE HOME MESSAGE

Multiparametric magnetic resonance imaging is a promising technique for evaluating renal diseases that may provide additional insights into kidney characterization and disease progression in AKI patients, not only for COVID-19-related AKI but for all patients with AKI. Larger studies are required to further evaluate mpMRI techniques for assessing renal changes that occur during the progression of AKI and assessing their applicability in early diagnosis and personalized clinical decision-making. Furthermore, using mpMRI in conjunction with other imaging modalities and biomarkers may improve AKI diagnosis and treatment accuracy, resulting in better patient outcomes and lower healthcare costs.

ARTICLE 25

Renal Outcomes according to Renal Replacement Therapy Modality and Treatment Protocol in the ATN and RENAL Trials

Naorungroj T, Neto AS, Wang A, Gallagher M, Bellomo R. Renal outcomes according to renal replacement therapy modality and treatment protocol in the ATN and RENAL trials.
Crit Care. 2022:26:269.

■ CLINICAL QUESTION OR PROBLEM

Does either the RRT modality viz. CRRT or intermittent hemodialysis (IHD) or the treatment protocols have an effect on the RRT dependence and patient outcomes in patients with AKI?

■ WHAT IS ALREADY KNOWN?

Renal replacement therapy is the primary supportive treatment for patients with severe AKI, needed in approximately 5–6% of critically ill patients. However, it is associated with high in-hospital mortality rates of 50–80%. Guidelines recommend either CRRT or IHD as a supportive strategy till the kidneys recover and the practices of RRT vary across centers.[5] A meta-analysis of pooled observational studies found higher RRT dependence with IHD than CRRT, but could not adjust for individual factors, such as illness severity, diagnosis, baseline physiological state, and premorbid characteristics. CRRT, which is often considered expensive, can actually be cost-effective when compared to initial IHD as it reduces the rate of long-term dialysis dependence among critically ill AKI survivors.[6] The current study aimed to compare the rate of persistent RRT dependence (defined as RRT dependence at 28 days after randomization) in patients first treated with CRRT versus patients first treated with IHD.

RENAL (Randomized Evaluation of Normal vs. Augmented Level of RRT) and ATN (Acute Renal Failure Trial Network) were two landmark multicenter RCTs comparing different intensities of CRRT for AKI in ICU in Australia and New Zealand (ANZ) and USA, respectively.[7,8] This study focuses on analyzing the treatment protocols and their association with renal and patient outcomes, including subjects from both trials.

■ STUDY DESIGN

To compare the rate of persistent RRT dependence (defined as RRT dependence at 28 days after randomization) in patients first treated with CRRT versus patients first treated with IHD among subjects, a pooled analysis of individual patient data from two trials was done:

- *Randomized Evaluation of Normal trial:* Multicenter RCT comparing two different intensities of CRRT (40 mL/kg/hour vs. 25 mL/kg/hour) for AKI in 35 ICUs in ANZ.
- *Acute Renal Failure Trial Network trial:* Multicenter RCT comparing the efficacy of two different intensities of RRT (35 mL/kg/hour vs. 20 mL/kg/hour) for AKI in 27 ICUs in the USA.

Inclusion criteria: Patients included in both RENAL and ATN trials were included in this analysis.
- *ATN:* Critically ill adults (18 years or older) who had
  - AKI clinically consistent with acute tubular necrosis (ATN) and requiring RRT
  - Failure of one or more nonrenal organ systems (defined as a nonrenal SOFA score ≥2)
  - Sepsis.
- *RENAL:* Adult patients who were critically ill, had AKI and required RRT and met at least one of the following criteria:
  - Oliguria (UO <100 mL in a 6-hour period) that was unresponsive to fluid resuscitation measures
  - Serum potassium concentration exceeding 6.5 mmol/L
  - Severe acidemia (pH <7.2)
  - Plasma urea nitrogen level >70 mg/dL (25 mmol/L)
  - Serum creatinine concentration >3.4 mg/dL (300 μmol/L)
  - The presence of clinically significant organ edema (e.g., pulmonary edema).

Exclusion criteria: Absence of sufficient information on the first modality of RRT after randomization.

■ POPULATION STUDIED

The study trials enrolled a total of 2,589 patients and after the exclusion of 47 patients with missing data, 2,542 patients were included with 2,175 (85.5%) in the CRRT-first group and 367 (16.5%) in the IHD-first group.

■ OUTCOME EVALUATED

Primary outcome was RRT dependence at day 28 after randomization, defined as the last date of RRT.

Secondary outcomes included RRT dependence at day 60, RRT dependence at day 28 and day 60 among survivors, RRT-free days at day 28 (patient alive and free of RRT), ICU, and hospital length of stay, and ICU, hospital, 28- and 60-day mortality.

- RRT dependence at day 28—on day 28 after recruitment, 320 (14.7%) CRRT-first patients and 113 (30.8%) IHD-first group were alive. On unadjusted analysis, CRRT-first patients had a lower risk of RRT dependence at day 28 [OR, 0.19 (95% CI 0.11–0.33); $p <0.001$]. After adjustment, however, this difference was not statistically significant.
- After sensitivity analysis adjustment, only the number of RRT-free days at day 28 remained significantly greater among CRRT-first patients [COR, 1.45 (95% CI 1.12–1.88); $p = 0.005$].
- Continuous renal replacement therapy exclusive patients had higher number of RRT-free days at day 28, and shorter ICU and hospital stay, but greater ICU and hospital mortality.
- Among patients who exclusively received CRRT, it was found that there were other relevant statistically non-significant findings. These included a lower risk of RRT dependence during the initial 3 days for survivors with a SOFA score of ≤2 who received CRRT as their first treatment modality.
- Patients with a cardiovascular SOFA score of ≥3 who received CRRT as the first treatment in two trials had multiple baseline differences, and subsequent dialytic care differed by protocol. The ATN protocol was associated with greater length of stay in the ICU, fewer RRT-free days, longer hospital stays, significantly greater mortality, and a greater than four-fold increase in RRT dependence at day 28 and day 60 among survivors.

AUTHORS' VIEWPOINT

- The study highlights the plausibility of relation between the first modality of RRT used and dependence on RRT.
- The study implies that participants of ATN and RENAL trials, who received CRRT as the first modality of RRT had more number of RRT-free days and a faster recovery (after sensitivity analysis).
- Among patients who survive to at least 28 days, having received IHD as the first RRT modality was independently associated with a significantly higher probability of persistent RRT dependence.
- Treatment protocol had a strong association with renal and patient outcomes.

STRENGTH OF THE STUDY

- Large observational study using pooled data from two high-quality large multicenter RCTs having a degree of internal and external validity.
- No conceivable ascertainment bias as the data collected independently for the purpose of the trials.
- One of the first studies to analyze the association between treatment protocol and renal and patient outcomes in CRRT-first patients.

DRAWBACKS OF THE STUDY

- Observational nature of study, so unmeasured confounding could have affected the results and thus the findings can establish at best an association that can be only considered hypothesis generating.
- There were 2,175 participants in the CRRT-first group and only 367 participants in the IHF-only group. This wide difference in population size could have affected the outcomes.
- While patients in the RENAL trial received only CRRT, in the ATN trial, they received both CRRT and IHD depending on their hemodynamic state creating additional bias.

- Time from ICU admission to randomization was longer in the ATN trial.
- Lack of consensus on the definition of persistent RRT dependence after AKI.
- Finally, the association between treatment protocol and renal and patient outcomes in CRRT—first patient may not reflect just the impact of the treatment protocol itself but also the impact of other unmeasured practice variation differences between the USA and ANZ.

■ REVIEWERS' VIEWPOINT

With many aspects of RRT in ICU patients remaining controversial including the effect of modality on renal recovery, it is clinically plausible that RRT modality might affect this outcome. Although the data has been taken from two very large RCTs, by virtue of being an observational study itself, the measured and unmeasured confounders may cause bias. Sensitivity analysis data combined without being weighted analyze data as being derived from a single sample and sometimes ignores characteristics of the subgroups, moreover, using methodology with a propensity score analysis, confounding factors may persist. The study showed that the treatment protocol had a strong association with renal and patient outcomes but a number of previous studies comparing IHD and CRRT as first modality seemed to convey no benefit in terms of survival or of kidney recovery and CRRT to be associated with less favorable outcome in patients with lesser severity of disease. The clinical decision for choosing the optimal RRT mode relies also on multiple other factors including practicability, availability of machines, and the existence of trained nurse for IHD. Hence, prospective randomized non-inferiority trial should be implemented to solve the persistent conundrum of the optimal RRT technique.

■ TAKE HOME MESSAGE

Continuous renal replacement therapy when used as primary RRT modality can have beneficial patient outcomes in terms of faster recovery, more RRT free days, and renal recovery.

ARTICLE 26

Impact of Continuous Renal Replacement Therapy Initiation on Urine Output and Fluid Balance: A Multicenter Study

White KC, Laupland KB, See E, Serpa-Neto A, Bellomo R. Impact of continuous renal replacement therapy initiation on urine output and fluid balance: a multicenter study.
Blood Purif. 2023;52(6):532-40.

■ CLINICAL QUESTION OR PROBLEM

Is there any effect of initiation of CRRT on UO and how this may relate to fluid balance shifts among patients admitted to ICU?

■ WHAT IS ALREADY KNOWN?

There are concerns of possible harm induced by early RRT leading to RRT-associated kidney injury due to intradialytic hypotension, myocardial injury, vascular access-related complications, coagulation-related complications and volume depletion inducing a negative fluid balance with associated decrease in UO. UO is identified as a universal real-time marker of kidney function and thereby a key component of the AKI definition globally. Previous research has identified increasing UO during CRRT as a predictor of successful discontinuation, demonstrating the importance of residual renal function in weaning from CRRT in critically ill patients.[2] However, the impact of CRRT commencement on UO has not been previously investigated.

STUDY DESIGN

A multicenter, retrospective cohort study, using the electronic clinical information systems, from two closed-model tertiary Australian ICUs of large academic institutions with statewide referrals for neurosurgical and trauma patients.

POPULATION STUDIED

All adult patients admitted to the participating ICUs who received CRRT between January 2015 and December 2020 were considered. 1,267 patients who received CRRT were eligible for inclusion.

Inclusion criteria
- All adult patients admitted to the participating ICUs who received CRRT.
- Record of UO data for at least 4 hours prior to CRRT and should be for 24 hours after CRRT commencement available.

Exclusion criteria
- Patients with chronic kidney disease requiring chronic dialysis
- Readmission episodes within the same hospital admission.

INTERVENTION STUDIED

Routinely collected data were obtained from both centers including the baseline demographics, admission diagnosis, severity of illness based on the Acute Physiology and Chronic Health Evaluation III (APACHE III) score, daily laboratory parameters, noradrenaline equivalent (NAE) score, the vasoactive inotrope score, hourly fluid balance, and the CRRT data.

OUTCOME EVALUATED

- Primary—UO (mL/kg) on the commencement of CRRT
- Secondary—impact of CRRT on fluid balance

The differences between patients who were oliguric post-CRRT commencement, defined as UO <0.5 mL/kg/hour, and those who were not oliguric, was assessed.

Continuous renal replacement therapy characteristics: The severity of illness as measured by the median APACHE III was 95 (IQR, 76–115), and the most common source of admission was the emergency department with the most common diagnostic categories being sepsis (263, 25.0%) and cardiovascular conditions (248, 23.6%).

The median time for the first CRRT session from admission was 17 hours (IQR, 5–49), and the median duration of CRRT was 67 hours (IQR, 29–169). 96.3% of patients received hemodiafiltration with regional citrate being the most prescribed anticoagulation technique (487, 47.4%). The median hourly fluid removal was 33.6 mL/hour (IQR, 5.0–102.7). In the 24-hour post CRRT, 36 (3.4%) patients received furosemide with a median hourly dose of 10.0 mg/hour (IQR, 7.3–20.0).

Urine output: In the 24-hour period prior to CRRT, the mean hourly UO was 60.2 mL (SD ± 142.8), i.e. 0.75 mL/kg/hour (SD ± 1.78). In patients who received furosemide, the mean hourly UO was 58.2 mL (SD ± 133) or 0.7 mL/kg/hour (SD ± 1.8). In the 24 hours after CRRT, the mean hourly UO was 34.3 mL/hour (SD ± 108.8) or 0.4 mL/kg/hour (SD ± 1.4). The absolute difference in mean hourly UO before and after CRRT was −27.0 mL/hour (95% CI −32.1 to −21.8; $p <0.01$).

The initiation of CRRT was associated with a rapid drop in UO (−0.122 mL/kg/hour; 95% CI −0.165 to −0.079; $p <0.01$); which remained depressed over the 24 hours after CRRT (−0.011 mL/kg/hours; 95% CI −0.015 to −0.009; $p <0.01$).

Fluid balance: The absolute difference in mean hourly fluid balance before and after CRRT was— 129 mL/hour (95% CI −169 to −133; $p <0.01$). It was observed that the hourly fluid balance became negative only after 22 hours of starting CRRT, and even after 24 hours, the cumulative fluid balance was still positive at 2,250 mL.

Association between urine output and fluid balance: Urine output and fluid balance were only weakly associated (r −0.29; 95% CI: −0.35 to −0.23; $p <0.01$). After the start of CRRT, there was a decrease in average hourly UO, which resulted in a more positive average hourly fluid balance. Only patients who were not affected by oliguria were evaluated.

Oliguria post-continuous renal replacement therapy commencement: A total of 806 (78.6%) of the cohort were oliguric post-CRRT commencement. Oliguric patients had a significantly higher net ultrafiltration rate (0.73 mL/kg/hour vs. 0.09 mL/kg/hour; $p<0.01$), a significantly higher NAE score (0.07 vs. 0.00; $p <0.01$) but had no difference in invasive ventilation requirement (79.7% vs. 75.3%, p 0.23).

■ AUTHORS' VIEWPOINT

Continuous renal replacement therapy initiation was associated with a rapid and sustained decrease in UO, even after adjusting for pre-CRRT UO trends, use of furosemide, and patient characteristics. Additionally, it was found that the pre-CRRT trend of fluid accumulation was not immediately reversed; however, there was a reduction in the mean hourly fluid balance after CRRT to a less positive value. Overall, a negative hourly fluid balance was not achieved until 22 hours after instigation of CRRT, and changes in fluid balance were not correlated with UO.

■ STRENGTH OF THE STUDY

- A robust study of a large cohort that included a wide array of ICU admissions in ICUs that encompass the full range of adult critical care services except for acute heart and lung transplants.
- The data collected were predominantly validated, complete, and given its collection by non-research staff represents a non-biased sample.
- A sensitivity analysis on furosemide use to determine its influence on UO was conducted, which did not alter the original findings of the study, thereby strengthening the data.
- The study population was remarkably similar to several recent large multinational CRRT trials with similar APACHE III scores, ventilation rates, vasopressor use, and hospital mortality rate.

■ DRAWBACKS OF THE STUDY

- The study cohort was entirely from two resource intensive hospitals, which may limit the study application to less resource intensive environments.
- Heterogeneity of the study population with unknown medical comorbidities and a wide range of admission diagnosis potentially modified the outcome analysis.

- Further exploration of subgroups within the study population will be required to assess for within population differences in UO after CRRT commencement.
- Continuous renal replacement therapy indication and hemodynamic variables, such as cardiac output and central venous pressure, were not collected, which could interact with the demonstrated association.
- Baseline weight was not available, thereby the fluid balance as a proportion of body weight could not be calculated, which would be a more accurate measure of fluid balance.

■ REVIEWERS' VIEWPOINT

Despite extensive use of CRRT in the critically ill, its impact on renal function remains uncertain but there are obvious concerns of possible harm leading to RRT-associated kidney injury. The study suggests a negative impact of CRRT on UO. Commencement of CRRT in critically ill patients resulted in a near 50% rapid decrease in UO with a simultaneous reduction in fluid balance to a less positive value but there was a demonstrable weak association between change in UO and change in fluid balance. UO being a universally accepted marker of renal function in AKI, it is plausible that the decrease in UO on CRRT signals harm to the already injured kidney. Overall, these observations imply a potentially harmful effect of CRRT on renal function that is not mediated by changes in fluid balance and suggest the presence of additional mechanisms which might be responsible for the decrease in UO which justifies further systematic investigations.

■ TAKE HOME MESSAGE

Continuous renal replacement therapy is usually associated with a decrease in UO which might result in RRT related chronic kidney disease.

ARTICLE 27

The Furosemide Stress Test predicts the Timing of Continuous Renal Replacement Therapy Initiation in Critically Ill Patients with Acute Kidney Injury: A Double-Blind Prospective Intervention Cohort Study

Zhang K, Zhang H, Zhao C, Hu Z, Shang J, Chen Y, et al. The furosemide stress test predicts the timing of continuous renal replacement therapy initiation in critically ill patients with acute kidney injury: a double-blind prospective intervention cohort study.
Eur J Med Res. 2023;28(1):149.

■ CLINICAL QUESTION OR PROBLEM

Does furosemide stress testing (FST) serve as an effective tool in identifying high-risk patients for CRRT in critically ill patients with AKI?

■ WHAT IS ALREADY KNOWN?

The incidence of AKI necessitating RRT in ICUs is increasing globally. Even with the development of CRRT and other medical advancements, the mortality rate for ICU patients with severe AKI remains high. Conservative and supportive methods with intermittent RRT are commonly used to treat AKI, while CRRT is the standard treatment for severe cases with hemodynamic instability and life-threatening conditions. The timing of initiation of RRT is much debated with most of the major trials finding no significant difference in mortality between the two strategies, except for the ELAIN trial which showed that early initiation of RRT resulted in lower mortality rates over the first 90 days as compared to delayed initiation. The ELAIN data also demonstrated that the combination of the KDIGO classification system and plasma neutrophil gelatinase-associated lipocalin (NGAL) can reliably detect patients with progressively deteriorating AKI. Clinical trials have found high heterogeneity of new biomarkers to predict RRT and there are several limitations associated with biomarker-based predictions, such as variable cutoffs, reliance on single measurements, and confounding from underlying comorbidities and clinical conditions. Furosemide stress testing may be a practical and beneficial instrument to predict AKI development as it has outperformed various new markers in predicting worse outcomes.[9] FST has also been suggested as a way to anticipate the requirement for RRT following a kidney transplant and in individuals with AKI.

■ STUDY DESIGN

- A double-blind, prospective cohort study; registered on the China Clinical Trial Registry website: www.chictr.org.cn (ChiCTR1800015734).
- Duration: February 2021 and August 2022.

■ POPULATION STUDIED

An independent study group screened patients admitted to the ICU for AKI.

- Inclusion criteria:
  - Patients admitted to the ICU meeting the AKI diagnostic criteria for KDIGO guidelines.
  - Appropriate blood volume and central venous pressure (CVP) ≥6 mm Hg.
  - Urine output ≤0.5 mL/kg/hour for 6 hours.
- Exclusion criteria for inclusion in the study are as follows:
  - Indications for emergency CRRT, including refractory hyperkalemia (serum potassium ≥6.5 mmol/L), refractory metabolic acidosis (pH ≤7.15), acute pulmonary edema due to fluid overload, and uremia-related complications like pericarditis and bleeding.
  - Age <18 years.
  - Pregnancy or lactation.
  - Chronic kidney disease or receiving RRT 30 days before inclusion.
  - Treatment with ECMO.
  - Pulmonary embolism.
  - Presence of postrenal obstruction factors
  - A primary disease that is irreversible or expected to lead to death within 24 hours.
- Furosemide stress testing was performed in 187 of 241 patients who satisfied the inclusion and exclusion criteria.
- After receiving 1 mg/kg intravenous administration of furosemide (1.5 mg/kg if loop diuretics were taken within the past 7 days), and receiving proper fluid resuscitation, the volume of urine was measured 2 hours later. If the urine volume was >200 mL after 2 hours, the patient was deemed FST-responsive. If not, the patient was classified as FST-nonresponsive.
- The study team ensured the physicians were blinded by covering the urine bag with an opaque paper bag for 2 hours, recording the 2-hour urine volume, and then disposing of the urine.

- The clinician decided if CRRT should be started based on clinical and laboratory data other than the FST data.
- Serum NGAL was assessed.
- All recruited study participants were followed up till the time CRRT was initiated or the patient was shifted out of the ICU.

The baseline data of 187 ICU patients with AKI was analyzed. NGAL levels were significantly higher in patients who received CRRT and although the proportion of patients with sepsis was equal in both groups, those who received CRRT had significantly higher SOFA and APACHE II scores.

OUTCOME EVALUATED

A total of 187 patients were given FST, and 48 patients had a positive response, while 139 patients had a negative response. 37.5% of the patients who responded received CRRT, while 89.2% of the nonresponding patients received CRRT. The groups receiving or those not receiving CRRT showed no significant difference in terms of overall health and medical history but after 2 hours of FST, the CRRT group had a notably lower urine volume compared to the non-CRRT group (35 mL vs. 400 mL; p <0.001). Patients who did not respond to FST were found to be 2.379 times more likely to need CRRT than those who did respond (95% CI 1.644–3.443, p <0.001). Patients who underwent CRRT had notably elevated levels of plasma NGAL but on multivariate analysis, it did not demonstrate a higher efficacy compared to FST. Urine production at 2 hours post FST had significantly greater predictive value than the serum creatinine and SOFA score.

AUTHOR'S VIEWPOINT

Furosemide stress testing has been used to assess proximal renal tubular cell injury and to predict the progression of AKI. In patients with AKI, FST is a safe and practical method to identify high-risk patients and determine the optimal timing for initiating CRRT with better performance as compared to NGAL.

STRENGTH OF THE STUDY

- The patients and physicians were blinded to the urinary volume and outcome of the FST.
- All patients who were diagnosed with AKI as per KIDIGO guidelines were recruited irrespective of the stage of AKI.
- Low attrition bias—outcome data from each outcome has been comprehensively reported for all recruited patients.
- Low reporting bias—all outcomes mentioned in the clinical trial registry (ChiCTR1800015734) were reported.

DRAWBACKS OF THE STUDY

- Single center, observational study.
- Small sample size.
- The study population may not represent the wide range of critically ill patients managed in an ICU with most patients having respiratory failure or shock, and only a small fraction hospitalized for trauma.
- Another offset in sample characteristic was 41.18% of participants had a malignancy.
- The investigators did not report or analyzed outcomes other than initiation of CRRT such as mortality, duration of ICU/hospital stay, long-term complications of AKI.
- The endpoint of the study and patient follow-up was limited to the initiation of CRRT or shifting out of ICU.

REVIEWERS' VIEWPOINT

Managing AKI in critical patients, particularly those with hemodynamic instability or life-threatening complications often involves the use of CRRT as a primary approach. The KDIGO guidelines recommend initiating CRRT as a supportive option immediately in patients with life-threatening fluid accumulation or greater disequilibrium in homeostasis. However, most critically ill AKI patients lack an absolute indication for CRRT. Early initiation can be beneficial by eliminating uremic toxins, achieving volume and solute control, and correcting electrolyte imbalances at an early stage of the disease. However, beginning early may be disadvantageous since some patients with AKI may recover spontaneously without requiring RRT. In this case, an early approach would mean an unnecessary therapy escalation exposing patients to unnecessary treatment-related complications. The main question is how we can identify patients at risk of disease progression and may require RRT, as these patients might benefit from early initiation of RRT.

Furosemide stress testing is an inexpensive, widely available, and easily interpretable bedside method which has been used to assess the severity of AKI and predict weaning from RRT in patients with AKI. The change in urine volume after FST partly reflects the reserve of renal function, especially being used in clinical scenarios to avoid the delayed initiation of CRRT. The study in review evaluated the efficacy of FST in predicting the initiation of CRRT in ICU patients with AKI and has reported high sensitivity and specificity for predicting the initiation of CRRT in these patients. The results from the study also show that FST is a better predictor than measuring NGAL levels. However, this study had several limitations and further multicenter trials are required to recommend FST as a reliable predictor of initiating CRRT in critically ill patients with AKI.

TAKE HOME MESSAGE

Furosemide stress testing can be a useful practical tool for deciding initiation of CRRT in critically ill patients with AKI.

ARTICLE 28

Prevalence of Systemic Venous Congestion Assessed by Venous Excess Ultrasound Grading System (VExUS) and association with Acute Kidney Injury in a General ICU Cohort: A Prospective Multicentric Study

Andrei S, Bahr PA, Nguyen M, Bouhemad B, Guinot PG. Prevalence of systemic venous congestion assessed by Venous Excess Ultrasound Grading System (VExUS) and association with acute kidney injury in a general ICU cohort: a prospective multicentric study.
Crit Care. 2023;27(1):224.

CLINICAL QUESTION OR PROBLEM

What is the prevalence of venous congestion in critically ill patients, evaluated using venous excess ultrasound (VExUS) score, and is there any correlation between VExUS grade of venous congestion and AKI?

WHAT IS ALREADY KNOWN?

Intensive care unit patients who experience fluid overload have a greater risk of morbidity and mortality. When venous congestion occurs, the arteriovenous gradient decreases, which ultimately impacts organ perfusion.

A dysfunctional endothelial barrier can cause capillary hydrostatic pressure to increase for a prolonged period leading to worsening interstitial edema. As a result, an increase in systemic venous pressure can cause a decrease in organ perfusion pressure, which can potentially injure capsulated end organs such as the kidney and brain. Further, any endothelial damage occurring can cause release of proinflammatory cytokines, triggering the tissue edema and impairing tissue oxygenation through diffusion.

There are caveats in calculating organ perfusion pressure, which is usually inaccurately calculated by subtracting CVP from MAP. Instead, organ's true perfusion is determined by subtracting postcapillary venular pressure from precapillary arteriolar pressure. Several venous ultrasound-based parameters including the inferior vena cava diameter, the portal pulsatility index and the renal venous flow pattern have been proposed as markers of venous congestion and have been associated with AKI.

In 2020, Beaubien-Souligny used point-of-care ultrasound (POCUS) to develop the venous excess ultrasound (VExUS) score, which was originally used to diagnose and grade systemic venous congestion in patients undergoing cardiac surgery but subsequently, a case series showed that VExUS can be utilized in other pathologies as well.[10] VExUS is a scoring system that quantifies systemic venous congestion by using ultrasound examination of the inferior vena cava diameter, the sub-hepatic vein flow, the portal pulsatility index, and the renal venous flow pattern, stratifying venous congestion from Grade 0 (absent) to Grade 3 (severe).

■ STUDY DESIGN

- Multicenter, prospective, observational study (ClinicalTrials.gov: NCT04680728) in four ICUs of university-affiliated and tertiary hospitals.
- Duration—from October 2020 to October 2022.
- Inclusion criteria—all adult patients within 24 hours of ICU admission.

Exclusion criteria were:
- Individuals not affiliated with national health insurance.
- Age <18 years.
- Pregnant or breastfeeding women.
- Poor echogenicity on ultrasound.
- Chronic atrial fibrillation.
- Mechanical cardiac assistance.
- Uncontrolled blood pressure (MAP <65 mm Hg).
- Patients were subjected to multiple assessments, including clinical, biological, echocardiographic, and venous ultrasound evaluations at four different intervals, during the first 24 hours of ICU admission, between 24 and 48 hours on day 1, between 48 and 72 hours on day 2, and finally, on the last day of the patient's stay in the ICU.
- The VExUS type C **(Fig. 1)** algorithm was utilized by the investigators to identify a connection with AKI for grade ≥2. The ultrasound parameters, performed by a board-certified physician, were averaged from five measurements without regard to the respiratory cycle.
- Primary outcome—prevalence of venous congestion defined as VExUS ≥2:
  - VExUS grade 1: considered as absence of venous congestion.
  - VExUS grade 2: defined as moderate congestion.
  - VExUS grade 3: defined as severe congestion.
- Secondary outcomes:
  - Acute kidney injury (as defined by the KDIGO criteria) during the first week in ICU.
  - 28-day mortality.

Nephrology

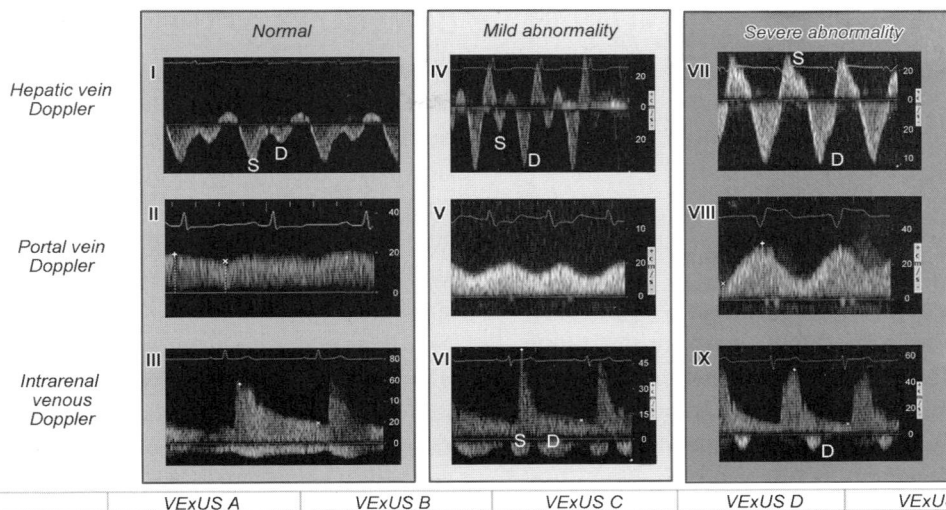

Fig. 1: Venous excess ultrasound (VExUS) grading system combines the diameter of the inferior vena cava (IVC) with the venous Doppler waveform of the portal, hepatic, and interlobular renal veins. Hepatic Doppler is mildly abnormal when S is lower than D but still toward the liver and severely abnormal when S is reversed toward the heart. Portal Doppler is mildly abnormal if there is a speed difference of 30–50% in the cardiac cycle and severely abnormal if it is equal to or >50%. Discontinuous intrarenal venous Doppler with only a diastolic phase is severely abnormal, while with both an S and D phase in discontinuity, it is mildly abnormal.

POPULATION STUDIED INCLUDING DEMOGRAPHICS

The study consisted of 185 patients, of which 40 (20%) were excluded due to incomplete echocardiographic data at inclusion.

OUTCOME EVALUATED

Primary outcome
A total of 20% of patients out of 145 had significant venous congestion (VExUS ≥2) on admission to ICU, and the proportion was nearly the same on day 1 (19%; n = 136). 26% of patients had venous congestion on day 2 (n = 111), which reduced to 10% at the time of ICU discharge (n = 96).

Secondary outcomes
- Out of 145 patients, 68 (47%) developed AKI, and 8% received renal replacement therapy. The logistic regression did not show any association between AKI and

VExUS grade at any point during the ICU stay.
- Of the 145 patients, 39 (28%) were deceased at 28 days. Higher VExUS scores were not associated with increased mortality at 28 days.

■ AUTHORS' VIEWPOINT

Moderate-to-severe systemic venous congestion was relatively uncommon among patients in the general ICU cohort. The early evaluation of systemic venous congestion did not show any correlation with AKI or 28-day mortality.

■ STRENGTH OF THE STUDY

- The study evaluated the effectiveness of VExUS, a novel scoring system, in detecting systemic venous congestion in a broader range of ICU patients, and its association with AKI and mortality, which had not been evaluated previously.
- Prospective, multicenter study design.
- High authenticity of ultrasound images acquisition; consistently performed by a board-certified physician using the Philips Envisor ultrasound system (Affinity ultrasound system Philips Medical System, Suresnes, France).
- Margin of error was low since the ultrasound parameters were calculated as the average of five measurements, regardless of the respiratory cycle.
- Low bias since data acquisition was reviewed offline by an experienced operator blinded to the study outcomes.
- Low reporting bias—all outcomes mentioned in the clinical trial registry (ClinicalTrials.gov: NCT04680728) have been reported by the authors.
- No funding source.

■ DRAWBACKS OF THE STUDY

- Observational study design.
- *Performance bias:* This was an unblinded study, where the VExUS grade was probably disclosed to the treating physician. Moreover, the researchers have not described if any therapeutic measures were taken by the clinicians based on the VExUS grading.
- *Small sample size:* During a 2-year period, all adult patients who were admitted to four different ICUs were studied by the researchers. However, the sample size was limited to only 145. There seems to be some inclusion bias.
- *High attrition bias:* Of the 145 patients, only 96 completed the study, and the researchers did not describe the reasons for this attrition.
- The researchers have reported the grading of venous congestion based on VExUS C protocol; however, as this is a prototype system, grading passed on other protocols could have led to different results.
- Study protocol mandated POCUS assessment and VExUS scoring to be done for the initial 72 hours and on the day of discharge. The rationale behind this arbitrary timing has not been explained. Moreover, venous congestion is a dynamic phenomenon, and results can vary significantly even after 3rd day of ICU management.
- The researchers dichotomized the VExUS grading into VExUS <2 and VExUS ≥2. Due to this, the association of AKI or mortality with severe congestion or VExUS Grade 3 was not analyzed.
- Outcomes of morbidity such as ICU/hospital length of stay have not been studied.

■ REVIEWERS' VIEWPOINT

Venous congestion is an under-recognized contributor to mortality in critically ill patients. Unfortunately, venous congestion is difficult to measure, and right heart catheterization (RHC) has been considered the most readily available means for measuring venous filling pressure. Research on venous congestion in critically ill patients without cardiac dysfunction and its association with organ failure, morbidity, or mortality is limited. Additionally, there is a lack of reliable and effective methods for accurately assessing the presence or severity of venous congestion. VExUS is a noninvasive scoring system that can be easily implemented for assessing venous congestion in ICUs without increasing healthcare costs with increased utilization of POCUS. The study under review has been the first to utilize VExUS for estimating venous congestion in ICU patients. The investigators report a relatively low prevalence of moderate-to-severe venous congestion on day 2 of ICU stay, to be 26%. However, this is a subjective assessment as several intensivists may consider this as a relatively high rate. Further high-quality research is required to assess the impact of venous congestion in critically ill patients and the efficacy of the VExUS scoring system.

■ TAKE HOME MESSAGE

With increased availability of POCUS in Indian ICUs, VExUS, a noninvasive scoring system, can be potentially used to assess the venous congestion in critically ill patients.

ARTICLE 29

Long-term Outcomes after Severe Acute Kidney Injury in Critically Ill Patients: The SALTO Study

Chaïbi K, Ehooman F, Pons B, Martin-Lefevre L, Boulet E, Boyer A, et al. Long-term outcomes after severe acute kidney injury in critically ill patients: the SALTO study.
Ann Intensive Care. 2023;13(1):18.

■ CLINICAL QUESTION OR PROBLEM

What are the long-term effects of severe AKI and RRT on survival, renal outcomes, and health-related quality of life (HRQOL)?

■ WHAT IS ALREADY KNOWN?

Earlier considered a totally reversible syndrome, AKI is lately recognized as a potential risk factor for chronic kidney disease and associated with long-term impacts affecting survival and quality of life. Most of the studies looking at impacts of AKI and RRT are retrospective and based on administrative database, not on actual patients and also on heterogeneous patient population with no defined AKI staging. With these limitations, prospective long-term follow-up of critically ill patients with severe AKI has been considered as a research priority.

■ STUDY DESIGN

The SALTO study is a prospective follow-up of patients included in the AKIKI (the Artificial Kidney Initiation in Kidney Injury) trial, which was an institutionally sponsored, unblinded, prospective, multicenter, open-label, and two-group RCT conducted in 31 intensive care units in France from September 2013 through January 2016.[11]

■ POPULATION STUDIED

Patients with severe AKI, defined by KDIGO stage 3 classification, compatible with the diagnosis of acute tubular necrosis in a context of ischemic or toxic aggression and receiving invasive mechanical ventilation and/or catecholamine infusion, were randomly allocated to one of the two RRT initiation strategies—an early strategy where RRT was initiated within 6 hours after AKI KDIGO 3 status was documented; and a delayed strategy where RRT was initiated if one or more of the following events occurred:

- Serum potassium concentration >6 mmol/L (or >5.5 mmol/L that persisted despite well-conducted medical treatment),
- A pH <7.15 in the context of pure metabolic or mixed acidosis,
- An acute overload pulmonary edema generating severe hypoxemia,
- A serum urea concentration >40 mmol/L,
- Oliguria or anuria for >72 hours.

■ INTERVENTION STUDIED

For the SALTO study, the duration of follow-up was extended from day 60 (the initial follow-up for each patient in AKIKI trial) from randomization; and survival, renal outcomes, and HRQOL were prospectively assessed at 2 months, 3 years, and 5 years.

■ OUTCOME EVALUATED

Of the 619 patients included in the AKIKI trial, 316 (51%) survived for at least 60 days (2 months) after randomization. 50 (16%) surviving patients had chronic kidney disease (CKD) at baseline. Five patients of 619 in the original study were lost to follow-up but long-term vital status for three was retrieved through administrative data.

Survival

Overall survival rate was 41.8% at 2 years and 39.4% at 3 years from inclusion. The survival did not differ with the RRT initiation strategy.

Renal Outcomes

Because CKD is defined by the persistence of kidney disease for a period of >90 days, all renal outcomes were assessed beyond this point. They included worsening renal function (WRF) which was defined differently according to CKD status at baseline.

- For non-CKD patients at baseline, WRF was defined by the occurrence of CKD (progression from stage 1 or 2 of KDIGO CKD nomenclature to a stage 3, 4, or 5)
- For CKD patients at baseline, WRF was defined by the progression from a stage 3 to a stage 4 or 5.

Values for serum creatinine concentration beyond day 90 were available in 175 of 280 patients who survived after day 90. The cumulative incidence of WRF was 8.5% and 20.6% at 3 years and 4 years after the severe AKI episode, respectively and 26.2% at the end of follow-up. The occurrence of WRF did not differ according to RRT initiation strategy.

The number of patients dependent on chronic dialysis was also assessed. Among the 280 patients who survived after day 90, six remained dialysis-dependent after their ICU stay. Five percent patients eventually remained chronic dialysis-dependent, after a median of 2.3 months. No patient received a kidney transplant.

Health-related Quality of Life

Out of the long-term survivors, 35% completed the EQ-5D questionnaire which assessed their mobility, self-care, usual activities, pain, and anxiety. The median index value reported was 0.67 (IQR 0.40–1.00), signifying a significant decline in their quality of life. The initiation strategy for RRT did not have any impact on their long-term outcome.

■ AUTHORS' VIEWPOINT

In critically ill patients, severe AKI was linked to significant mortality within the first 2 months. However, this association was less pronounced during long-term follow-up. A noticeable decline in quality of life was experienced by a quarter of long-term survivors who suffered from WRF. However, the initiation strategy of renal replacement therapy did not have an impact on long-term outcomes.

■ STRENGTH OF THE STUDY

- Prospective follow-up of a multicentric study.
- Long duration of follow-up—extended follow-up of >3 years, with some patients followed for >7 years.
- The long duration of follow-up allowed to identify definitive worsening renal function; avoiding overestimation of WRF with short-term follow-up.
- All renal outcomes defined beyond 90 days as the CKD is defined by the persistence of kidney disease for a period of >90 days—decreasing the bias.
- Although significant missed data on HRQOL but data missed completely at random with patients and families contact information missing at admission—bias in data collection is unlikely.

■ DRAWBACKS OF THE STUDY

- Substantial proportion of data on kidney function and HRQOL was not available at the time of follow-up leading to missing data that might have affected the precision of the results.
- They did not perform a population-based study with non-AKI matched cohort.
- No hazard ratio for risk of death, WRF, and HRQOL impairment provided.
- Urinary sediment or proteinuria was not assessed, although it is an important information for CKD staging in KDIGO guidelines.

■ REVIEWERS' VIEWPOINT

Patients who are critically ill may face considerable long-lasting consequences due to an episode of AKI. Current research mostly concentrates on short-term consequences, and the available limited evidence about long-term outcomes is mostly retrospective and derived from administrative databases. The study in review did a prospective follow-up of patients included in a large multicenter clinical trial on RRT. The present study documents significant long-term outcomes of critically ill patients with severe AKI with significant death rate, high progression rate to CKD, and HRQOL impairment >3 years after. There was no difference in outcomes according to RRT initiation strategy.

The RENAL trial reported comparable figures (long-term survival of 38% with most deaths occurring in the first 3 months). These observations are consistent with the hypothesis that comorbidities become the most impacting entity on life expectancy after recovery from an episode of AKI. The study results differ from ELAIN trial reporting that an early initiation of RRT during AKI was associated with a considerably lower mortality rate after 90 days in the early strategy group as compared with the delayed one. But study had many limitations.

■ TAKE HOME MESSAGE

Even a single episode of AKI in a critically ill patient is detrimental and causes high mortality in the early recovery period with WRF and quality of life in the future. AKI in ICU should be anticipated and avoided at all costs. It is still open to debate whether the decision to initiate RRT affects long-term outcomes or not.

ARTICLE 30

Independent Risk Factors of Acute Kidney Injury among Patients receiving Extracorporeal Membrane Oxygenation

Chen W, Pei M, Chen C, Zhu R, Wang B, Shi L, et al. Independent risk factors of acute kidney injury among patients receiving extracorporeal membrane oxygenation.
BMC Nephrol. 2023;24:81.

■ CLINICAL QUESTION OR PROBLEM

What are the risk factors of AKI in patients undergoing ECMO support?

■ WHAT IS ALREADY KNOWN?

Extracorporeal membrane oxygenation is being increasingly used as a bridge therapy for critically ill patients with respiratory failure and cardiogenic shock. AKI is a common serious complication among patients treated with ECMO, with an overall incidence of around 70–85%, and mortality among patients developing AKI during or after ECMO can be as high as 80%.[12] AKI may also be associated with adverse clinical outcomes including prolonged ECMO duration, increased risk of CKD and in-hospital mortality. The reported risk factors of AKI during ECMO vary from the severity of illness to inflammatory biomarkers and hemodynamic instability. Therefore, it is imperative to identify the risk factors for AKI during ECMO comprehensively.

■ STUDY DESIGN

A retrospective observational cohort study conducted in a Chinese provincial hospital between June 2019 and December 2020 on adult patients (>18 years) on ECMO who had AKI.

■ POPULATION STUDIED

A total of 104 people were treated with ECMO from June 2019 to December 2020.

Exclusion criteria
- Patients younger than 18 years of age
- Duration of ECMO <48 hours
- Dying within 48 hours after admission
- Patients with CKD or receiving CRRT before admission
- Cancer
- Lack of complete data.

The clinical data recorded included the demographic data, comorbidities, severity of illness including acute physiology and chronic health evaluation II score (APACHE II score) and SOFA score, laboratory examination, cause of ECMO support, mode of ECMO, duration of ECMO support, oxygenation index (OI), Vasoactive drug index (VIS), and echocardiogram data before and after initiation of ECMO support.

After following the exclusion criteria, eventually 84 patients were enrolled in the study.

■ INTERVENTION STUDIED

The primary endpoint was the occurrence of AKI within 48 hours after ECMO implementation. AKI was defined as an increase in serum creatinine (S Cr) by ≥0.3 mg/dL (≥26.5 μmol/L) within the first 48 hours or urine volume <0.5 mL/kg/hour for 6 hours after initiation of ECMO support according to the KDIGO criteria.

■ OUTCOME EVALUATED

Among the 84 adult patients, the overall incidence of AKI within 48 hours after initiation of ECMO support was 53.57% ($n = 45$).

Risk Factors for Acute Kidney Injury

The significant risk factors of post-ECMO AKI determined by univariate analysis included the APACHE II score, SOFA score, creatinine at 24 hours and 48 hours after ECMO initiation, Blood urea nitrogen (BUN) at 24 hours and 48 hours after ECMO initiation, lactate before ECMO initiation and at 24 hours and 48 hours after ECMO initiation and LVEF before ECMO initiation and at 24 hours and 48 hours after ECMO initiation. After multivariate logistic regression analysis, only three independent risk factors associated with AKI occurrence during hospitalization were identified including SOFA score before ECMO initiation (OR 1.41; 95% CI 1.16–1.71; $p = 0.001$), LVEF before ECMO initiation (OR 0.80; 95% CI 0.70–0.90; $p < 0.001$), and serum lactate at 24 hours after ECMO initiation (OR 1.27; 95% CI 1.09–1.47; $p = 0.002$). All the three risk factors were not related to baseline serum creatinine. The area under receiver operating characteristics of the model was 0.879 showing that the fitted risk model was effective in predicting the development of AKI with a sensitivity of 0.933 and a specificity of 0.667.

■ AUTHORS' VIEWPOINT

The overall incidence of AKI in patients undergoing ECMO in the present study was 53.6%. SOFA score, LVEF before ECMO initiation, and lactate at 24 hours after ECMO initiation were independent risk factors of AKI, with all three having good performance in predicting AKI. The overall in-hospital mortality was 58.1%, which is similar to 42.9–70.2% mortality rates reported by multicenter cohort studies.

■ STRENGTH OF THE STUDY

- Good methodology
- Strong statistical analysis

■ DRAWBACKS OF THE STUDY

- Single center study
- Small sample size
- Retrospective data analysis
- Being a retrospective study, insufficient data may have led to underestimation of the prevalence of risk factors.
- Due to the rapid progression of the disease and the pressing time for rescue, collected data are limited on study population.
- Because of the retrospective design of the study, notwithstanding multivariable analysis residual confounding is likely.
- Some patients needed CRRT treatment after AKI, which may affect the judgment on the classification of AKI.

■ REVIEWERS' VIEWPOINT

Acute kidney injury is extremely common and associated with severe complications and worse short-term and long-term outcomes in patients receiving ECMO. Severe preoperative organ dysfunction, hemodynamic instability caused by decreased cardiac output before ECMO initiation and microcirculation hypoxia at early stage after ECMO initiation increase the risk of AKI development. The risk factors for AKI during ECMO therapy need to be identified so as to prevent the occurrence. Multiple risk factors have been postulated as per existing literature including the patient related factors—older age, preexisting and ECMO related factors-comorbidities, severity of underlying disease, delay in ECMO institution, cardiac dysfunction before ECMO initiation, the blood lactate level at 24 hours after ECMO initiation and longer duration of ECMO therapy. The study has shown in corroboration that three factors including higher SOFA score, low LVEF, and lactate levels are independent risk factors for development of AKI on ECMO patients. Patients in AKI group having higher SOFA scores indicate severe status of organ failure. Higher LVEF is a protective factor for AKI, with every 1% increase in LVEF, the risk of AKI decreases by 20%. Lower LVEF values before ECMO might be suggestive of decreased cardiac output and low arterial perfusion pressure, with more severe cardiac failure and shock before initiation of ECMO support therapy, often implying a worse perfusion status.

■ TAKE HOME MESSAGE

Pre-ECMO SOFA score, LVEF before ECMO initiation, and lactate level at 24 hours after ECMO implementation are independent risk factors of AKI in the early phase among patients receiving ECMO treatment. Thereby, it is imperative that patients with these clinical characteristics should be paid more attention during ECMO so as to prevent AKI.

ARTICLE 31

Association of Anticoagulation Use during Continuous Kidney Replacement Therapy and 90-Day Outcomes: A Multicentre Study

Lau YH, Li AY, Lim SL, Woo KL, Ramanathan K, Chua H-R, et al. Association of anticoagulation use during continuous kidney replacement therapy and 90-day outcomes: a multicentre study.
Ann Acad Med Singap. 2023;52:390-7.

■ CLINICAL QUESTION OR PROBLEM

Is there any association between anticoagulant use and outcomes (90-day-mortality and dialysis dependence) in critically ill patients with AKI on CRRT?

■ WHAT IS ALREADY KNOWN?

Continuous renal replacement therapy is a common treatment for critically ill patients with acute kidney injury AKI in the ICU. Unlike traditional renal replacement therapies, CRRT can provide solute clearance and acid-base regulation for patients with unstable hemodynamic status. However, extracorporeal circuit clotting can occur during CRRT, leading to potential blood loss, hemodynamic instability, and increased treatment costs. Anticoagulation is commonly used in conjunction with other strategies, such as catheter choice and blood flow rate, to prevent clotting of the circuit.

In clinical settings, different anticoagulation options are utilized, with unfractionated heparin (UFH) being the most commonly used due to its affordability, ease of monitoring, and simple reversal.[5] However, there is an increased risk of bleeding and heparin-induced thrombocytopenia (HIT), which may lead to serious complications. Another commonly used anticoagulation option for CRRT is RCA, which has been recommended for its longer circuit life and safety, even in patients with liver dysfunction. Nevertheless, critically ill patients may experience potential disturbances such as citrate toxicity, metabolic alkalosis, and hypocalcemia. Low-molecular-weight heparin (LMWH), nafamostat mesylate (NM), prostaglandin I2 (PGI2), and regional-UFH are among other anticoagulation options available during CRRT. Despite the use of various anticoagulation options during CRRT, the efficacy and safety of these anticoagulants are still a subject of debate.

STUDY DESIGN

- Nationwide multicenter retrospective observational study.
- Duration: 1 April 2017 to 30 September 2017

POPULATION STUDIED INCLUDING DEMOGRAPHICS

- *Inclusion criteria:* All critically ill patients with AKI who have underwent CRRT.
- *Exclusion criteria:*
  - Preexisting end stage renal disease
  - Patients on intermittent hemodialysis, sustained low-efficiency dialysis (SLED), or peritoneal dialysis
  - Incomplete data
- *Data sources:* Information regarding the first RRT plan and the progression of the patient's illness was retrieved from electronic and physical medical records. The primary investigator gathered and anonymized the patient particulars at each respective location before being consolidated.
- *Primary outcome evaluated:* Dialysis dependence or death within 90 days of ICU admission.

Demographic and Baseline Characteristics

- During the study period 398 critically ill patients received CRRT amongst all the study centers.
- An analysis was conducted on the records of 276 patients from 14 ICUs located in six hospitals in Singapore.
- 130 (47.1%) did not receive anticoagulants.
- Of the 146 (52.9%) patients who received anticoagulation during CRRT, 100 (36.2%) received RCA and 46 (16.7%) received UFH.
- Mean age 64.2 years; mean APACHE II score: 27.3. 85.5% patients were on mechanical ventilation.
- Most common cause of AKI—sepsis (54.7%).
- Most common indication for dialysis—acidosis (72.5%).
- Baseline characteristics were not significantly different between patients who received anticoagulation and those who did not.

OUTCOME EVALUATED

- For the 276 individuals who underwent CRRT while in the ICU, anticoagulation was linked to lower rates of mortality and dialysis dependence at 90 days [adjusted odds ratio (AOR) of 0.47, with a 95% CI of 0.27–0.83, and a p value of 0.009].

- The logistic regression analysis was repeated, using anticoagulation as a three-level indicator variable. The results showed that citrate anticoagulation was associated with a reduced mortality rate (AOR 0.46, 95% CI 0.25–0.83, $p = 0.011$). However, heparin showed the same trend in reducing mortality, but without any significant difference (AOR 0.51, 95% CI 0.23–1.14, $p = 0.102$).

■ AUTHORS' VIEWPOINT

For individuals with AKI in critical condition, the utilization of anticoagulation during CRRT resulted in a decrease in the need for dialysis or death within 90 days of ICU admission. This was particularly noteworthy in the case of RCA and showed a positive trend in the same direction for systemic heparin anticoagulation. Two-thirds of patients with new onset AKI in ICU progress to develop chronic dialysis or death within 90 days of ICU admission. Mortality was highest amongst patients who did not receive anticoagulation with heparin or citrate. It is recommended that anticoagulation be utilized during CRRT whenever feasible.

■ STRENGTH OF THE STUDY

- The data collected came from various surgical, cardiac, and medical units, making it more applicable to a broader range of situations.
- Multicenter study.
- Most of the baseline characteristics such as age, comorbidities, APACHE II score, and proportion of patients were similar in both groups.

■ DRAWBACKS OF THE STUDY

- Retrospective study design
- 122 cases were excluded due to incomplete records.
- Only the first RRT session was included in data collection; subsequent sessions were ignored, that could have an impact on the outcomes.
- Outcomes such as bleeding, citrate accumulation and filter changes were not evaluated.
- Reason for not using anticoagulation was not studied.

■ REVIEWERS' VIEWPOINT

Current research into the use of anticoagulants during CRRT primarily revolves around assessing the risks of bleeding complications and filter lifespan. However, there is a dearth of information regarding the comparison of long-term outcomes, such as mortality or dialysis dependence, between patients who undergo anticoagulation and those who do not, particularly in critically ill AKI patients. The study has evaluated patients on CRRT from 14 ICUs in Singapore to evaluate the CRRT practices and the impact of anticoagulation on mortality and dialysis dependence after 90 days. The results showed that anticoagulation during CRRT was associated with lower mortality and dialysis dependence at 90 days. This retrospective analysis offers valuable insights that can help inform future randomized trials on this subject.

■ TAKE HOME MESSAGE

Anticoagulation during CRRT should be considered whenever possible. Further studies can be designed to look at the association of anticoagulation modalities with patient-centered outcomes, and also explore the reasons for omitting anticoagulation.

■ REFERENCES

1. Wu MY, Hsu YH, Bai CH, Lin YF, Wu CH, Tam KW. Regional citrate versus heparin anticoagulation for continuous renal

replacement therapy: a meta-analysis of randomized controlled trials. Am J Kidney Dis. 2012;59(6): 810–8.
2. Mishra RC, Sodhi K, Prakash KC, Tyagi N, Chanchalani G, Annigeri RA, et al. ISCCM Guidelines on Acute Kidney Injury and Renal Replacement Therapy. Indian J Crit Care Med 2022;26(S2):S13-S42.
3. Khwaja A. KDIGO clinical practice guidelines for acute kidney injury. Nephron Clin Pract. 2012;120(4):c179-84. doi: 10.1159/000339789. Epub 2012 Aug 7. PMID: 22890468.
4. Tu MY, Hong S, Lu J, Liu YH, Deng M. Effect of strict intraoperative blood pressure management strategy on postoperative acute kidney injury in non-cardiac surgery: a meta-analysis of randomised controlled trials. Int J Clin Pract. 2021;75(11): e14570.
5. Sodhi K, Phillips A, Mishra RC, Tyagi N, Dixit SB, Chaudhary D, Singla MK, Kowdle PC, Kapoor PM. Renal Replacement Therapy Practices in India: A Nationwide Survey. Indian J Crit Care Med. 2020 Sep;24(9):823-831. doi: 10.5005/jp-journals-10071-23554. PMID: 33132567; PMCID: PMC7584823.
6. Schneider AG, Bellomo R, Bagshaw SM, Glassford NJ, Lo S, Jun M, et al. Choice of renal replacement therapy modality and dialysis dependence after acute kidney injury: a systematic review and meta-analysis. Intensive Care Med. 2013;39(6):987–97.
7. Bellomo R, Cass A, Cole L, Finfer S, Gallagher M, Lo S, et al. Intensity of continuous renal-replacement therapy in critically ill patients. N Engl J Med. 2009;361(17):1627–38.
8. Palevsky PM, Zhang JH, O'Connor TZ, Chertow GM, Crowley ST, Choudhury D, et al. Intensity of renal support in critically ill patients with acute kidney injury. N Engl J Med. 2008;359(1):7–20.
9. Koyner JL, Davison DL, Brasha-Mitchell E, Chalikonda DM, Arthur JM, Shaw AD, Tumlin JA, Trevino SA, Bennett MR, Kimmel PL, et al. Furosemide stress test and biomarkers for the prediction of AKI severity. J Am Soc Nephrol. 2015;26(8):2023–31.
10. Beaubien-Souligny W, Rola P, Haycock K, Bouchard J, Lamarche Y, Spiegel R, et al. Quantifying systemic congestion with Point-Of-Care ultrasound: development of the Venous Excess Ultrasound Grading System. Ultrasound J. 2020;12:16.
11. Gaudry S, Hajage D, Schortgen F, Martin-Lefevre L, Tubach F, Pons B, et al. Comparison of two strategies for initiating renal replacement therapy in the intensive care unit: study protocol for a randomized controlled trial (AKIKI). Trials. 2015;16:170.
12. Sodhi K, Chandwani J. Acute kidney injury during ECMO; in ISCCM Manual of RRT and ECMO in ICU: A Reference Book for Practicing Intensivists; Editors: Mishra R, Sodhi K, Prakash KC, Gupta V.

Section 6

Infections and Antibiotics

Section Editor: Sumesh Arora

ARTICLE 32

Hydrocortisone in Severe Community-Acquired Pneumonia

Dequin PF, Meziani F, Quenot JP, Kamel T, Ricard JD, Badie J, et al. Hydrocortisone in Severe Community-Acquired Pneumonia.
N Engl J Med. 2023;388(21):1931-41.

CLINICAL QUESTION OR PROBLEM

Whether the use of corticosteroids in patients with community-acquired pneumonia (CAP) results in decreased mortality.

This is not a new question. It has been extensively studied. A meta-analysis of seven randomized trials on the use of CAP has shown improvement in some respects (time to achieve clinical stability and hospital length of stay), but not in mortality.[1]

WHAT IS ALREADY KNOWN?

- We know that the proinflammatory cytokine levels are raised in CAP, particularly in pneumococcal pneumonia.[2]
- However, currently, steroids are not recommended for treatment of CAP in the absence of septic shock. Steroids are recommended for patients with septic shock, and that includes the patients who have CAP as a diagnosis. In 2019, the Infectious Diseases Society of America and the American Thoracic Society published guidelines on CAP. These guidelines did not recommend use of glucocorticoids in patients with CAP due to poor quality of overall evidence.[3] The guidelines, however, endorsed the use of glucocorticoids in patients with septic shock.
- The role of glucocorticoids in severe coronavirus disease-2019 (COVID-19) has become established over the last few years.[4]

STUDY DESIGN

The salient features of the design are outlined in **Table 1**.

POPULATION STUDIED INCLUDING DEMOGRAPHICS

Inclusion Criteria

Patients over the age of 18 years with diagnosis of severe CAP. Pneumonia was labeled as

Infections and Antibiotics

TABLE 1:	Study design CAPE COD trial.
Country	France, 31 intensive care units (ICUs)
Randomizing	Centralized, web-based, stratified to trial center, and use of mechanical ventilation
Blinding	Yes. Identical packaging of the drug in the intervention and the control group
Control group	1:1 Control and Intervention group
Enrolment	2015–2020
Termination	After planned second interim analysis

severe if at least one of the following criteria were met.
- Mechanical ventilation [positive end-expiratory pressure (PEEP) >5]
- Use of high flow nasal cannula, with fraction of inspired oxygen (FiO_2) >50% and P:F ration <300
- For patients on nonrebreather mask, P:F ratio <300
- Pneumonia severity index >130.

Exclusion Criteria

The notable exclusion criteria were:
- *Septic shock:* This is an important criterion to note. Those following the surviving sepsis campaign guidelines will use steroids in patients who have CAP with associated septic shock.
- *Influenza:* It is thought that steroids may make outcome in influenza worse. Therefore, patients with influenza test were excluded. It should be noted that the sensitivity of influenza test varies with the sampling technique, the quality of sample, the kit used, etc.
- Do not intubate orders.

■ INTERVENTION(S) STUDIED

Intervention Group

Continuous infusion of hydrocortisone, 200 mg/day for 4 days. On day 4, the medical team decided on the duration of steroids based on a predefined criteria—8 days or 14 days.

The steroids were weaned based on a predefined criterion.

If the patient was discharged before the planned end date for steroids, the treatment was discontinued.

Control Group

Identically packaged saline.

■ COMPARATOR USED

Saline, packaged identically to the study drug.

■ OUTCOMES EVALUATED

Primary

Death from any cause on day 90.

Secondary

- Death by day 90 from any cause.
- Length of intensive care unit (ICU) stay.
- Among patients not receiving mechanical ventilation at baseline: Need for endotracheal intubation or noninvasive ventilation.
- Among patients receiving noninvasive ventilation at baseline: Need for endotracheal intubation.
- Vasopressor therapy by day 28 (note that septic shock was an exclusion criterion, therefore the patients were not on vasopressors at baseline).
- Ventilator-free days (VFDs) at day 28.
- Vasopressor-free days at day 28.

Beginners may question why VFDs, and not ventilator days. The VFD is better described as "number of days alive and free of

Infections and Antibiotics

TABLE 2: Results CAPE COD trial.

Parameter	Intervention group (hydrocortisone, 200 mg/day continuous infusion)	Placebo	Treatment effect [95% confidence interval (CI)]	p value
Primary outcome				
Death by day 28	6.2%	11.9%	−9.6 to −1.7	0.006
Secondary outcomes				
Death by 90 days	9.3%	14.7%	−9.9 to −0.8	
Need for endotracheal tube (no mechanical ventilation at baseline)	18%	29%	Hazard ratio 0.59 CI (0.40–0.86)	
Need for noninvasive ventilation (no mechanical ventilation at baseline)				

ventilator at day 28". For example, if a patient needs ventilation for 2 days, and survives to day 28, the number of VFD is 26 (28 − 26 = 2). Another patient, who needed ventilation for 2 days, but died on day 2 while on ventilator, the number of VFD is 0.

Result

Primary Outcome

There was reduced 28-day mortality with the intervention **(Table 2)**.

Secondary Outcomes

The mortality benefit persisted at day 90. In addition, there was lower need to start mechanical ventilation (among patients not receiving any at baseline) or vasopressors.

Safety Outcomes

No difference in the risk of ventilator-acquired pneumonia, bloodstream infections, or gastrointestinal bleeding. More insulin was required for patients in the intervention group.

■ AUTHORS VIEWPOINT

The authors conclude that the results of the study demonstrate that use of hydrocortisone, 200 mg/day as a continuous intravenous (IV) infusion reduced the risk of death in patients admitted to the ICU with severe CAP. The treatment is safe.

■ STRENGTH OF THE STUDY

This is a well-conducted, randomized, double-blind, and multicenter study. There is minimal selection bias and minimal loss to follow-up. Adherence to treatment protocol was high and only 6% of the patients received open label steroids.

Inclusion criteria are very specific. The study does not try to bundle up all comers with CAP. The included patients had severe CAP, but not shock, and did not have influenza. The inclusion criteria narrow the scope of the patients, but it still represents a large group of admissions to the ICU.

■ DRAWBACKS OF THE STUDY

A trial of this nature is very hard to conduct. In correspondence to this article, Friedrich and Bogossian raised a very important point which highlighted this difficulty.[5] After enrolment in the study, some participants developed shock and required vasopressors. It is reasonable to believe that in most cases in the setting of CAP would have been labeled as septic shock. Ordinarily, most of these patients would have received steroids, including those in the placebo arm. Is the mortality benefit the result of harm to the patients in the placebo group, who did not receive steroids? It is a question that merits answer, but it is very hard to answer in clinical research.

In another letter to the editor, van Geffen and Zijlstra pointed out that about 30% of the patients in this study had chronic obstructive pulmonary disease (COPD) in the placebo group, who may have qualified for steroids.[5] It is a valid point and highlights the difficulties in conducting a large and pragmatic study of this nature.

■ REVIEWERS' VIEWPOINT

The treatment for every patient needs to be individualized. While I present my viewpoint, it is important to note that not every factor that influences my decision may be penned here. Keeping in mind the results of this study, I hope to practice as follows:

- In patients with CAP, who are not in shock, but merit admission to ICU nonetheless, and who have a negative influenza rapid test (influenzae A and B), I will use hydrocortisone, 200 mg/day. In my practice, I will use it as intermittent bolus, 50 mg, and 6th hourly. Continuous infusion will require an additional cannula or may influence the need for a central venous catheter. I do not think that I am ready to insert do that for hydrocortisone infusion.

My practice is, however, likely to evolve over coming years as new studies come up, because of the following reasons:

- This is not the first study to evaluate steroids in CAP. Another study, published by Meduri et al. on behalf of the ESCAPe study group, in the year 2022, in intensive care medicine evaluated the use of methylprednisolone in CAP, and showed no effect on mortality.[6] This trial failed to show an improvement in mortality. It is, however, not directly comparable to CAPE COD trial. The patients in the trial by the ESCAPe study group were overwhelmingly men (96%), had 72 hours to been rolled in the study, and the trial was halted early due to slow recruitment. Nonetheless, the results of the CAPE COD are yet to be duplicated in other studies, or registry observations.
- In future, we are likely to see more studies on the level of biomarkers, and possibly on the use of bedside tests for cytokines levels in critically ill. Such studies may give us a better guide to selecting patients who may benefit from the use of steroids.

■ IMPACT ON CURRENT PRACTICE AND TAKE HOME MESSAGE

The Infectious Diseases Society of America and the American Thoracic Society published guidelines on CAP in 2019. These guidelines did not recommend use of glucocorticoids in patients with CAP due to poor quality of overall evidence.[3] It is likely to change in the future guidelines by these and other organizations.

ARTICLE 33

Ceftobiprole for Treatment of Complicated *Staphylococcus aureus* Bacteremia

Holland TL, Cosgrove SE, Doernberg SB, Jenkins TC, Turner NA, Boucher HW, et al: ERADICATE Study Group. Ceftobiprole for Treatment of Complicated *Staphylococcus aureus* Bacteremia.

N Engl J Med. 2023. 389(15):1390-401.

CLINICAL QUESTION OR PROBLEM

Ceftobiprole, a cephalosporin, is effective in treatment of complicated *Staphylococcus aureus* bacteremia, including that due to methicillin resistant *S. aureus*.

WHAT IS ALREADY KNOWN?

Staphylococcus aureus bacteremia is common in both community settings and hospital settings, and carries high mortality, in the range of 20–40%.[7] Methicillin-resistant *S. aureus* (MRSA) bacteremia may carry higher mortality than that due to methicillin-sensitive *S. aureus* (MSSA). Treatment failure is common, and its consequences may be devastating.[8,9] Prolonged antibiotic therapy is generally required to prevent treatment failure.[10]

Daptomycin was approved over 15 years ago for treatment of *S. aureus* bacteremia.[11] Ceftobiprole is a new drug, and this trial is a phase III study to evaluate its safety and efficacy.

STUDY DESIGN

This was a phase 3, double-blind, double dummy (method of blinding), noninferiority trial comparing ceftobiprole with daptomycin in a 1:1 allocation.

The sample size was calculated assuming 40% success rate from antibiotic treatment in both groups, a noninferiority margin of 15%, with 80% power and one-sided alpha of 0.025, 350 patients were required for intention to treat analysis.

POPULATION STUDIED INCLUDING DEMOGRAPHICS

Inclusion Criteria

Adult patients, >18 years of age were recruited if they had *S. aureus* in at least one positive blood culture within 72 hours before randomization, and evidence of complicated *S. aureus* bacteremia. Note that patients with both MSSA and MRSA were eligible for the study. The criteria for complicated *S. aureus* bacteremia were:

- Persistent bacteremia for ≥3 days despite appropriate antibiotics
- Right sided native valve endocarditis
- Cerebral or epidural abscess
- Intra-abdominal abscess
- Articular or bone infection
- Bacteremia arising from soft tissue source
- Bacteremia associated with maintenance hemodialysis
- Septic pulmonary embolism.

After randomization, investigations were continued for the next 7 days to establish the diagnosis of complicated *S. aureus* bacteremia.

Exclusion Criteria

- Unremovable infected hardware (e.g., a bony prosthesis)
- Pneumonia (because daptomycin activity is inhibited by the pulmonary surfactant)

- Effective antibiotics for *S. aureus* for >48 hours in the preceding 7 days.

INTERVENTION(S) STUDIED
- Ceftobiprole, 500 mg, 6th hourly for 8 days
- Then, ceftobiprole, 500 mg, 8th hourly for the rest of the treatment duration
- Plus, patient received dummy infusion of daptomycin (containing placebo).

COMPARATOR USED
- Daptomycin 6 mg/kg body weight, once a day
- Dose up to 10 mg/kg was allowed if dictated by institutional practices
- Plus, patient received dummy infusion of ceftobiprole (containing placebo).

OUTCOMES EVALUATED
Blood cultures were taken daily for 3 days, and then every 48–72 hours, until two cultures were negative, 24 hours apart.

Primary Outcome
The primary outcome measure was treatment success at 70 days. Treatment success was defined as consisting of all the following:
- Survival
- Symptom improvement
- Clearance of bacteremia
- Absence of new complications from *S. aureus* bacteremia
- No use of other potentially effective antibiotics.

Secondary Efficacy Outcomes
- Death from any cause
- Overall treatment success at day 70 as per-protocol analysis
- Bacteremia clearance rate.

Safety Outcomes
Analysis of the potential drug side effects.

Results
About 390 patients were randomized. 192 were assigned to receive ceftobiprole and 198 to receive daptomycin. Of these, the numbers included in the per-protocol analysis were 163 in the ceftobiprole group and 167 in the daptomycin group. The median duration of treatment was 21 days. 69.8% patients in the ceftobiprole group and 68.7% patients in the daptomycin group experienced treatment success (adjusted difference, 2%; 95% confidence interval, –7.1 to 11.1). This suggests noninferiority of ceftobiprole to daptomycin. There were no differences in the two groups for treatment failure. Microbiological clearance was obtained in 82% in ceftobiprole group and 77.3% in daptomycin group, but the difference did not reach statistical significance.

Both ceftobiprole and daptomycin achieved similar clearance for MRSA and MSSA.

Ceftobiprole had to be discontinued in 4.7%, mostly for allergy or gastrointestinal upset. In contrast, daptomycin had to be discontinued in 1.5% of patients, due to eosinophilic pneumonia (two patients) and myopathy (one patient). One patient in the ceftobiprole group may have had seizure due to the study drug.

AUTHORS' VIEWPOINT
In this randomized, double-blind trial, ceftobiprole was noninferior to daptomycin in treating complicated *S. aureus* bacteremia and achieved similar clearance to daptomycin for both MRSA and MSSA.

While the trial was not powered to investigate the difference between clearance rate for MRSA and MSSA in the two groups, similar clearance of MRSA in the two groups is an important finding, because that it likely to be the most important indication for ceftobiprole.

■ STRENGTH OF THE STUDY

This is a large, multinational, and well-conducted study. The patients included are those at highest risk of treatment failure. Even after randomization, the patients were investigated to ensure that they fulfil the eligibility criteria. For a new drug, it is important to understand both the results of intention to treat and per-protocol analysis.

■ DRAWBACKS OF THE STUDY

The most important indication for this drug is likely to be MRSA infections. In this study, however, only about a quarter of the patients had MRSA infections. While this trial confirms safety and noninferiority of ceftobiprole overall, studies specifically looking at MRSA remains to be done. It will, obviously, be the next step in research for this antibiotic.

Patients with pneumonia were excluded from this study. Efficacy of ceftobiprole in S. aureus bacteremia from pneumonia remains to be seen.

■ REVIEWERS' VIEWPOINT

This is a very important study. Infections due to S. aureus are common and difficult to treat. We have not had any new antibiotics to treat S. aureus infection in over a decade. While there are good treatment options for MSSA, treatment of MRSA is more difficult. Vancomycin is a large molecule and does not penetrate several compartments of the body well (e.g., respiratory secretions).[12] Linezolid may be associated with severe side effects (e.g., leukopenia)[13] and daptomycin is inhibited by pulmonary surfactant.[14] Because of the latter, pneumonia was an exclusion criterion.

Therefore, having ceftobiprole in the arsenal when the current agents cannot be used is a welcome addition. This is the first phase III study. Indeed, there will be many more, particularly in patients with pneumonia and MRSA infection.

It should be noted that this is a noninferiority trial. Its result indicates that ceftobiprole is at least as good as daptomycin but may be better. Proving the latter will of course require conduction superiority trials.

■ IMPACT ON CURRENT PRACTICE AND TAKE HOME MESSAGE

Before ceftobiprole may be used clinically, it needs to be approved by the regulatory authorities. At the time of writing this review of the article, ceftobiprole is not approved for clinical use yet. We hope to see an approval followed by more clinical studies on this important antibiotic.

ARTICLE 34

Continuous vs. Intermittent Meropenem Administration in Critically Ill Patients With Sepsis: The MERCY Randomized Clinical Trial

Monti G, Bradic N, Marzaroli M, Konkayev A, Fominskiy E, Kotani Y, et al.: MERCY Investigators. Continuous vs Intermittent Meropenem Administration in Critically Ill Patients with Sepsis: The MERCY Randomized Clinical Trial.
JAMA. 2023;330(2):141-51.

■ CLINICAL QUESTION OR PROBLEM

The MERCY trial was done with to answer the following question (Published verbatim from the article): Does continuous administration of meropenem reduce a composite of mortality and emergence of drug-resistant bacteria among critically ill patients with sepsis compared with intermittent administration?

■ WHAT IS ALREADY KNOWN?

Minimum inhibitory concentration (MIC) of a drug refers to the concentration that prevents in vitro growth of the bacteria or fungi. It is the first step before grading the susceptibility of a microorganism. There are predefined breakpoints, defined by organizations like Clinical and Laboratory Standards institute (CSLI, USA) or European Committee on Antimicrobial Susceptibility Testing (EUCAST, Europe). Beta lactam antibiotics exhibit time-dependent killing.[15] Time-dependent killing refers to the observation that the prolonged exposure to drug above MIC is the most important factor in clearance of microorganism. The duration of time spent above MIC between the dosing interval is referred to as time above MIC (t > MIC). It is a predictor of outcome for antibiotics that display time-dependent killing. To prolong t > MIC, for drugs with short half-life, the drug either has to be administered frequently or as a continuous infusion.

Prolonged infusion of beta lactams may improve mortality and cure rate, particularly in critically ill patients. A pooled analysis of 1,876 patients suggested that all-cause mortality improved if antipseudomonal antimicrobials were administered as a continuous infusion.[16] Another analysis suggested the same for piperacillin-tazobactam (a beta lactam and beta lactamase combination).[17]

■ STUDY DESIGN

The silent features of the MERCY trial are outlined in **Table 3**.

■ POPULATION STUDIED INCLUDING DEMOGRAPHICS

Patients with sepsis or septic shock, >18 years older, and who needed to be started on meropenem as determined by the treating team. Sepsis or septic shock was defined as per the Sepsis-3 definitions.[18]

■ INTERVENTION(S) STUDIED

For patients in sepsis or septic shock, after appropriate cultures, including three sets of blood cultures had been withdrawn, the patient received a 1 g loading dose of meropenem. After that, the following intervention was studies. Dose adjustment for renal failure was prespecified.

TABLE 3:	Study design MERCY trial.
Setting	International, multicenter (31 centers)
Countries	Croatia, Italy, Russia, and Kazakhstan
Blinding	Yes, double-blind. Double-dummy technique, in which each patient received continuous infusion as well as intermittent infusion, with one of the two being the placebo, and other meropenem
Randomization	Yes, central web based
Informed consent	Yes. If the participant died before consent, data was collected if allowed by the local ethics board
Sample size calculation	For a 12% reduction in primary outcome, 300 patients per arm would achieve 80% power to detect a difference at an alpha of <0.05
Primary outcome analysis	Intention to treat

Intervention Arm

Meropenem 3 g/day continuous infusion (the available preparation with longest stability after reconstitution was used).

Control Arm

Meropenem, 1 g, IV, and three times a day. Each dose was administered over 30–60 minutes.

■ COMPARATOR USED

Meropenem, 1 g, IV, and three times a day. Each dose was administered over 30–60 minutes as outlined earlier.

■ OUTCOMES EVALUATED

Primary Outcome

The primary outcome was a composite of all-cause mortality and emergence of pan drug-resistant or extensively drug-resistant bacteria at day 28.

Pan drug resistance was defined as resistance to all available antibiotics. Extensive drug resistance was defined as resistance to all but 1–2 classes of antibiotics.

Secondary Outcomes

These were:
- Days alive and free of antibiotics at day 28
- Days alive and free of ICU at day 28
- All-cause mortality at day 90.

Post-Hoc Exploratory Outcomes

- All-cause mortality at day 28
- Emergence of new pan drug-resistant or extensive drug-resistant organisms at day 28.

A blinded investigator did the follow-up at day 28 and day 90.

Results

About 607 patients were recruited in the study (303 in the intervention arm and 304 in the control arm). All completed 28 and 90 day follow-up. Median time from hospital admission to recruitment was 9 days, and median duration of meropenem therapy was 11 days. Sixty-seven percent of patients had septic shock. At 28 days, primary outcome occurred in 47% and 49% of patients in the intervention (continuous infusion of meropenem) and control group (intermittent infusion of meropenem) [relative risk, 0.96 (95% CI, 0.81-1.13), $p = 0.60$, no significant difference between the groups]. At 90 days, mortality was 42% in both groups [42% in both groups; relative risk, 1.00 (95% CI, 0.83 to 1.21), $p = 0.97$].

There were no differences in the primary or any of the secondary outcome measures.

AUTHORS VIEWPOINT

In critically ill patients with sepsis or septic shock who needed meropenem on clinical grounds, administration as a continuous infusion did not reduce the incidence of composite outcome of mortality and emergence of pan-resistant or extensively drug-resistant bacteria at day 28. The authors have refrained from making any further hypothesis in their conclusion (e.g., if the results should be applicable to other beta lactams or not).

STRENGTH OF THE STUDY

This is a well-conducted study. Its strengths include:
- Multinational and multicenter design.
- Rigorous double-blinding (including the double dummy technique, as outlined in **Table 3**).
- A high proportion of patients had septic shock (67%).
- Blood cultures before any antibiotics were administered.
- No loss to follow-up.

DRAWBACKS OF THE STUDY

The patients were in the hospital for a mean of 9 days before they were recruited. It is likely that they received other antibiotics before recruitment. It is, however, a real-world problem for running a trial on meropenem. Being a broad-spectrum antibiotic, it should not, and it was not used at admission.

REVIEWERS' VIEWPOINT

The editorial to the MERCY trial suggests that the trial is unlikely to influence guidelines given that there is little downside to continuous infusion.[19] While that may be the case in a patient who is immobile and has an indwelling central line with an unused lumen. Running continuous infusion of a drug in a patient with peripheral cannulas will require a dedicated cannula for the duration of therapy. IV cannulas have side effects, and need for dedicated cannula is not a trivial thing. Continuous infusions also mean that while mobilizing, the patient requires an IV infusion pump, and this may restrict mobilization, and result in associated complications of immobility.

On the other hand, advances in drug delivery solutions, e.g., elastomeric pumps and home infusion devices may improve the ability to deliver ambulators antibiotic treatment with such antibiotics.

IMPACT ON CURRENT PRACTICE AND TAKE HOME MESSAGE

Continuous infusion of meropenem is not proven to be better than intermittent infusion, but there are theoretical arguments to support its use. Therefore, when possible, I may use continuous infusion or prolonged infusion of meropenem. But in circumstances where IV access is limited or if patient mobility is compromised, intermittent infusion may be just as effective. Results of future trials, e.g., BING III are awaited to add to the current knowledge.[20]

ARTICLE 35

Effect of Selective Decontamination of the Digestive Tract on Hospital Mortality in Critically Ill Patients Receiving Mechanical Ventilation: A Randomized Clinical Trial

The SuDDICU Investigators for the Australian and New Zealand Intensive Care Society Clinical Trials Group; Myburgh JA, Seppelt IM, Goodman F, Billot L, Correa M, Davis JS, et al. Effect of Selective Decontamination of the Digestive Tract on Hospital Mortality in Critically Ill Patients Receiving Mechanical Ventilation: a Randomized Clinical Trial.
JAMA. 2022;328(19):1911-21.

■ CLINICAL QUESTION OR PROBLEM

Does the use of selective decontamination of digestive tract (SDD) reduces the mortality in mechanically ventilated critically ill patients?

■ WHAT IS ALREADY KNOWN?

Mechanically ventilated patients in the ICU are at risk of ventilator-associated pneumonia (VAP). Gram-negative bacteria are among the most common group of organisms to cause VAP. Selective decontamination of the digestive tract refers to use of enteral, nonabsorbable antibiotics, and antifungal agents; plus, a short course of IV antibiotics to reduce the burden of gram-negative bacteria in the digestive tract.[21]

■ STUDY DESIGN

The salient features of the study are outlined in **Tables 4 and 5**.

■ POPULATION STUDIED INCLUDING DEMOGRAPHICS

The participating hospitals had medical and surgical ICUs, capable of having mechanically

TABLE 4: SuDDICU trial design—selective decontamination of digestive tract controlled trial arm.

Design feature	Comment
Cluster randomized	Meaning that the participating hospitals were randomized. If there are 10 hospitals in the study, 5 hospitals in intervention arm and 5 in the control arm. All patients in a particular hospital get the same treatment. This is an appropriate design for studies of this nature
Crossover	For 12 months, a hospital is in the intervention arm. Then, after a 3 month gap, moves to the control arm for the next 12 months and vice versa
Country	Australia
Sample size	• 6,000 patients from 20 intensive care units (ICUs) to achieve 4.2% decrease in mortality from 29% baseline, at alpha = 0.05 and 80% power • For ecological survey, 20 ICUs had 90% power to reject noninferiority margin of 3%
Blinding	No. Such studies are difficult to be conducted as blinded. It is appropriate that this was not blinded
Informed consent for intervention or ecological assessment	No. Waived by the ethics research board. For the duration of the study, this was the standard practice of the unit

Infections and Antibiotics

TABLE 5: SuDDICU trial—ecological assessment arm.	
Sample	All patients in the intensive care unit (ICU) at the time, except those who were included in the intervention arm [i.e., received selective decontamination of digestive tract (SDD)]
Duration	One week
Time	During five windows: 1. Pretrial period 2. First intervention period (12 months) 3. Interperiod gap 4. Second intervention period (12 months) 5. Post-trial period

ventilated patients. 19 ICUs participated in the study. For the patients, the eligibility criteria were:
- Mechanical ventilation through an endotracheal tube at admission to the ICU
- Predicted to be ventilated for 48 hours at admission.

There were 2,791 participants were randomized in the intervention group and 3,191 in the control group.

■ INTERVENTION(S) STUDIED

Selective decontamination of the digestive tract with the following:
- *Oral:* 6th hourly application of 0.5 g paste consisting of:
  - 10 mg colistin
  - 10 mg tobramycin
  - 125,000 units of nystatin
- *Nasogastric:* 6th hourly administration of 10 mL of suspension containing:
  - 100 mg colistin
  - 80 mg tobramycin
  - 2,000,000 units of nystatin
- *Intravenous:* 4-day course of ceftriaxone or ciprofloxacin, unless on IV antibiotics that cover gram-negative organisms.

Oral and IV antibiotics were continued for the duration of mechanical ventilation or 90 days, whichever was first.

■ COMPARATOR USED

The earlier mentioned intervention was compared to placebo.

■ OUTCOMES EVALUATED

Primary Outcome
All-cause mortality at 90 days.

Secondary Outcomes
Clinical
- ICU mortality
- Days alive and free of ventilator, ICU admission and hospital admission at 90 days.

Microbiological
- Results of all blood cultures
- New *Clostridioides difficile*
- Incidence of predefined multiresistant organisms on blood cultures
- Total antibiotic use.

Ecological Survey Data
- Results of all blood cultures
- New *C. difficile*
- Incidence of predefined multiresistant organisms on blood cultures.

In addition, a cohort microbial metagenomic analysis was conducted but not reported in the study.

Results

There were 2,791 patients in the SDD group and 3,191 patients in the control group. The participants received the intervention for 87% of the days.

Primary Outcome

About 90-day mortality was 27.0% in the intervention arm (SDD) and 29.1% in the control arm (odds ratio 0.91, confidence interval 0.82–1.02).

Secondary Outcome

There was no difference between the two groups in any of the secondary outcomes.

Ecological Survey Data

About 8,599 patients were included in the ecological survey. There were no significant differences between the two groups.

The SDD group was noninferior to control arm in terms of:
- Number of positive blood cultures
- *C. difficile* infections
- Positive blood cultures with multiresistant organisms.

The adverse events were not different in the two groups.

■ AUTHORS VIEWPOINT

The use of SDD did not reduce the risk of ICU mortality, duration of mechanical ventilation, ICU length of stay, or hospital length of stay.

■ STRENGTH OF THE STUDY

It is a multicenter trial, with an unblinded and cluster randomization design, which is appropriate for such studies. The intervention drug was commercially manufactured, rather than prepared in the hospital pharmacy. The study design was as per the best practice for such studies in the past.

■ DRAWBACKS OF THE STUDY

Overall, the study was conducted as per the established best practices on this topic. This is not the first study on the topic, and there is a significant body of experience to run a well-designed study on SDD. The intervention arm had slightly more patients, and it is outside the power of the researchers to control that.

■ REVIEWERS' VIEWPOINT

The impact of SDD on mechanically ventilated critically ill patient is an exceedingly complex subject to study.

Why use Selective Decontamination of Digestive Tract

The first question is why do the decontamination of digestive tract? The answer lies in two observations—firstly, in hospitalized patients, the normal flora in the oropharyngeal tract gets replaced by pathogenic gram-negative organisms within a few days. Secondly, VAP is commonly caused by gram-negative pathogens. Based on these two observations, it has been hypothesized that removing the gram-negative organisms from the oropharynx and the digestive tract may reduce the risk of VAP. This has been studied in multiple studies, particularly in immunocompromised patients, e.g., with neutropenia or in patients with trauma. There is some evidence that SDD may reduce mortality.

In this study, the authors used mortality as the primary endpoint. The use of SDD is proposed to reduce the risk of VAP. However, the diagnosis of VAP in an unblinded study like this may introduce bias. Therefore, studies on SDD often choose mortality as a primary endpoint. It should be noted that the correlation between SDD and mortality is not direct. In this study, VAP was neither a primary nor secondary endpoint.

However, despite the evidence, clinicians are wary of using SDD because of fears of selecting organisms resistant to antimicrobials. Proponents of SDD argue that emergence of resistance has never been proven.

Impact of Antibiotics on Human Microbiome

In recent years, the research on human microbiome and its importance in maintaining health has grown significantly. Even a single dose of antibiotic may have long-lasting effects on the microbiome. Antibiotics result in reduced microbial diversity, altered metabolome, and clinical diseases like *C. difficile* infection. Imbalance of microbiome has been linked to antibiotic resistance, obesity, irritable bowel syndrome, and mental health disorders among others.[22] The basic premise of using SDD is that it should kill the enteric gram-negative organisms without an impact on the healthy microflora, primarily the anerobes. This study does not report any impact that the SDD had on the microflora.[21] The authors mention that a cohort metagenetic analysis was done, but it has not been reported. Instead, the authors have chosen a very narrow ecological assessment—*C. difficile* colonization and positive blood cultures with multiresistant organisms. In my opinion, this is not enough information about ecological impact of SDD. There are many methods for assessment on microflora, e.g., microbial gene count and investigating the chemical composition of feces (e.g., concentration of bile acids or sugars like arabinitol).[23,24]

Before further studies on SDD can be undertaken, preclinical studies on the impact on microflora (either in bench studies or animal studies) must be undertaken. The correlation between antibiotic exposure and emergence of resistance is well established. With modest benefits, if any, the risk of long-term harm is substantial. Many authors have commented about the human race going back to the preantibiotic dark ages because of the emerging resistance among the bacteria, and an approach like SDD may bring us closer to that reality.

Until more data is available on safety, in my opinion, SDD is not a safe long-term approach for critically ill mechanically ventilated patients.

IMPACT ON CURRENT PRACTICE AND TAKE HOME MESSAGE

The current study fails to show a benefit in mortality from SDD and does not quite go far enough in determining impact on the ecological safety. Therefore, in my opinion, SDD cannot be recommended as a treatment strategy for critically ill mechanically ventilated patients.

A reader interested in a primer to the effect of antibiotics on microbiome is referred to an excellent article by Ramirez listed in the references.[22]

ARTICLE 36

Burden of Typhoid and Paratyphoid Fever in India

John J, Bavdekar A, Rongsen-Chandola T, Dutta S, Gupta M, Kanungo S, et al. NSSEFI Study Team. Burden of Typhoid and Paratyphoid Fever in India.
N Engl J Med. 2023;388(16):1491-500.

The National Surveillance System for Enteric Fever in India Study

■ CLINICAL QUESTION OR PROBLEM

Enteric fever, also known as typhoid fever, is relatively common in India. The incidence of enteric fever in South Asia, including India, has been estimated to be about 500–700 cases per 100,000 population, which is the highest in the world.[24] There is, however, a lack of contemporary data on the burden of the problem. The study personnel were involved in the establishment of the "Surveillance for Enteric Fever in India (SEFI)" and conducted the "National Surveillance System for Enteric Fever in India" study. The aim of this study is to estimate the burden of enteric fever in India, in both rural and urban communities.

■ WHAT IS ALREADY KNOWN?

Enteric fever includes disease caused by *Salmonella typhi* and *Salmonella* paratyphi A and paratyphi B. *S. typhi* is thought to cause about 70% of the global cases of enteric fever. It is transmitted by fecal–oral route, and poor hygienic conditions contribute to its spread. The use of proton pump inhibitors increases the risk and presence of human immunodeficiency virus (HIV) increases may increase the severity of the disease.[25,26] Complications of enteric fever may be severe (e.g., intestinal perforation or infective endocarditis) and may result in admission to the ICU. Resistance to antibiotics is emerging.

For patients admitted to the ICU in India with gastrointestinal disease, enteric fever is often a part of the diagnosis and it is important that the treating physicians have an appreciation of the epidemiology of the disease in the country.

A typhoid conjugate vaccine is now available, and it reduces the risk of infection from *S. typhi*. The World Health Organization recommends the use of the vaccine in countries with high incidence or in areas where the risk of antibiotic resistance is high. India qualifies for both these indications, but the uptake of vaccine remains low.

This study does not have a significant direct impact on a physician working in ICU in India. Its importance, however, cannot be overstated. It is an immense effort, a large public health study undertaken in India, and published in the New England Journal of Medicine. In addition to providing important epidemiological information to Indian physicians, it will provide guidance to physicians all over the world caring for travelers returning from India.

■ STUDY DESIGN

The salient features of the study are outlined in **Table 6**.

■ POPULATION STUDIED INCLUDING DEMOGRAPHICS

The study included two phases—a tier 1 surveillance and a tier 2 surveillance. The details of the methods used are as follows:

TABLE 6: Study design—the NSSEFI study.

Country	India
Design	Prospective, community-based active surveillance (tier 1) and hospital-based active surveillance (tier 2)
Informed consent	Yes
Blinding, randomization, and control group	Not applicable
Sample size and subjects	• Tier 1—6,000 children, followed up for 24 months • Tier 2—hospital
Enrolment	2017–2020
Ethics review board	Christian Medical College, Vellore
Funding	Bill and Melinda Gates Foundation (Grant OPP1159351)

Tier 1—Community-based Active Surveillance (From 2017 to 2018)

The tier 1 was a community-based active surveillance in three urban communities (Delhi, Kolkata, and Vellore) and one rural community (near Pune). 6,000 eligible children were enrolled between the age of 6 months and 13 years at each site. These four sites were chosen to represent four geographical regions of the country (Delhi in the north, Pune in west, Vellore in south, and Kolkata in east). These children were followed for 24 months. They were called every week and 1 monthly visit was conducted. They were provided with a digital thermometer and a fever diary. If any of the children developed fever, it triggered a home visit. If fever continued for more than 3 days, it was a potential enteric fever. Blood cultures were then drawn to look for presence of S. typhi and S. paratyphi. The incidence of acute febrile illness, potential enteric fever, and infection with S. typhi and S. paratyphi per 100,000 child year were calculated at the end of the observation period. Prior antibiotic use was not a contraindication for blood culture, and the incidence was adjusted assuming that the blood culture is 60% sensitive.

Tier 2—Hospital-based Active Surveillance (2018–2020)

The tier 2 was a hospital-based active surveillance at six hospitals. The hospitalized patients were screened for patients, at least 6 months in age, for fever. After written consent, a blood culture was drawn. An independent agency conducted healthcare utilization surveys in the catchment area for each hospital to estimate the percentage of the population that used the surveillance hospitals for fever-related hospitalization. From the data from the hospital and the community; and from tier 1, the incidence of typhoid and paratyphoid fever was calculated. Monte Carlo simulation, a mathematical technique that uses past data from repeat random sampling to predict future outcomes, was used to account for uncertainty in adjusted estimates.

Results

Tier 1—Community-based Active Surveillance (From 2017 to 2018)

A total of 24,062 children were enrolled across four sites, and 21,470 completed the study (6% had data censored at age 15 years while 4.8% were lost to follow-up). 76,000 febrile episodes were observed over 47,000 children years. Overall incidence of culture proven typhoid fever (due to S. typhi) was *637 episodes per 100,000 children years*, and that of paratyphoid fever (due to S. paratyphi) was 68 episodes per 100,000 children years. Households with more crowding, without access to clean water or a toilet had children at higher risk. The clinical characteristics of typhoid and paratyphoid were similar.

Tier 2—Hospital-based Active Surveillance (2018–2020)

The incidence of typhoid fever ranged from 12 to 1,622 cases per 100,000 children years, after adjustment for surveillance coverage, study adherence, disease severity, and the sensitivity of the blood cultures. The incidence of paratyphoid fever ranged from 10 to 696 cases per 100,000 children years.

■ AUTHORS VIEWPOINT

The authors concluded that:
- In India, the incidence of typhoid fever and paratyphoid fever remains high.
- The incidence is like what it was between 1995 and 2006.
- While the reported incidence from the hospitals has come down, the incidence in the community remains low. Mathematical modeling of hospital reported cases to estimate the incidence of cases in the community underestimates the burden of the disease.
- In India, the incidence of typhoid fever is above the threshold where the conjugate vaccine for prevention of typhoid should be highly cost-effective. They propose that the policymakers and public health officials should work toward that.

■ STRENGTH OF THE STUDY

This is a remarkable study in its size and complexity. The authors should be congratulated on their efforts and results. It provides strong baseline data for healthcare planners and provides them with a recommendation regarding vaccination to reduce the burden of this dreadful disease in the community. The strengths of study include:
- Inclusion of sites from diverse regions in India, one each from north, east, south, and west
- Very little loss to follow-up.
- Robust design.

The study was funded by the Bill and Melinda Gates Foundation. A large study of this nature cannot be conducted without adequate funding. The foundation should also be congratulated for its achievements.

■ DRAWBACKS OF THE STUDY

It is possible that the prior use of antibiotics, before blood culture could have been drawn, may have reduced the sensitivity of the blood cultures. The researchers had no control over the timing of the blood culture. And indeed, awaiting the study personnel to attend to the child in the community may have resulted in dangerous delay in antibiotics administration. Similarly, the sensitivity of the blood cultures may be low, but the authors have taken it into account in their mathematical modeling. Such drawbacks represent problems in running a study like this in the real world and are to be expected.

■ REVIEWERS' VIEWPOINT

This is an excellent study. In India, enteric fever is an important public health problem, and there was a lack of good quality baseline data. Dr John has provided us that and made a strong recommendation to increase the use of vaccine for *S. typhi*.

Bacterial cultures are a highly resource intensive method for determining the burden of enteric fever. Future studies may look at surveillance sampling from sewage water or serological studies.

While vaccination may reduce the burden of the disease, the goal should be provision of safe water and improvement in sanitation. India has made immense progress in this regard in recent years through the Swachh Bharat Mission, and the incidence of acute diarrheal disease outbreaks may be decreasing.[27]

IMPACT ON CURRENT PRACTICE AND TAKE HOME MESSAGE

For public health improvement activities, the first thing is to have high quality baseline data, and the next step is to implement the recommendations based on that data. Dr John has provided us with high-quality baseline data. It is now up to the public health officials and health planners to implement the recommendations. Improvement in sanitation and provision of safe drinking water is a complex task and will take years of work to improve upon. Under the Swachh Bharat Mission, India has already done a lot of work in that direction. The implementation of a good vaccination program for *S. typhi* is the most obvious recommendation of this study and should be implemented.

As an expatriate who treats returning travelers from India from time to time, it is an important study. Enteric fever should be a differential in managing patients who have recently been to India and present with acute febrile illness.

REFERENCES

1. Briel M, Spoorenberg SMC, Snijders D, Torres A, Fernandez-Serrano S, Meduri GU, et al. Corticosteroids in Patients Hospitalized With Community-Acquired Pneumonia: Systematic Review and Individual Patient Data Metaanalysis. Clin Infect Dis. 2018; 66(3):346-54.
2. Endeman H, Meijvis SC, Rijkers GT, van Velzen-Blad H, van Moorsel CH, Grutters JC, et al. Systemic cytokine response in patients with community-acquired pneumonia. Eur Respir J. 2011;37(6):1431-8.
3. Metlay JP, Waterer GW, Long AC, Anzueto A, Brozek J, Crothers K, et al. Diagnosis and Treatment of Adults with Community-acquired Pneumonia. An Official Clinical Practice Guideline of the American Thoracic Society and Infectious Diseases Society of America. Am J Respir Crit Care Med. 2019;200(7):e45-67.
4. Horby P, Lim WS, Emberson JR, Mafham M, Bell JL, Linsell L, et al. Dexamethasone in Hospitalized Patients with Covid-19. N Engl J Med. 2021;384(8):693-704.
5. Friedrich JO, Gouvêa Bogossian E. Hydrocortisone in Severe Community-Acquired Pneumonia. N Engl J Med. 2023; 389(7):670-1.
6. Meduri GU, Shih MC, Bridges L, Martin TJ, El-Solh A, Seam N, et al. Low-dose methylprednisolone treatment in critically ill patients with severe community-acquired pneumonia. Intensive Care Med. 2022;48(8):1009-23.
7. Bai AD, Lo CKL, Komorowski AS, Suresh M, Guo K, Garg A, et al. *Staphylococcus aureus* bacteraemia mortality: a systematic review and meta-analysis. Clin Microbiol Infect. 2022;28(8):1076-84.
8. Lodise TP, Graves J, Evans A, Graffunder E, Helmecke M, Lomaestro BM, et al. Relationship between vancomycin MIC and failure among patients with methicillin-resistant *Staphylococcus aureus* bacteremia treated with vancomycin. Antimicrob Agents Chemother. 2008;52(9):3315-20.
9. Shurland S, Zhan M, Bradham DD, Roghmann MC. Comparison of mortality risk associated with bacteremia due to methicillin-resistant and methicillin-susceptible *Staphylococcus aureus*. Infect Control Hosp Epidemiol. 2007;28(3):273-9.
10. Holland TL, Raad I, Boucher HW, Anderson DJ, Cosgrove SE, Aycock PS, et al. Effect of Algorithm-Based Therapy vs Usual Care on

Clinical Success and Serious Adverse Events in Patients with Staphylococcal Bacteremia: A Randomized Clinical Trial. JAMA. 2018;320(12):1249-58.
11. Fowler VG, Boucher HW, Corey GR, Abrutyn E, Karchmer AW, Rupp ME, et al. Daptomycin versus standard therapy for bacteremia and endocarditis caused by *Staphylococcus aureus*. N Engl J Med. 2006;355(7):653-65.
12. Yang W, He B, Deng CH. Population pharmacokinetics of vancomycin from severe in patients with lower respiratory tract infection. Zhonghua Jie He He Hu Xi Za Zhi. 2017;40(3):205-9.
13. Moraza L, Leache L, Aquerreta I, Ortega A. Linezolid-induced haematological toxicity. Farm Hosp. 2015;39(6):320-6.
14. Silverman JA, Mortin LI, Vanpraagh AD, Li T, Alder J. Inhibition of daptomycin by pulmonary surfactant: in vitro modeling and clinical impact. J Infect Dis. 2005;191(12):2149-52.
15. MacVane SH, Kuti JL, Nicolau DP. Prolonging β-lactam infusion: a review of the rationale and evidence, and guidance for implementation. Int J Antimicrob Agents. 2014;43(2):105-13.
16. Vardakas KZ, Voulgaris GL, Maliaros A, Samonis G, Falagas ME. Prolonged versus short-term intravenous infusion of antipseudomonal β-lactams for patients with sepsis: a systematic review and meta-analysis of randomised trials. Lancet Infect Dis. 2018;18(1):108-20.
17. Rhodes NJ, Liu J, O'Donnell JN, Dulhunty JM, Abdul-Aziz MH, Berko PY, et al. Prolonged Infusion Piperacillin-Tazobactam Decreases Mortality and Improves Outcomes in Severely Ill Patients: Results of a Systematic Review and Meta-Analysis. Crit Care Med. 2018;46(2):236-43.
18. Singer M, Deutschman CS, Seymour CW, Shankar-Hari M, Annane D, Bauer M, et al. The Third International Consensus Definitions for Sepsis and Septic Shock (Sepsis-3). JAMA. 2016;315(8):801-10.
19. Shappell CN, Klompas M, Rhee C. Do Prolonged Infusions of β-Lactam Antibiotics Improve Outcomes in Critically Ill Patients With Sepsis? JAMA. 2023;330(2):126-8.
20. Lipman J, Brett SJ, De Waele JJ, Cotta MO, Davis JS, Finfer S, et al. A protocol for a phase 3 multicentre randomised controlled trial of continuous versus intermittent β-lactam antibiotic infusion in critically ill patients with sepsis: BLING III. Crit Care Resusc. 2019;21(1):63-8.
21. Wittekamp BHJ, Oostdijk EAN, Cuthbertson BH, Brun-Buisson C, Bonten MJM. Selective decontamination of the digestive tract (SDD) in critically ill patients: a narrative review. Intensive Care Med. 2020;46(2):343-9.
22. Ramirez J, Guarner F, Bustos Fernandez L, Maruy A, Sdepanian VL, Cohen H. Antibiotics as Major Disruptors of Gut Microbiota. Front Cell Infect Microbiol. 2020;10:572912.
23. Choo JM, Kanno T, Zain NM, Leong LE, Abell GC, Keeble JE, et al. Divergent Relationships between Fecal Microbiota and Metabolome following Distinct Antibiotic-Induced Disruptions. mSphere. 2017;2(1): e00005-17.
24. GBD 2017 Typhoid and Paratyphoid Collaborators. The global burden of typhoid and paratyphoid fevers: a systematic analysis for the Global Burden of Disease Study 2017. Lancet Infect Dis. 2019;19(4):369-81.
25. Bavishi C, Dupont HL. Systematic review: the use of proton pump inhibitors and increased susceptibility to enteric infection. Aliment Pharmacol Ther. 2011;34(11-12):1269-81.
26. Keddy KH, Sooka A, Smith AM, Musekiwa A, Tau NP, Klugman KP, et al. Typhoid Fever in South Africa in an Endemic HIV Setting. PLoS One. 2016;11(10):e0164939.
27. Dandabathula G, Bhardwaj P, Burra M, Rao PVVP, Rao SS. Impact assessment of India's Swachh Bharat Mission—Clean India Campaign on acute diarrheal disease outbreaks: Yes, there is a positive change. J Family Med Prim Care. 2019;8(3):1202-8.

Section 7

Sepsis

Section Editor: Jaicob Varghese
Associate Editors: Nilanjan Umesh, Melwin George

ARTICLE 37

CLOVERS trial: Should We adopt an Early Restrictive or Liberal Fluid Strategy in Sepsis induced Hypotension?

Early restrictive or liberal fluid management for Sepsis- Induced hypotension. National Heart, Lung, and Blood Institute Prevention and Early Treatment of Acute Lung Injury Clinical Trials Network, Shapiro NI, Douglas IS, et al. Early Restrictive or Liberal Fluid Management for Sepsis-Induced Hypotension.
N Engl J Med. 2023;388(6):499-510.

Sepsis has always been a hotly debated topic with a large data worldwide and several ongoing clinical research projects. Though last surviving sepsis guidelines were updated in 2021, there have been some important trials in the past 1 year which are noteworthy.

■ WHAT IS ALREADY KNOWN?

Resuscitation with intravenous fluids is commonly used in the initial treatment of patients with septic shock and sepsis-induced hypotension. Previous trials have all adopted a liberal fluid strategy for sepsis-induced hypotension[1,2] and the recent surviving sepsis guidelines have advocated a fluid bolus of 30 mL/kg of crystalloid. However, liberal amounts of fluids have been attributed to cause increase in peripheral edema, organ failure, and fluid overload.[3] Recently the CLASSIC[4] trial was published, and it showed that with regard to 90 day mortality, there was no difference in adopting a restrictive fluid strategy as compared to standard care. A similar trial was conducted in the US to address the confusion regarding liberal or restrictive fluid strategy.[5]

■ STUDY DESIGN

The study was an unblinded superiority trial which was conducted in 60 centers in the US, and patients were randomly assigned to either a restrictive fluid strategy or a liberal fluid strategy for a 24-hour period.

■ POPULATION STUDIED INCLUDING DEMOGRAPHICS

A total of 1,563 patients were enrolled, with 782 assigned to the restrictive fluid group and 781 to the liberal fluid group. Adult patients (≥18 years of age) who were suspected to be in sepsis (broadly defined as the administration or planned administration of antibiotic agents) and sepsis-induced hypotension [systolic blood pressure, <100 mm Hg in spite of administering ≥1L of intravenous (IV) fluids] were included. Patients with an elapse of >4 hours since the meeting of the criteria for hypotension refractory to the intravenous administration of at least 1,000 mL of fluid or an elapse of >24 hours since presentation at the hospital were excluded from the study. Those who received >3 L of intravenous fluid during this episode (including prehospital administration of fluid by emergency medical services), the presence of fluid overload, and severe volume depletion from non-sepsis causes were also excluded.

■ INTERVENTION STUDIED

The restrictive fluid protocol mainly used vasopressors in case of hypotension, with "rescue fluids" being permitted in certain cases that suggested severe intravascular volume depletion, severe hypotension or certain prespecified conditions as and when felt by the treating team. Once mean arterial pressure (MAP) reached target, then fluids were restricted to medications and nutrition. The liberal fluid protocol used an initial 2-L intravenous infusion of isotonic crystalloid, followed by fluid boluses administered based on clinical parameters (e.g., tachycardia) with "rescue vasopressors" in case of severe hypotension in prespecified conditions.

■ COMPARATOR USED

Analysis of the primary outcome used Kaplan-Meier 90-day mortality point estimates involving all the patients who were discharged home or were still alive at day 90, with data censored at day 91.

■ OUTCOME EVALUATED

The primary outcome was death before discharge to home by day 90, occurred in 109 patients (14.0%) in the restrictive fluid group and in 116 patients (14.9%) in the liberal fluid group (estimated difference, −0.9 percentage points; 95% CI, −4.4 to 2.6; $p = 0.61$. There was no significant difference in days free from organ support therapy by day 28, days free from ventilator use at 28 days, days out of intensive care unit (ICU) from day 1-28, acute respiratory distress syndrome (ARDS) onset between day 1 and day 7 or serious adverse events in both the groups.

■ AUTHORS' VIEWPOINT

A restrictive fluid strategy (with earlier vasopressor use) did not result in significantly increase (or decrease) mortality before discharge to home by day 90 than a liberal fluid strategy. Thus, reducing the amount of fluid should be considered even in sepsis induced hypotension.

■ STRENGTH OF THE STUDY

The trial was randomized with excellent adherence to the protocol and had broad inclusion criteria. The groups used common clinical characteristics and volume assessment was done routinely to trigger protocol-directed actions for vasopressor and fluid administration. The study also succeeded in separation of fluids received within initial 24 hours. Also excellent safety outcome was reported.

■ DRAWBACKS OF THE STUDY

It was a single country study, unblinded and both groups received nearly equivalent amounts of fluids at day 7 and over 2L of fluids before randomization. Also there were potentially important subgroups (patients with specific coexisting conditions for which data were not collected in this trial) that were not assessed. Moreover, large numbers were eligible but not enrolled which might have led to selection bias. Fluids were not administered according to weight or age and dynamic methods to monitor fluid responsiveness were not used.

■ REVIEWERS' VIEWPOINT

The study was done in a single country and unblinded. Moreover, over 2 L of IV fluids were given in both groups prior to randomization which itself is a significant amount. Also a weight-based fluid bolus would have been a more accurate way to understand the impact of "rescue fluids". Hence, the restrictive fluid strategy does not seem really "restrictive" and we often use much lesser amounts of fluids in our patients in the initial 24 hours.

■ IMPACT ON CURRENT PRACTICE AND TAKE HOME MESSAGE

Considering the two recent trials, we should consider individualizing fluid therapy and vasopressors in sepsis-induced hypotension based on dynamic hemodynamic monitoring parameters rather than adopting a 30 mL/kg bolus for all patients.

ARTICLE 38

Can Early Adjunctive Methylene Blue reduce Time to Vasopressor Discontinuation in Patients with Septic Shock?

Early adjunctive Methylene blue in patients with septic shock: a randomized control trial. Ibarra-Estrada M, Kattan E, Aguilera-González P, et al. Early adjunctive methylene blue in patients with septic shock: a randomized controlled trial.
Crit Care. 2023;27:110.

■ WHAT IS ALREADY KNOWN?

Methylene blue (MB) is a compound which specifically inhibits inducible nitric oxide synthase (iNOS) and its downstream enzyme soluble guanylate cyclase (sGC). Through its indirect vasopressor effects, it has been shown to restore vasoregulation in conditions of NO upregulation.[6,7] Only 50% patients respond to fluid challenges, that too transiently. Noradrenaline is the vasopressor of choice but using high doses increases the risk of adverse effects such as tachyarrhythmia, myocardial dysfunction, peripheral ischemia, and even immunosuppression.[8] Thus, there is a need for adding catecholamine-sparing agents to a multimodal strategy. Earlier also studies have seemingly demonstrated an acute vasopressor effect of MB in refractory septic shock.[9,10]

■ STUDY DESIGN

The study conducted was an investigator-initiated, parallel, double blinded, and randomized controlled trial at an academic referral center in Mexico, in a medical-surgical ICU.

■ POPULATION STUDIED INCLUDING DEMOGRAPHICS

Inclusion criteria: Patients aged ≥18 years with septic shock as defined by Sepsis-3 criteria (highly suspected or confirmed infection, requiring norepinephrine to maintain a MAP ≥65 mm Hg, and serum lactate >2 mmol/L after adequate fluid resuscitation).

Patients >24 hours since initiation of norepinephrine, pregnancy, concurrent hemorrhagic, obstructive or hypovolemic shock, probable damage control surgery, having major burn injury, personal or familiar history of glucose-6-phosphate dehydrogenase (G6PD) deficiency, allergy to methylene blue, phenothiazines, or other food dyes and recent intake (4-weeks) of selective serotonin reuptake inhibitors were major exclusion criteria.

■ INTERVENTION STUDIED

Random allocation of patients to receive MB using a predetermined randomization sequence prepared in sealed opaque envelopes was done. The study was triple blinded. Patients assigned to MB group received an IV infusion of 100 mg of MB in 500 mL of NS over 6 hours once daily for a total of three doses. Patients assigned to control group received the same dose of 500 mL of 0.9% sodium chloride without MB. In patients of both groups, vasopressin was initiated at a dose of 0.03 IU/minute if norepinephrine dose reached ≥0.25 µg/kg/minute; and fluid responsiveness was assessed at least three times each day as long as vasopressors were needed.

■ COMPARATOR USED

Fischer's exact test was used for comparing numeric data. Continuous data from different groups were compared using Mann–Whitney U test or Student's T test.

■ OUTCOMES EVALUATED

Among 91 patients randomized, 45 were assigned to MB and 46 to placebo. Those who received MB had a shorter time to vasopressor discontinuation (69 hours) versus (94 hours); ($p < 0.001$), an additional day vasopressor-free at day 28 ($p = 0.008$), a shorter ICU duration by 1.5 days ($p = 0.039$) and shorter duration of hospitalization by 2.7 days ($p = 0.027$) compared to patients in the control group. Among adverse events, the most common was green-blue discoloration of urine in 42 of 45 (93%) patients in the MB group. Methemoglobin saturation was significantly higher in patients of the MB group [2.9% (IQR 2.2–3.3) vs. 0.5% [IQR 0.4–0.7]; $p < 0.001$].

■ AUTHORS' VIEWPOINT

In this single-center RCT, adjunctive MB administered within 24 hours of septic shock diagnosis reduced the time to vasopressor discontinuation, and importantly, no severe adverse effects were detected. The results might shift the current understanding of MB as a rescue therapy to an adjunctive one at earlier stages of the disease.

■ STRENGTH OF THE STUDY

This is the largest RCT ever published comparing MB with placebo in patients with septic shock. MB also had a good safety profile, wider availability and lower cost than other catecholamine-sparing agents.

■ DRAWBACKS OF THE STUDY

It was a single center study. Most patients were managed in other departments at the moment of septic shock identification before admission to ICU. Hence, the lack of trained healthcare staff and resources might have led to suboptimal resuscitation and poor patients' status, as shown by the relatively higher doses of norepinephrine compared to other larger RCTs of patients with septic shock. The trial also took many years to complete in view of the coronavirus disease (COVID-19) pandemic and the SSC guidelines were updated in the midst. Cytokine or nitrate/nitrite serum levels to confirm the mechanism of the effects of MB were not measured.

REVIEWERS' VIEWPOINT

Methylene blue is definitely worth trying in refractory septic shock. Continuous research of MB as an early adjunctive therapy in patients with septic shock should be done to confirm the potential benefit in larger multicenter randomized clinical trials. This trial adds on to a long list of growing evidences in favor of MB.

IMPACT ON CURRENT PRACTICE AND TAKE HOME MESSAGE

Early use of MB in refractory septic shock would be encouraged in light of the clinical evidence, especially because of a relatively good safety profile, easy availability, and relative inexpensiveness.

ARTICLE 39

Association between Combination Antibiotic Therapy as opposed as Monotherapy and Outcomes of ICU patients with Pseudomonas Aeruginosa Ventilator-associated Pneumonia: An Ancillary Study of the iDIAPASON Trial

Foucrier A, Dessalle T, Tuffet S, Federici L, Dahyot-Fizelier C, Barbier F, et al. Association between combination antibiotic therapy as opposed as monotherapy and outcomes of ICU patients with Pseudomonas aeruginosa ventilator-associated pneumonia: an ancillary study of the iDIAPASON trial.
Crit Care. 2023;27(1):211.

WHAT IS ALREADY KNOWN?

Ventilator-associated pneumonia (VAP) is one of the most common ICU-acquired infections. *Pseudomonas aeruginosa* (*P. aeruginosa*) is one of the most common bacteria causing VAP. The US guidelines[11] suggest combination therapy for patients with PA-VAP (*Pseudomonas aeruginosa* ventilator-associated pneumonia) leading to septic shock or those at high risk of death, whereas the French guidelines suggest monotherapy.[12] The randomized controlled trial iDIAPASON was conducted to evaluate optimal duration of antibiotic treatment in PA-VAP. Non-inferiority of 8-day group compared to the 15-day group was not demonstrated for the primary outcome combining mortality and PA-VAP recurrence occurring during the ICU stay until day 90. This ancillary study investigated a well-defined cohort of prospectively included patients whether the use of monotherapy or combination therapy antibiotic regimen was associated with an increased risk of mortality or PA-VAP recurrence.

STUDY DESIGN

The iDIAPASON trial was a prospective, multicenter, randomized controlled trial which compared a composite endpoint combining mortality and PA-VAP recurrence occurring during the ICU stay until day 90, according to an 8-day or 15-day duration of antibiotic therapy in ICU patients with PA-VAP. The above trial was an ancillary study of the same.

POPULATION STUDIED INCLUDING DEMOGRAPHICS

Adults were included in the study if there was a clinical suspicion of infection and confirmation by a *P. aeruginosa* positive quantitative culture of a respiratory sample. Patients, who were pregnant, immunosuppressed and had extrapulmonary *P. aeruginosa* infection and chronic colonization, were excluded.

■ INTERVENTION STUDIED

Empirical antibiotics were started without waiting for bacterial sample analysis. The choice of antibiotics was left to the discretion of the treating physician based on multiple factors. The primary outcome was the mortality rate at day 90. The secondary outcomes included PA-VAP recurrence rate, invasive mechanical ventilation duration, ICU stay duration, antibiotic exposure duration, number and types of extrapulmonary infections, and acquisition of multidrug-resistant organisms (MDR) pathogens.

■ COMPARATOR USED

The primary outcome of the 2 groups of the iDIAPSON trial were compared using a Chi-square test. Time from appropriate antibiotic therapy to death or cure at day 90 was represented using Kaplan–Meier survival curves and compared between groups using a log-rank test.

■ OUTCOME EVALUATED

A total of 169 patients were included and the median duration of appropriate antibiotic therapy was 14 days. At day 90, 37 patients (21.9%) died. 17 patients had received monotherapy and 20 of them received a combination therapy ($p = 0.180$). Monotherapy and combination therapy were similar for VAP recurrence, the number of extrapulmonary infections, or the acquisition of MDR organisms during the ICU stay. An increase in duration of mechanical ventilation was observed in the combination antibiotic group.

■ AUTHORS' VIEWPOINT

Optimal antibiotic management for the treatment of VAP has always been controversial and only few randomized controlled trials have addressed the issue. The ancillary study showed no difference with respect to 90-day mortality or secondary outcomes in using monotherapy or combination therapy for PA-VAP and interestingly there was not an increase in resistance using monotherapy.

■ STRENGTH OF THE STUDY

It was a prospective multicentric trial and baseline characteristics of both the groups were well matched.

■ DRAWBACKS OF THE STUDY

Only patients who had early onset VAP and did not have MDR risk factors were started on narrow spectrum antibiotics while all other cases were started on combination antibiotics. Also the iDIAPASON protocol had de-escalation of antibiotics as soon as antimicrobial susceptibility testing (AST) of Pseudomonas was obtained as a primary strategy.

■ REVIEWERS' VIEWPOINT

Monotherapy was mostly used in early VAP and also in those without MDR risk factors. In this era of multiple comorbidities and numerous hospitalizations it is difficult to confidently start empirical monotherapy for PA-VAP.

■ IMPACT ON CURRENT PRACTICE AND TAKE HOME MESSAGE

In light of current guidelines favoring combination therapy in PA-VAP and also the limited number of patients in whom monotherapy was used, perhaps we should still continue combination antibiotic therapy in most cases.

ARTICLE 40

Identification of Indications for Albumin Administration in Septic Patients with Liver Cirrhosis

Hu W, Chen H, Ma C, Sun Q, Yang M, Wang H, et al. Identification of indications for albumin administration in septic patients with liver cirrhosis.
Crit Care. 2023;27(1):300.

WHAT IS ALREADY KNOWN?

Liver cirrhosis patients with sepsis have a worse outcome among other subset of patients. Cirrhotic patients with sepsis constitute a distinct population regarding clinical course and prognosis, which is characterized by marked hemodynamic instability, reduced colloid oncotic pressure, and hypoalbuminemia. Recent studies investigating the efficacy of albumin in septic patients with liver cirrhosis focused on the resuscitation stage,[13] neglecting the impact on the prognosis of dynamic albumin administration throughout the entire clinical course of the illness. Also the well-designed ALBIOS trial[14] could not substantiate the advantages of albumin infusion. The study was conducted to identify indications of albumin usage in septic patients with liver cirrhosis.

STUDY DESIGN

A retrospective analysis of the MIMICIV (2.0) database, which contains comprehensive information about patients admitted to ICUs at Beth Israel Deaconess Medical Center between 2008 and 2019. The primary outcome was 28-day mortality and secondary outcomes included ICU-free days at day 28, hospital-free days at day 28, and in-hospital mortality.

POPULATION STUDIED INCLUDING DEMOGRAPHICS

Critically ill adult patients with liver cirrhosis who met the Sepsis 3.0 criteria were included. Patients with an ICU stay <24 hours or >100 days and those who were identified as sepsis 12 hours before or 24 hours after ICU admission were excluded. Furthermore, only first ICU stay of patients was analyzed who were admitted to ICU more than once.

INTERVENTION STUDIED

Daily administration of IV albumin throughout the ICU stay was evaluated. All manners of administering albumin were considered and the infusion time of albumin, solution concentration, and the total amount of albumin administered were recorded from the database.

COMPARATOR USED

The study population was categorized into those treated with albumin (albumin group) and those who did not receive albumin during the entire ICU stay (non-albumin group). Comparisons between groups were made using the X^2 test or Fisher's exact test for categorical variables and Student's t-test or Mann–Whitney U test for continuous variables as was found appropriate.

OUTCOMES EVALUATED

A total of 2,265 septic patients with liver cirrhosis were included in the final analysis. During the 28-day follow-up, 670 patients died (29.6%). Out of this, 1,093 patients (48.3%) received albumin infusion at least once during their ICU stay. Albumin administration was associated with a reduced mortality across the follow-up of 28 days. Albumin administration was particularly associated with lower 28-day mortality in patients with model for end-stage liver disease (MELD) score ≥20 [HR 0·68 (95% CI 0·54–0·84)], septic shock [HR 0·65 (95% CI 0·48–0·89)], and a total bilirubin ≥3.0 mg/dL.

AUTHORS' VIEWPOINT

Dynamic albumin administration provided a significant better survival benefit at 28 days in patients of sepsis with liver cirrhosis, especially in certain sub-cohorts. Serum albumin levels, serum lactate, MAP, and dose of vasopressors used were found to be modifiers of treatment effectiveness and should be considered when deciding to initial albumin infusion.

STRENGTH OF THE STUDY

A large database was taken. Also subgroup analysis was done in detail. The data also confirmed that patients with higher severity of illness would benefit from daily albumin administration.

DRAWBACKS OF THE STUDY

The study was based only on electronic healthcare records of routine clinical practice with frequent missing data and outliers. Also as the data was collected over a long period of time, the findings might be influenced by changes in the guidelines for sepsis and liver cirrhosis that occurred during this period. Another point was whether the benefits observed are primarily attributed to sepsis management, cirrhosis-related complications, or an amalgamation of both and the same was not addressed.

REVIEWERS' VIEWPOINT

The study certainly has a large database and targets a very specific subgroup of septic patients. It emphasizes the use of albumin not just for resuscitation but also for daily administration in certain sub-cohorts. The results are clear and convincing.

IMPACT ON CURRENT PRACTICE AND TAKE HOME MESSAGE

The results further underline the importance of albumin in liver cirrhotic patients and would convince us to use it on a daily basis in patients of sepsis, especially if they have an increased severity of illness or a higher MELD score. However, cost would be an important factor in the Indian setting.

Some interesting trials have hence been put forth the past year. We have seen more evidence coming in for restricting fluids in sepsis and using albumin in septic cirrhotic patients while medications like methylene blue seem to be gaining momentum. Using antibiotic monotherapy for PA-VAP is also an interesting proposal. We hope more evidence comes in favor of the same.

REFERENCES

1. Rivers E, Nguyen B, Havstad S, Ressler J, Muzzin A, Knoblich B, et al. Early goal-directed therapy in the treatment of severe sepsis and septic shock. N Engl J Med. 2001;345(19):1368-77.
2. Angus DC, Barnato AE, Bell D, Bellomo R, Chong CR, Coats TJ, et al. A systematic review and meta-analysis of early goal-directed therapy for septic shock: the ARISE, ProCESS and ProMISe Investigators. Intensive Care Med. 2015;41(9):1549-60.
3. Hansen B. Fluid overload. Front Vet Sci. 2021;8:668688.
4. Meyhoff TS, Hjortrup PB, Wetterslev J, Sivapalan P, Laake JH, Cronhjort M, et al.

Restriction of intravenous fluid in ICU patients with septic shock. N Engl J Med. 2022;386(26):2459-70.
5. Self WH, Semler MW, Bellomo R, Brown SM, deBoisblanc BP, Exline MC, et al. Liberal versus restrictive intravenous fluid therapy for early septic shock: rationale for a randomized trial. Ann Emerg Med. 2018;72(4):457-66.
6. Puntillo F, Giglio M, Pasqualucci A, Brienza N, Paladini A, Varrassi G. Vasopressor-sparing action of methylene blue in severe sepsis and shock: a narrative review. Adv Ther. 2020;37:3692-706.
7. Ibarra-Estrada M, Kattan E, Aguilera-González P, Sandoval-Plascencia L, Rico-Jauregui U, Gómez-Partida CA, et al. Early adjunctive methylene blue in patients with septic shock: a randomized controlled trial. Crit Care. 2023;27(1):110.
8. Stolk RF, van der Pasch E, Naumann F, Schouwstra J, Bressers S, van Herwaarden AE, et al. Norepinephrine dysregulates the immune response and compromises host defense during sepsis. Am J Respir Crit Care Med. 2020;202:830-42.
9. Andresen M, Dougnac A, Díaz O, Hernández G, Castillo L, Bugedo G, et al. Use of methylene blue in patients with refractory septic shock: Impact on hemodynamics and gas exchange. J Crit Care. J Crit Care. 1998;13(4):164-8.
10. Abd-Alhameed AE, Hamed AM, Omran AS. Methylene blue: role in early management of septic shock patients?. Ain-Shams J Anaesthesiol. 2014;7:327-35.
11. Kalil AC, Metersky ML, Klompas M, Muscedere J, Sweeney DA, Palmer LB, et al. Management of adults with hospital-acquired and ventilator-associated pneumonia: 2016 clinical practice guidelines by the infectious diseases society of America and the American thoracic society. Clin Infect Dis. 2016;63(5):e61-111.
12. Leone M, Bouadma L, Bouhemad B, Brissaud O, Dauger S, Gibot S, et al. Hospital-acquired pneumonia in ICU. Anaesth Crit Care Pain Med. 2018;37(1):83-98.
13. Maiwall R, Kumar A, Pasupuleti SSR, Hidam AK, Tevethia H, Kumar G, et al. A randomized-controlled trial comparing 20% albumin to plasmalyte in patients with cirrhosis and sepsis-induced hypotension [ALPS trial]. J Hepatol. 2022;77(3):670-82.
14. Caironi P, Tognoni G, Masson S, Fumagalli R, Pesenti A, Romero M, et al. Albumin replacement in patients with severe sepsis or septic shock. N Engl J Med. 2014;370(15):1412-21.

Section 8

Hematology

Section Editor: Deven Juneja
Associate Editor: Sahil Kataria

ARTICLE 41

Prehospital Tranexamic Acid for Severe Trauma

PATCH-Trauma Investigators and the ANZICS Clinical Trials Group; Gruen RL, Mitra B, Bernard SA, McArthur CJ, Burns B, et al. Prehospital tranexamic acid for severe trauma.
N Engl J Med. 2023;389(2):127-36.

CLINICAL QUESTION OR PROBLEM

In adults at risk for trauma-induced coagulopathy, can early administration of 1 g of tranexamic acid (TXA) followed by an infusion of 1 g over 8 hours improve survival and functional outcomes at 6 months compared to placebo?

WHAT IS ALREADY KNOWN?

Trauma is the primary factor contributing to mortality among young individuals, with a significant proportion of preventable fatalities resulting from bleeding. In a subset of patients (10–25%), trauma-induced coagulopathy further exacerbates bleeding, manifesting as hyperfibrinolysis that can be identified upon admission to the hospital.

Tranexamic acid, an antifibrinolytic, inhibits plasminogen activation competitively and, at far higher concentrations, inhibits plasmin in a non-competitive manner. Multiple clinical trials have evaluated the efficacy of TXA in individuals with traumatic injuries. The CRASH-2 trial, which took place in 2010, provided evidence that administering TXA within 3 hours of injuries can effectively decrease mortality rates in trauma patients with suspected bleeding.[1] A post hoc review of the CRASH-2 trial revealed an unanticipated rise in the probability of death owing to bleeding when TXA was administered after 3 hours of injury. Furthermore, the CRASH-3 trial demonstrated a decrease in mortality rates notably among those with mild-to-moderate traumatic brain injury.[2] However, it is important to note that the patients were not monitored beyond 28 days in both these trials, and no data regarding functional outcomes were provided. Furthermore, majority of study participants were enlisted from nations that had not yet established comprehensive trauma treatment systems at a regional level. The generalizability of these findings may be limited in nations with more advanced trauma systems that have provided quick access to critical care, blood products, surgical procedures, and interventional radiology. Further, the STAAMP and ROC trials included trauma victims from high-income nations.[3,4] Neither trial demonstrated a survival advantage in patients receiving TXA. However, the STAAMP study indicated a benefit for those who received the intervention within 1 hour after the injury. However, administration of TXA is not without its own set of dangers, as seen in the TAMPITI experiment.[5] This research revealed that the dosage of TXA had no impact on real-time coagulation but instead showed a dose-dependent increase in the risk of venous thromboembolism.

STUDY DESIGN

A 7-year double-blinded, placebo-controlled, randomized controlled experiment was conducted between July 2014 and September 2021. The trial involved the participation of 15 emergency medical services (EMS) and 21 hospitals in Australia, New Zealand, and Germany.

The patients underwent screening at the trauma site, and if they satisfied the specified inclusion criteria, randomization was conducted using a smartphone application that determined their group assignment. Patients were randomly assigned 1:1 to receive TXA or placebo using computer-generated numbers based on their initial Glasgow Coma Scale (GCS, <9 or ≥9) and national or state jurisdiction. The acquisition of consent was not immediately obligatory, but it was promptly pursued by the patient or their next of kin, as soon as it was feasible. Blinding was made possible by storing the placebo medication in a tamper-proof foil pack and wrapping it in an identical 10 mL glass vial. The allocation was concealed from patients, doctors, and follow-up evaluators. The study was overseen by a data and safety monitoring committee, which assessed the suitability of continuing the trial at two specific time intervals, throughout the study. The primary outcome was evaluated by a standardized telephone interview.

POPULATION STUDIED INCLUDING DEMOGRAPHICS

Potential study participants included adult patients with severe traumatic injuries who were treated on the spot and then transported to trauma centers.

Inclusion criteria:
- Patients over 18 years with suspected serious traumatic injuries as determined by prehospital professionals (paramedics or physicians).
- High risk of trauma-induced coagulopathy as indicated by a COAST score of three or more **(Table 1)**.

TABLE 1: Coagulopathy of severe trauma (COAST) score.

Variable	Value	Score
Entrapment (e.g., in vehicle)	Yes	1
	No	0
Systolic blood pressure (mm Hg)	>100	0
	<100	1
	<90	2
Temperature (°C)	>35	0
	<35	1
	<32	2
Major chest injury likely to require intervention (e.g., decompression, chest tube)	Yes	1
	No	0
Likely intra-abdominal or pelvic injury	Yes	1
	No	0

- Before hospitalization, the patient should have received the initial dose of TXA or a placebo within 3 hours after the injury.

Exclusion criteria: Patients who were pregnant or residents of an assisted living facility or nursing home.

Subgroups: Age (<50), GCS (<9), initial systolic blood pressure <75 mm Hg, injury type (blunt/penetrating/burn), and delay between injury and first TXA dosage (<1 hour, <2 hours, and <3 hours).

Baseline characteristics: The intervention and control groups had comparable characteristics at the beginning of the study. *Age and gender:* The average age of the participants in the study was around 44 years, with males comprising around 70% of the population studied.

Injury type: Around 92% of the patients experienced blunt trauma.

Baseline GCS score: 34% had a GCS score of <9.

Injury severity score: The median injury severity score was 29.

INTERVENTION STUDIED

Tranexamic acid: One gram of TXA was given as soon as possible, either at the scene of the trauma or en route to the hospital (n = 661), as a slow push over 10 minutes. Subsequently, 1 g of TXA was administered in a solution of 1 L of 0.9% saline over a period of 8 hours.

COMPARATOR USED

Matching placebo: The control group participants were administered a placebo consisting of 0.9% saline, which was delivered as a bolus over a period of 10 minutes followed by an 8-hour infusion of 1 L of 0.9% saline.

Management common to both groups:
- Both patient groups were provided with standard medical treatment during pre-hospital, in-hospital, and post-hospital phases of their illness.
- If a suspected adverse reaction occurred during medication administration, prompt cessation of the drug was warranted. Alternatively, if an exclusion criterion was identified, discontinuation of drug administration was done.
- In case the consent was revoked, administration of any additional medication was halted.
- In case survival proved unattainable, the administration of the medicine was discontinued.
- On admission, coagulation profiles and lactate levels were measured, as well as after 8 and 24 hours.
- Doppler ultrasonography was conducted around the 7th day to check for the presence of any evidence of deep vein thrombosis.

OUTCOME EVALUATED

Tranexamic Acid versus Placebo Comparisons (Table 2)

Primary outcome:
- Survival with a favorable functional outcome at 6 months, based on the Glasgow Outcome Scale-Extended (GOS-E >5)—no significant difference in the primary outcome **(Table 3)**.
  53.7% versus 53.5%; risk ratio, 1.0, 95% CI, 0.90–1.12; $p = 0.95$; ARR, 0.2%; 95% CI, −5.6–6.0.

Secondary outcomes:
- Mortality:
  - At 24 hours—significantly reduced in TXA group
    9.7% (64/657) versus 14.1% (90/640) – (RR: 0.69; 95% CI, 0.51–0.94)
  - At 28 days—significantly reduced in TXA group

Hematology

TABLE 2: Study outcomes.

Outcome	Tranexamic acid (n = 657)	Placebo (n = 643)	Risk ratio/Hazard ratio with 95% CI
Primary outcome			
Survival with favorable outcome	307/572 (53.7%)	299/559 (53.5%)	1.00 (0.90–1.12)
Secondary outcomes			
24-hour mortality	64/657 (9.7%)	90/640 (14.1%)	0.69 (0.51–0.94)
28-day mortality	113/653 (17.3%)	139/637 (21.8%)	0.79 (0.63–0.99)
6-month mortality	123/648 (19.0%)	144/629 (22.9%)	0.83 (0.67–1.03)
Mortality attributable to bleeding	36/123 deaths (29.3%)	52/244 deaths (36.1%)	
Vascular occlusive events	155/657 (23.6%)	126/641 (19.7%)	1.2 (0.97–1.48)

TABLE 3: The Glasgow Outcome Scale-Extended (GOS-E).

Clinical state	Name	Score
	Death	1
Lack of awareness of self and environment	Persistent vegetative state	2
Needs full assistance in performing activities of daily living	Lower severe disability	3
Needs partial assistance in performing activities of daily living	Upper severe disability	4
Independent, but unable to work/schooling or all previous social activities	Lower moderate disability	5
Reduced work capacity; resumes <50% of the pre-injury level of social and leisure activities	Upper moderate disability	6
Minor problems that affect daily life; resumes >50% of the pre-injury level of social and leisure activities	Lower good recovery	7
Full recovery or minor symptoms that do not affect daily life	Upper good recovery	8

A score of 5 or higher was considered a favorable functional outcome.

- 17.3% (113/653) versus 21.8% (139/637) (RR: 0.79; 95% CI, 0.63–0.99).
- At 6 months—no significant difference 19% (123/648) versus 22.9% (144/629) (RR: 0.83; 95% CI, 0.67–1.03).
- Bleeding as a cause of death within 6 months after injury.
- 29.3% versus 36.1% (HR 0.66; 95% CI 0.43–1.01).
- Vascular occlusion—no significant difference:
  - All: 23.6% versus 19.7% (RR: 1.20; 95% CI, 0.97–1.48)

Subgroup analysis:
- There was no statistically significant difference observed among subgroups when considering variables such as age, time to first dose of TXA, systolic blood pressure, mechanism of injury, GCS, or injury severity score.

AUTHORS' VIEWPOINT

In advanced trauma systems, prehospital administration of TXA followed by an 8-hour infusion did not improve outcomes for adults with major trauma and suspected trauma-induced coagulopathy. However, TXA administration improved early survival rates at 24-hour and 28-day marks, consistent with the outcomes observed in the CRASH-2 study.

■ STRENGTH OF THE STUDY

- The study was well implemented with blinding procedures, ensuring a minimum probability of bias.
- The utilization of intention-to-treat and per-protocol analyses enhanced the validity of the study.
- The present study's results have enhanced relevance and applicability to complex trauma situations compared to prior investigations, such as the CRASH-2 trial.
- The study used an objective grading system to identify severe trauma patients who might benefit from TXA.
- The between-group baseline balance is satisfactory.
- In contrast to previous clinical trials, the primary outcome emphasizes functional outcomes, not mortality.

■ DRAWBACKS OF THE STUDY

- A total of 13% of the patients included in the study were found to have missing primary outcome data, predominantly due to a loss of follow-up. Although, in order to address this issue, the researchers chose to augment the sample size from 1,184 to 1,316.
- There were variations in dosing across patients, whereby certain individuals did not get the intended amounts of TXA. In contrast, others were administered open-label TXA, which deviated from the established study protocol.
- Using the dosage strategy of TXA in the present study from CRASH-2/CRASH-3 trials does not completely rule out the possibility of harm or benefit from using different dosing strategies.
- When administered intravenously, TXA's half-life is approximately 2 hours. However, no information is available regarding the effect of transit time or the interval between the initial bolus and subsequent infusion on its pharmacokinetics. Consequently, it remains unclear if a delay in the infusion of TXA could have influenced the patient outcomes.
- The study may lack sufficient statistical power to detect clinically significant variations in treatment response within subgroups such as penetrating trauma and other subgroups with small sample sizes.

■ REVIEWERS' VIEWPOINT

The study's findings are consistent with those of the CRASH-2 trial, which suggests that the use of TXA in prehospital settings lowers the risk of early death secondary to bleeding in patients with severe injuries. Moreover, there is no significant rise in the vascular-occlusive events associated with the administration of TXA. Nevertheless, it is crucial to acknowledge that the TXA group demonstrated a greater percentage of individuals who survived but still encountered adverse neurological outcomes. This unquestionably has a significant impact on patients' overall health and welfare while also carrying substantial implications for their families and society in terms of the financial burden associated with providing care for individuals with significant dependencies.

■ IMPACT ON CURRENT PRACTICE AND TAKE HOME MESSAGE

In our perspective, it is recommended to uphold the utilization of prehospital TXA in individuals with substantial trauma who possess a heightened susceptibility to the development of coagulopathy. Ultimately, the early use of TXA increases the number of early survivors who might benefit from other interventions to enhance functional outcomes. The potential for future improvements in the functionality suggests that incorporating extended-term results (12 months) might contribute to full comprehension and evaluation of this study and augment the current findings.

ARTICLE 42

Efficacy and Safety of Early Administration of 4-Factor Prothrombin Complex Concentrate in Patients with Trauma at Risk of Massive Transfusion: The PROCOAG Randomized Clinical Trial

Bouzat P, Charbit J, Abback PS, Huet-Garrigue D, Delhaye N, Leone M, et al. Efficacy and Safety of Early Administration of 4-Factor Prothrombin Complex Concentrate in Patients with Trauma at Risk of Massive Transfusion: The PROCOAG Randomized Clinical Trial.
JAMA. 2023;329(16):1367-75.

■ CLINICAL QUESTION OR PROBLEM

Can administration of 4-factor prothrombin complex concentrate (4F-PCC) to trauma patients at high risk of requiring a massive transfusion result in reduced blood product consumption during the initial 24-hour period?

■ WHAT IS ALREADY KNOWN?

The leading factor in fatalities from severe traumatic injuries is hemorrhage. Implementing several interventions, such as early hemorrhage control, administration of TXA within 3 hours of an injury, minimizing the use of crystalloid fluids, and applying a balanced ratio blood product transfusion, has demonstrated significant enhancements in the outcomes of trauma patients.[6] Nevertheless, the mortality rate remains elevated due to trauma-induced coagulopathy, distinguished by a diminished fibrinogen concentration and frequently augmented fibrinolytic activity. About 33% of individuals at the hospital following severe trauma exhibit a coagulopathic condition. The timely identification and intervention of coagulopathy in individuals who have experienced trauma play a pivotal role in enhancing overall outcomes.

Four-factor prothrombin complex concentrate is made up of proteins S and C and factors II, VII, IX, and X. It is often used to stop severe bleeding caused by anticoagulants like warfarin and direct oral anticoagulants. Although this can potentially enhance thrombin generation and decrease the need for blood products, there is still some concern regarding an elevated risk of thromboembolic events. Based on limited observational data, the efficacy of 4F-PCC has been established with evidence of reduced hematoma formation in patients with traumatic head injuries.[7] Recent meta-analyses comparing fresh frozen plasma (FFP) alone versus FFP plus PCC in the treatment of trauma-induced coagulopathy found that adding PCC significantly reduced the need for packed red blood cell and FFP transfusions, and lowered mortality, without any increase in thromboembolic side effects. However, it is essential to note that this meta-analysis was constrained by its inclusion of only three retrospective studies, including 840 individuals.[8] Further research is required to validate the meta-analysis findings, establish the efficacy of using FFP plus PCC in a more extensive and diverse patient population, and explore the most effective dosage and time for administering PCC to maximize its benefits and minimize potential risks.

STUDY DESIGN

This was a superiority-randomized, placebo-controlled, intention-to-treat clinical investigation conducted at 12 French level 1 trauma sites from December 2017 to August 2021. The patients were allocated randomly into groups of 2–6, with stratification by center using a randomization procedure. The randomization occurred within the 1st hour of the patient's arrival at the trauma bay. The clinician investigator, patient care team, data management staff, and statistical analysts were blinded to the treatment, whereas the site and the supporting pharmacy were not.

POPULATION STUDIED INCLUDING DEMOGRAPHICS

Consecutive patients with trauma were potential candidates for enrolment in the study.

Inclusion criteria:
- Patients aged 18 years or older who have sustained a traumatic injury are transported directly from the injury site to a participating trauma center with the highest level of trauma activation.
- Patients who were considered at risk for massive transfusions which was defined as:
  - At least one unit of packed red blood cell transfusion (pRBC) transfused before hospitalization or within the 1st hour of admission or
  - An assessment of blood consumption score **(Table 4)** of at least two or more or
  - The attending physician determines that the patient is at risk for massive transfusion by clinical assessment, where *massive transfusion* was defined as >3 pRBC within 1 hour of admission or >10 pRBC within the first 24 hours.

Exclusion criteria:
- Pre-randomization traumatic cardiac arrest
- Critically injured patients anticipated to die within an hour of admission
- Secondary hospitalization
- Treatment with anticoagulants prior to injury
- Obstetric patients
- Known hypersensitivity to 4F-PCC and any analogues of it

TABLE 4: Assessment of blood consumption score.

Component	Score
Penetrating mechanism of injury	1
Systolic pressure <90 mm Hg in emergency department	1
Heart rate >120/minute in emergency department	1
Positive focused assessment with sonography for trauma	1

Scores ≥2 were likely to require massive transfusion, with sensitivity and specificity ranging from 75% to 90% and 67% to 88%, respectively.

- Individuals needing a legal guardian
- Any participation in a different trial during the last 30 days
- Pre-injury terminal illness
- Patients who did not have health insurance (according to French law).

Baseline characteristics:
Both groups had comparable characteristics such as age, gender distribution, prehospital and admission vital signs, and baseline coagulation profiles.
- *Median age:* 39 years
- *Demographics:* Male predominance, around 71%
- *Mode of injury:* 82% blunt trauma, 18% penetrating trauma.

INTERVENTION STUDIED

Four-factor prothrombin complex concentrate: At a dosage of 25 IU of factor ix per kilogram (1 mL/kg).

COMPARATOR USED

Matching placebo: 0.9% saline solution at the dosage of 1 mL/kg.

Management common to both groups
Within 1 hour of arrival, patients were randomized to intervention ($n = 160$) and control group ($n = 160$). Both PCC and placebo were given in a radiopaque syringe at the rate of 120 mL/hour, as soon as possible after admission.

Trauma resuscitation care was provided for all patients, which included the following:
- Limiting crystalloid fluid administration
- Initiating transfusions early with a ratio of 1:1–2:1 (PRBCs/FFP)
- Conforming to the CRASH-2 trial, intravenous TXA was given 3 hours after injury with a 1 g loading dose and 1 g over 8 hours.
- The use of platelet transfusions to maintain platelet counts above $50 \times 10^9/L$
- Administration of concentrated fibrinogen in cases where either viscoelastic criteria or a fibrinogen level of <1.5 g/L was present, indicating a functional deficiency.
- Controlling hemorrhage as soon as possible.
- The occurrence of thromboembolic events, whether arterial or venous, was documented up until day 28. Only passive monitoring methods (ultrasonography and/or contrast-enhanced computed tomography scan) were utilized to validate each clinical suspicion of a thromboembolic event.

OUTCOMES EVALUATED

Four-Factor Prothrombin Complex Concentrate Versus Placebo Comparisons (Table 5)

Primary outcome:
- Total quantity of all blood product units (pRBC, FFP, and platelets) used during the first 24 hours following arrival in the trauma bay.
  - 12 units versus 11 units (difference 0.2%, 95% CI: –2.99–3.33), $p = 0.72$

Secondary outcomes:
- The consumption of individual units of blood products within the initial 24-hour period.
  - Median pRBC utilization
    6 units versus 6 units (difference –0.3%, 95% CI: –1.8–1.3), $p = 0.93$
  - Median FFP utilization
    4 units versus 4 units (difference 0.1%, 95% CI: –1.3–1.5), $p = 0.56$
  - Platelet concentrate utilization

TABLE 5: Study outcomes.

Outcome	4F-PCC (n = 164)	Placebo (n = 160)	Absolute difference (95% CI), %	P value
Primary outcome				
Total blood product consumption, median (IQR)	12 (5–19)	11 (6–9)	0.2 (−2.99–3.33)	0.72
Secondary outcomes				
Red blood cell consumption, median (IQR)	6 (3.5–10)	6 (4–10)	−0.3 (−1.8–1.3)	0.93
Fresh frozen plasma consumption, median (IQR)	4 (1–8)	4 (2–8)	0.1 (−1.3–1.5)	0.56
Platelet concentrate consumption, median (IQR)	1 (0–1)	1 (0–1)	0.0 (−0.3–0.3)	0.83
Time to PTr <1.5, median (IQR) [No.], minute	0 (0–60) [154]	0 (0–60) [145]	−8.5 (−48.9–32.0)	0.86
Mortality at 24 hours	18 (11)	20 (13)	−2 (−9–5)	0.67
Mortality at 28 days	26 (17)	30 (21)	−3 (−12–5)	0.48
Time to achieve anatomic hemostasis, median (IQR) [No.], minute	300 (203–423) [131]	288 (210–404) [128]	22 (−73.3–73.8)	0.96
Hospital-free days through day 28, median (IQR)	6.5 (0–22.5)	7 (0–22)	−0.15 (−1.65–1.35)	0.78
Ventilator-free days through day 28, median (IQR)	4 (0.5–7)	4 (0–8)	0.33 (−1.0–1.6)	0.51
ICU-free days through day 28, median (IQR)	6.5 (0–22.5)	7 (0–22)	1.22 (−5.93–8.37)	0.78
Glasgow Outcome Scale-Extended score, median (IQR) [No.]	3 (3–4) [36]	3 (3–5) [27]	−0.5 (−1.91–0.91)	0.45

- 1 unit versus 1 unit (difference 0, 95% CI: −0.3–0.3), $p = 0.83$
- The time required for the prothrombin time (PT) to be <1.5 (median (IQR, minutes)
  - 0 (0–60) versus 0 (0–60) (difference −8.5%, CI: (−48.9–32.0), $p = 0.86$
- Time required to control bleeding (median (IQR, minutes) 300 (203–423) versus 288 (210–404) (difference 22%, CI:−73.3–73.8), $p = 0.96$
- Mortality rates at 24 hours and 28 days.
  - Mortality at 24 hours 11% versus 13% (difference −2%, 95% CI:−9–5), $p = 0.67$
  - Mortality at 48 hours 17% versus 21% (difference −3%, 95% CI: −12–5), $p = 0.48$
- Hospital, ventilator, and intensive care unit-free days till day 28, median (IQR).
  - Hospital-free days (0–22.5) versus 7 (0–22) (difference −0.15%, CI: −1.65–1.35), $p = 0.78$
  - Ventilator-free days 4 (0.5–7) versus 4 (0–8) (difference 0.33%, CI: −1.0–1.6), $p = 0.51$
  - Intensive care unit free days (0–22.5) versus 7 (0–22) (difference 1.22%, CI: −5.93–8.37), $p = 0.78$

- The 28-day hospitalization status:
  - Remained hospitalized
    33% versus 35% (difference 0%, CI: −10–10)
  - Intensive care unit
    28% versus 23% (difference 5%, CI: −5–16)
  - Home
    23% versus 23% (difference −3%, CI: −12–6)
  - Dead
    17% versus 21% (difference −3%, CI: −12–5)
  - Rehabilitation
    14% versus 18% (difference −2%, CI: −14–9)
  - Other
    2% versus 1% (difference 1%, CI: −2–3)
  - Unknown
    3% versus 4%
- Glasgow Outcome Scale-Extended score in computed tomography-demonstrated brain injury patients (Abbreviated Injury Scale score >2).
  - 3(3–4) versus 3(3–5), (difference −0.5%, CI: −1.91–0.91), $p = 0.45$

Safety outcome:
Thromboembolic events
- Patients in the 4F-PCC group had a statistically significant higher thromboembolic event from those in the placebo group [56 (35%) vs. 37 (24%); absolute difference 11% (95% CI, 1%–21%); relative risk 1.48 (CI, 1.04–2.10); $p = .03$].
- A post hoc study found that 4F-PCC patients with PT >1.2 had more thromboembolic events.

AUTHORS' VIEWPOINT

There was not a substantial reduction in 24-hour blood product consumption after administration of 4F-PCC among patients with trauma who were at risk of massive transfusion; however, thromboembolic events were more likely. This does not support the systematic use of 4F-PCC in massive transfusion-risk patients.

STRENGTH OF THE STUDY

- A randomized, placebo-controlled superiority trial:
  - Patients, investigators, and data analysts were unaware of the treatment assignment.
  - The nurse who prepared 4F-PCC and placebo in a protected space was not involved in patient resuscitation or care.
  - The administration of 4F-PCC and placebo was carried out using opaque syringes to prevent unblinding.
- After the trial began, there were no significant alterations to the protocol or results.
- Both groups were fairly similar in prehospital interventions, admission vital signs, laboratory parameters, and surgical/radiologic hemorrhage control.
- To prevent survivor bias for the primary outcome, the authors confirmed that the two groups spent the same amount of time in the study (up to 24 hours) before data analysis.
- Pragmatic inclusion criteria, recruited patients with severe bleeding who may benefit most from 4F-PCC, improving generalizability, and external applicability.

DRAWBACKS OF THE STUDY

- While the findings of this multicenter study conducted within a specific country are valuable, it is important to acknowledge that the generalizability of these results may be limited due to variations in healthcare systems across different countries.
- The primary outcome, namely using blood products within 24 hours, does not align with patient-centered outcomes.

- Only passive surveillance was implemented to detect thromboembolic events. This could have resulted in a lower-than-accurate reporting of thromboembolic events.
- In the placebo group, FFP was delayed despite randomization by 20 minutes, which may have affected the outcomes.
- Commercially available PCC may have different clotting factor ratios, affecting external validity.
- In the placebo group, more patients received TXA before hospital arrival (86% vs. 76%) and a higher median total dose of fibrinogen concentrate, which may have affected 4F-PCC's efficacy.
- The trial involved administering a combination of 4F-PCC and FFP, rather than 4F-PCC alone, without first confirming the presence of coagulopathy. This situation potentially exposed patients without coagulopathy to the hazard of excessive coagulation factor dosage.

REVIEWERS' VIEWPOINT

The randomized controlled trial conducted did not provide evidence to support the empirical administration of 4F-PCC in patients at risk of requiring massive transfusions. Furthermore, the administration of 4F-PCC was associated with a significantly increased incidence of thromboembolic events compared to placebo. Further randomized controlled trials are necessary to investigate the potential efficacy and safety of administering 4F-PCC as a standalone treatment in a specific subgroup of patients presenting with traumatic coagulopathy upon admission. Additionally, it may be necessary to modify the dosage of 4F-PCC in order to mitigate the potential occurrence of thromboembolic events, while simultaneously managing coagulopathy in patients who are at high risk of necessitating massive blood transfusions.

IMPACT ON CURRENT PRACTICE AND TAKE HOME MESSAGE

Four-factor prothrombin complex concentrate should not be used empirically in trauma patients. The utilization of fixed-ratio blood product transfusion and prompt hemorrhage control continues to be widely regarded as the optimal approach in caring for trauma patients with severe bleeding.

ARTICLE 43

Platelet Transfusion before CVC Placement in Patients with Thrombocytopenia

van Baarle FLF, van de Weerdt EK, van der Velden WJFM, Ruiterkamp RA, Tuinman PR, Ypma PF, et al. Platelet transfusion before CVC placement in patients with thrombocytopenia.
N Engl J Med. 2023;388(21):1956-65.

CLINICAL QUESTION OR PROBLEM

In patients with thrombocytopenia (10,000–50,000/mm^3) undergoing ultrasound-guided central venous catheter (CVC) placement, is no platelet transfusion non-inferior to prophylactic platelet transfusion in terms of catheter-related bleeding risk?

Hematology

WHAT IS ALREADY KNOWN?

The placement of a CVC is a frequently performed medical intervention in an intensive care unit (ICU) that enables monitoring and treatment of patients. The occurrence of bleeding complications during the placement of CVCs is infrequent, yet it poses a potentially significant risk in certain individuals. An elevated risk of bleeding is observed in patients with thrombocytopenia. The current approach involves increasing the platelet count beyond a predetermined threshold through platelet transfusions to mitigate the risk of substantial bleeding resulting from CVC insertion.[9,10] However, this practice varies widely across different ICUs. There is a lack of robust and reliable evidence to determine the most effective threshold for platelet transfusion, ensuring safe placement of CVC. Clinicians encounter a state of ambiguity regarding determining the optimal threshold for platelet count and the necessity of platelet transfusion. It is crucial to acknowledge that blood transfusions can have adverse consequences, including circulatory overload, acute lung injury, and alloimmunization. Furthermore, it is imperative to consider the limited availability and high cost associated with blood transfusions, specifically due to the relatively short shelf-life of platelet concentrates (5 days) compared to other blood products.

Prior research conducted retrospectively has demonstrated that ultrasound guidance for CVC insertion is deemed a safe practice, even when the platelet count is <20,000/mm^3. There is a lack of comprehensive, randomized research that has conclusively demonstrated the non-inferiority of omitting prophylactic platelet transfusions in thrombocytopenic patients undergoing CVC placement. As a result, individuals may be exposed to the potential risks linked to platelet transfusion without any apparent clinical benefits. The current scrutiny surrounding routine prophylactic transfusions has raised doubts about their necessity despite widespread adoption.

STUDY DESIGN

This study was an open-label, randomized, controlled, non-inferiority trial carried out in 10 hospitals across the Netherlands between February 2016 and March 2022. The non-inferiority margin was established as a 2.5% rise in the absolute risk of Grade 2–4 bleeding **(Table 6)**. The statistical power to detect the non-inferiority of the non-transfusion strategy was 80%, with a significance level (alpha) of 0.05. Before ultrasound-guided CVC placement, thrombocytopenic (10,000–50,000 per cubic milimeter) patients were randomized 1:1 to receive or withhold one unit of platelet concentrate for prophylactic platelet transfusion. The participants were stratified based on the trial center and the type of catheter used, explicitly distinguishing between large-bore dialysis catheters and regular CVCs. The patients were unblinded, while the operators, whenever feasible, were kept unaware of the trial assignment. The study encompassed various types of CVCs, including tunneled catheters, and incorporated a range of placement sites. Obtaining informed consent prior to randomization was preferred. However, deferred consent was permitted in emergencies. The bleeding and any treatments were noted immediately following CVC insertion, 1 and 24 hours later.

POPULATION STUDIED INCLUDING DEMOGRAPHICS

A total of 411 CVCs were initially randomized, but only 393 CVC placements (involving 358

Hematology

TABLE 6: Central venous catheter-related bleeding.

Bleeding grade	Definition
Grade 0	No bleeding
Grade 1	Oozing, hematoma, or bleeding requiring <20 minutes of physical compression to cease
Grade 2	Bleeding that necessitates minimal interventions to achieve hemostasis, such as prolonged manual compression lasting >20 minutes
Grade 3	Bleeding that necessitates radiologic or elective surgical intervention, or the administration of red-cell transfusion, in the absence of hemodynamic instability
Grade 4	Bleeding that is accompanied by significant hemodynamic instability, characterized by hypotension (defined as a reduction of >50 mm Hg or 50% in either systolic or diastolic blood pressure), together with tachycardia (an increase in heart rate of >20% for a duration of 20 minutes), and leading to an increased need for red-cell transfusion or fatal bleeding

patients) were ultimately included in the intention-to-treat analysis.

Inclusion criteria:
- Patients requiring CVC receiving treatment in the hematology ward or ICU and having severe thrombocytopenia (platelet count 10,000–50,000/mm^3) within the previous 24 hours.
- Central venous catheter to be in place for at least 24 hours, after the procedure.

Exclusion criteria:
- Patients already on therapeutic anticoagulants
- Congenital or acquired coagulation factor deficiency
- International Normalized Ratio (INR) >1.5 (originally, the upper limit was changed to 3 as a result of new evidence)
- Prior inclusion in the study within the previous 24 hours (the authors permitted multiple inclusions of patients who had already been enrolled in the study, provided each procedure was carried out 24 hours apart).

Baseline characteristics:
Patient traits were well-balanced when comparing transfusion (n = 188) and no transfusion (n = 185) groups.
- Age: 58 versus 59 years
- Female: 34 versus 38%
- Median platelet count: 30,000 per cubic milimeter
- Median INR values: 1.1
- The median activated partial thromboplastin time values were 29 and 31, respectively.
- Prior platelet transfusion <6 hours before randomization: 9 versus 10%.
- Location:
  - Hematology ward 57.4 versus 56.2%
  - ICU: 42.6% versus 43.8%
- Catheter type:
  - CVC: 82.4% versus 83.8%
  - Dialysis: 17.6% versus 16.2%
- Catheter Site:
  - Internal jugular 49.5 versus 50.3%
  - Subclavian: 37.8% versus 37.8%
  - Femoral: 12.8% versus 11.9%

■ INTERVENTION STUDIED

Prophylactic transfusion of one unit platelet concentrates before the procedure.

■ COMPARATOR USED

No transfusion.

Management common to both groups:
- The utilization of ultrasound guidance for CVC insertion.

Hematology

- The operator was required to have conducted a minimum of 50 CVC placements.
- Whenever feasible, catheters were inserted around 1 hour following the process of randomization.
- Otherwise, CVCs were inserted in line with regional clinical convention.

■ OUTCOME EVALUATED

Comparing prophylactic platelet concentrate transfusion versus no transfusion (Table 7)

Primary outcome:
- Grade 2–4 catheter-related bleeding:
  - The rate of transfusion was found to be 4.8% in the transfusion group, while it was 11.9% in the group that did not get transfusion.
- An absolute risk reduction of 7.1% (90% CI: 1.3–17.8%) and a relative risk of 2.45 (90% CI: 1.27–4.70).

Selected secondary outcomes:
- The transfusion group exhibited a significant difference in platelet count compared to the non-transfusion group in:
  - Platelet count at 1 hour and 24 hours after CVC placement: 54,000 versus 26,000 after 1 hour; 36,000 versus 26,000 after 24 hours
  - Median ICU LOS: 9 versus 7 days
- No significant difference in:
  - The risk of grade 3–4 catheter-related bleeding (2.1% vs. 4.9%)
  - Hematoma occurrence (12.2% vs. 18.9%)

TABLE 7: Study outcomes.

Outcome	Tranexamic acid (n = 657)	Placebo (n = 643)	(90% or 95% CI)
Primary outcome			
Grade 2–4 catheter-related bleeding	9/188 (4.8)	22/185 (11.9)	2.45 (1.27–4.70)
Secondary outcomes			
Catheter-related bleeding			
Grade 3–4	4/188 (2.1)	9/185 (4.9)	2.43 (0.75–7.93)
Grade 1	88/188 (46.8)	106/185 (57.3)	1.22 (0.91–1.61)
Hematoma	23/188 (12.2%)	35/185 (18.9%)	1.62 (0.94–1.86)
Rate of platelet transfusion in ≤24 hours	0.48 ± 0.76	0.49 ± 0.75	1.02 (0.76–1.37)
Median platelet count after CVC placement (IQR) — per mm^3			
After 1 hour	54,000 (42,000–66,000)	26,000 (18,000–37,000)	-26.8 (−31.4 to −22.3)
After 24 hours	36,000 (27,000–49,000)	26,000 (18,000–40,000)	−9.5 (−13.9 to −5.1)
Median length of stay (IQR)—days			
In ICU	9 (3–17)	24 (9–33)	0.84 (0.76–0.91)
In hospital	24 (13–34)	24 (9–33)	0.94 (0.90–0.98)
Death			
In ICU	38/67 (56.7)	43/83 (51.8)	0.92 (0.59–1.42)
In hospital	50/177 (28.2)	57/180 (31.70)	0.99 (0.84–1.16)

- Rate of red-cell transfusion in ≤24 hour (0.48 vs. 0.49)
- Allergic transfusion reaction (1% vs. 0.5%)
- ICU mortality (57% vs. 52%)
- Hospital mortality (28% vs. 32%).

Subgroup and other outcomes:
- Subgroup analysis favored transfusion if patient had:
  - Non-tunneled catheter
  - Subclavian vein
  - Hematology ward
- ICU patients had similar bleeding outcomes regardless of transfusion (4% vs. 5%)
- Non-transfusion group received more platelet transfusions in the 24 hours after CVC placement
- Pre-CVC platelet count was used to determine the rate of platelet transfusion in the 24 hours following CVC placement. The non-transfusion group received more platelet transfusions during this time.
  - Platelet count 10–19: 0.19 versus 0.67
  - Platelet count 20–29: 0.12 versus 0.58
  - Platelet count 30–39: 0.11 versus 0.35
  - Platelet count 40–50: 0.15 versus 0.16
- The overall costs associated with transfusion and bleeding events were found to be significantly higher in the transfusion group, with a total cost difference of $410 (95% CI: 285–545).

■ AUTHORS' VIEWPOINT

Withholding prophylactic platelet transfusion before CVC placement in patients with a platelet count of 10,000–50,000 per cubic milimeter did not meet the predefined margin for non-inferiority and led to more CVC-related bleeding than prophylactic platelet transfusion in patients with severe thrombocytopenia.

Patients who were admitted to the hematology wards and were undergoing treatment with tunneled catheters, along with those exhibiting a platelet count ranging from 10,000 to 20,000 per cubic milimeter, had the highest occurrence of bleeding. Therefore, it is strongly recommended that these patients be given careful consideration for preventive transfusions. The subgroup analysis indicated a tendency toward reduced bleeding in individuals who received prophylactic transfusions at the subclavian (2.8% vs. 18.6%) and femoral sites (0% vs. 9.1%), although this trend did not reach statistical significance.

■ STRENGTH OF THE STUDY

- A multicenter, randomized controlled trial.
- Statistical analyses and trial procedure were released before-hand.
- A non-inferiority trial design with a pertinent primary endpoint for safety.
- Intent-to-treat analysis.
- The utilization of broad inclusion criteria is indicative of a widely adopted approach.
- Few protocol violations and no follow-up loss
- Cost-analysis.
- Pragmatic approach and featured various CVC insertions, including locations, and catheter type.
- Background comorbidities and acute physiology are comparable to general ICU patients.

■ DRAWBACKS OF THE STUDY

- The inclusion of only one country in the study may restrict the generalizability of the findings to lower-income countries.
- Operators were not entirely blinded, which could provide a Hawthorne effect

when comparing these bleeding rates to routine practice, given that they were aware that this trial was looking at rates of bleeding issues.
- One unit of platelets may not be enough for certain people, especially those with lower platelet counts (10,000–20,000 per cubic milimeter), making extrapolation of above results difficult.
- The incidence of bleeding events varies between patients in an ICU and those admitted to a hematological ward. The findings of this study indicate that the hematology subgroup had a greater susceptibility to bleeding compared to ICU, potentially serving as a confounding variable.
- The primary outcome data were unavailable for 7% of the population.
- This trial showed a significantly higher bleeding rate than earlier studies. However, this may be owing to this RCT's prospective and organized bleeding evaluation, unlike earlier research, which was retrospective.

REVIEWERS' VIEWPOINT

In thrombocytopenic patients undergoing ultrasound-guided CVC placement, no prophylactic platelet transfusions to reduce bleeding risk have been proven superior to prophylactic transfusions. Nevertheless, it is imperative to contemplate a more individualized strategy wherein administering prophylactic platelets must be given significant consideration to patients exhibiting a platelet count of <30,000 per cubic milimeter, individuals admitted to hematological wards, and those undergoing placement of tunneled catheters. On the other hand, refraining from administering prophylactic platelets to ICU patients may be justifiable, given the observed trends of reduced bleeding risk and enhanced surveillance for bleeding events. Subsequent trials ought to conduct further investigations to ascertain the potential advantages of administering multiple units of platelets to individuals with a platelet count <20,000 per cubic milimeter, as their susceptibility to bleeding remains elevated after the administration of a single unit of platelets, as per the present study.

IMPACT ON CURRENT PRACTICE AND TAKE HOME MESSAGE

The results of this study highlight the significance of maintaining sufficient platelet counts to prevent bleeding associated with CVC insertion. In accordance with the findings of the study, it may be recommended to administer a prophylactic platelet transfusion to individuals presenting with thrombocytopenia and platelet counts <50,000/mm^3. Furthermore, it is important to consider the differences in the study population. Patients with hematologic malignancies who require long-term platelet transfusions are distinct from ICU patients who experience temporary decrease in platelet counts and receive more intensive monitoring. The former group is likely to derive greater benefit from prophylactic platelet transfusion prior to CVC placement compared to the latter group. Nonetheless, given their high transfusion rate, hematologic patients are more likely to experience transfusion-related side effects. The risk/benefit ratio for an intervention, in this example a platelet transfusion, is best evaluated at the patient level, as is the case with many medical situations.

REFERENCES

1. Roberts I, Shakur H, Coats T, Hunt B, Balogun E, Barnetson L, et al. The CRASH-2 trial: a randomised controlled trial and economic evaluation of the effects of tranexamic

acid on death, vascular occlusive events and transfusion requirement in bleeding trauma patients. Health Technol Assess. 2013;17(10):1-79.
2. CRASH-3 trial collaborators. Effects of tranexamic acid on death, disability, vascular occlusive events and other morbidities in patients with acute traumatic brain injury (CRASH-3): a randomised, placebo-controlled trial. Lancet. 2019;394(10210):1713-23.
3. Guyette FX, Brown JB, Zenati MS, Early-Young BJ, Adams PW, Eastridge BJ, et al. Tranexamic acid during prehospital transport in patients at risk for hemorrhage after injury: a double-blind, placebo-controlled, randomized clinical trial. JAMA Surg. 2021;156(1):11-20.
4. Rowell SE, Meier EN, McKnight B, Kannas D, May S, Sheehan K, et al. Effect of out-of-hospital tranexamic acid vs placebo on 6-month functional neurologic outcomes in patients with moderate or severe traumatic brain injury [published correction appears in JAMA. 2020 Oct 27;324(16):1683]. JAMA. 2020;324(10):961-74.
5. Spinella PC, Thomas KA, Turnbull IR, Fuchs A, Bochicchio K, Schuerer D, et al. The immunologic effect of early intravenous two and four gram bolus dosing of tranexamic acid compared to placebo in patients with severe traumatic bleeding (TAMPITI): a randomized, double-blind, placebo-controlled, single-center trial. Front Immunol. 2020;11:2085.
6. Cole E, Weaver A, Gall L, West A, Nevin D, Tallach R, et al. A decade of damage control resuscitation: new transfusion practice, new survivors, new directions. Ann Surg. 2021;273(6):1215-20.
7. Zeeshan M, Hamidi M, Feinstein AJ, Gries L, Jehan F, Sakran J, et al. Four-factor prothrombin complex concentrate is associated with improved survival in trauma-related hemorrhage: A nationwide propensity-matched analysis. J Trauma Acute Care Surg. 2019;87(2):274-81.
8. Kao TW, Lee YC, Chang HT. Prothrombin complex concentrate for trauma induced coagulopathy: a systematic review and meta-analysis. J Acute Med. 2021;11(3):81-9.
9. Estcourt LJ, Birchall J, Allard S, Bassey SJ, Hersey P, Kerr JP, et al. Guidelines for the use of platelet transfusions. Br J Haematol. 2017;176(3):365-94. Erratum in: Br J Haematol. 2017 Apr;177(1):157.
10. Kaufman RM, Djulbegovic B, Gernsheimer T, Kleinman S, Tinmouth AT, Capocelli KE, et al. Platelet transfusion: a clinical practice guideline from the AABB. Ann Intern Med. 2015;162(3):205-13.

Section 9

Sonography/Imaging

Section Editor: Shrikanth Srinivasan
Associate Editors: NVSN Prasant, Velmurugan Selvam, Magesh Parthiban, Vetriselvan P, Vadhan Prasanna S

ARTICLE 44

The Effects of Preoperative Focused Cardiac Ultrasound in High-risk Patients: A Randomised Controlled Trial (PREOPFOCUS)[1-4]

Pallesen J, Bhavsar R, Fjølner J, Bakke SA, Krog J, Andersen MAS, et al. The effects of preoperative focused cardiac ultrasound in high-risk patients: A randomised controlled trial (PREOPFOCUS).
Acta Anaesthesiol Scand. 2022;66(10):1174-84.

■ CLINICAL QUESTION OR PROBLEM

Will information obtained from a preoperative focused cardiac ultrasound (FOCUS) prior to noncardiac surgery in high-risk patients change the postoperative outcomes?

■ WHAT IS ALREADY KNOWN?

- Postoperative morbidity and mortality are high after noncardiac surgery in American Society of Anesthesiologists (ASA) 3 and 4 patients.
- This is attributed to a mismatch between supply and demand of the myocardium, making surgery the third leading cause of mortality worldwide.
- Preoperative FOCUS has been shown to both step-up and step-down patient monitoring and management in retrospective studies. However, results have been conflicting and differ substantially between the studies.
- Two smaller and one large retrospective study showed either a higher or similar mortality in the group with a full echocardiography.
- The ECHONOF-2 was a pilot study done on 100 patients with hip fractures. It is the only randomized controlled trial (RCT) on preoperative FOCUS and showed no difference between the groups.
- Currently there is no recommendation for routine preemptive FOCUS prior to surgery.

■ STUDY DESIGN

- This trial was a randomized, active-controlled, multicentric trial.
- Patients were randomized 1:1 ratio to FOCUS versus no FOCUS using randomized table generated in Stata (USA), with stratification for age (65–74 years/≥75 years), surgical subspeciality, and study site.

- Ethical approval was obtained from regional committees of both central and southern Denmark region.
- Informed consent from all participants or their legal authorized representatives was obtained prior to enrollment.
- Sample size was calculated using a 3-month data from Randers Hospital, Denmark.
- A reduction by one-third of the primary end point from 33% was taken for sample size calculation.
- A total of 724 patients were required to achieve a power of 90% and alpha of 0.05, and to account for study site heterogeneity, it was increased by 10% to 800 patients.

SETTING

- Patients were recruited from two hospitals from different regions in Denmark, the Randers Regional Hospital and the Hospital of Southern Jutland.
- Study period—May 1st, 2018 (Randers Hospital) and September 1st, 2018 (Hospital of Southern Jutland) to August 31st, 2020.

POPULATION STUDIED INCLUDING DEMOGRAPHICS

Inclusion

- All patients aged 65 years or more admitted for emergency (<6 hours) or urgent surgery (<24 hours)
- ASA classification 3 or 4
- Scheduled for general or neuraxial anesthesia.

Exclusion

- Patients who had a surgery prior during the same admittance
- Low-risk surgery
- Refused to consent
- FOCUS not possible due to logistic reasons, and prior participation in the same study were excluded.

Baseline Characteristics

A total of 762 patients were screened for eligibility, after exclusion 338 patients were randomized. Eleven patients were excluded after randomization due to refusal for further participation or were randomized twice. Final analysis was done for the remaining 327 patients who were randomized to FOCUS group ($n = 163$) and no FOCUS group ($n = 164$). One patient in the FOCUS group and three patients in the control group did not undergo surgery. Demographics were similar between the groups (control group vs. FOCUS group).

- *Age:* 81(±8) years versus 81(±8) years
  - 65–74 years: 24% versus 22%
  - ≥75 years: 76% versus 78%
- *Gender:* Females 59% versus 58%
- *Body mass index (BMI):* 24.6(±5.1) versus 25.4(±5.0)
- ASA 3–89% versus 92%; ASA 4–11% versus 8%
- Comorbidities including hypertension, coronary artery disease, diabetes mellitus, etc., were similar between the groups.
- *Surgery type:* Orthopedic surgery 85% versus 85%; abdominal surgery 15% versus 15%
- *Hospital admittance:* Randers versus Hospital of Southern Jutland: 162 versus 165 patients.

INTERVENTION

Focused cardiac ultrasound was performed with Focused Assessed Transthoracic Echocardiography protocol (FATE). All data recorded and views were fed into REDCap and using a software algorithm, specifically designed for this study, a categorical report was obtained and made available to the anesthesiologist prior to surgery.

■ COMPARATOR
No FOCUS done.

■ OUTCOMES EVALUATED
- Control group versus FOCUS group
- *Primary composite end point:* Hospital stay >10 days or death within 30 days: (35/164) 21% versus (41/163) 25%; odds ratio (OR) 1.23 [95% confidence interval (CI): 0.74–2.07]; adjusted OR: 1.37 (95% CI: 0.86–2.30), $p = 0.36$
- *Secondary end points, other clinical complications:*
  - No significant difference in 30-day or 90-day mortality, adjusted OR: 1.06 (95% CI: 0.48–2.36), $p = 0.44$ and 1.37 (95% CI: 0.70–2.70), $p = 0.36$, respectively
  - Length of hospital stay: 4 (3–7) days versus 4 (3–8) days; adjusted OR: 0.10 (−0.07–0.28), $p = 0.24$
  - Length of intensive care unit (ICU) stay: 65 (12–141) days versus 55 (19–99) days; adjusted OR: 0.31 (−0.70–1.32), $p = 0.53$
  - Postoperative ICU transfers: 12 (7%) versus 14 (9%); adjusted OR: 1.27 (0.55–2.93), $p = 0.57$
  - Readmission within 90 days: 40 (24%) versus 50 (31%); adjusted OR: 1.40 (0.86–2.30), $p = 0.18$
  - Acute kidney injury: 14 (9%) versus 17 (10%); adjusted OR: 1.17 (0.54–2.56), $p = 0.69$
  - Postoperative mechanical ventilation: 6 (4%) versus 6 (4%); adjusted OR: 1.00 (0.31–3.28), $p = 1.00$
  - New-onset cardiac arrhythmias: 11 (7%) versus 15 (9%); adjusted OR: 1.33 (0.57–3.09), $p = 0.51$
  - Pneumonia: 17 (10%) versus 13 (8%); adjusted OR: 1.27 (0.57–2.73), $p = 0.55$
  - Postoperative hemorrhage: 20 (12%) versus 20 (12%); adjusted OR: 1.08 (0.54–2.18), $p = 0.82$.

■ INFORMATION FROM FOCUS
- *New information provided by FOCUS:* 45% (74/163)
- *Left ventricular ejection fraction (LVEF):* 23%
- *Aortic valve pathology:* 20%
- *Volume status:* 20%
- *Mitral valve pathology:* 10%

■ CHANGES IN PREOPERATIVE MANAGEMENT
- *Preoperative transfer to ICU/central ward for optimization:* 3 (2%) versus 7 (4%); adjusted OR: 2.41 (0.61–9.48), $p = 0.21$
- *Surgery deferred:* 12 (7%) versus 13 (8%); adjusted OR: 1.10 (0.49–2.48), $p = 0.82$.
- *Surgery cancelled:* 3 (2%) versus 1 (1%); OR: 3.30 (0.34–32.1), $p = 0.30$
- *Formal echocardiography ordered:* 5 (3%) versus 8 (5%); adjusted OR: 1.49 (0.48–4.68), $p = 0.49$
- *Formal echocardiography performed:* 5 (3%) versus 7 (4%); adjusted OR: 1.43 (0.44–4.59), $p = 0.55$
- *Fluids administered prior to surgery:* 9 (7%) versus 11 (8%); adjusted OR: 1.25 (0.50–3.09), $p = 0.64$.

■ CHANGES IN ANESTHESIA
- *Changes in anesthesia strategy:* 16 (10%) versus 16 (10%); adjusted OR: 1.05 (0.50–2.23), $p = 0.89$
- *Changes in anesthetic and vasoactive drugs used:* 16 (10%) versus 24 (15%); adjusted OR: 1.49 (0.72–3.10), $p = 0.28$
- *Step-up in monitoring:* 6 (4%) versus 35 (21%); adjusted OR: 6.59 (2.84–15.3), $p ≤ 0.001$

■ AUTHORS' VIEWPOINT

In ASA 3 and 4 patients ≥65 years of age and admitted for acute, high-risk orthopedic or abdominal surgery information from routine FOCUS to the perioperative team does not reduce clinical end points including admission to hospital for >10 days or death within 30 days. However, these findings should be interpreted cautiously due to the premature termination and low sample size.

■ STRENGTH OF THE STUDY

- Multicentric RCT
- Low rate of protocol violations
- Trial protocol and statistical analysis plans were published prior
- FATE protocol was used in this study and all operators had a minimum 1-day course in FOCUS, used point-of-care ultrasound (POCUS) routinely and were screened for technical adequacy; thus, increasing the overall applicability of the results.
- Use of software for automated interpretation report
- Pragmatic trial, as the perioperative team had no restrictions imposed regardless of group allocation.

■ DRAWBACKS OF THE STUDY

- Study was conducted in a single country, may limit external validity.
- Prematurely terminated due to coronavirus disease 2019 (COVID-19) pandemic, thus underpowering the results.
- Event rate in the study is lower than the previous 3-month data, although it could be attributed to random variation, however, a larger sample size would be required to show same relative effect.
- Only ASA 3 and 4 patients were enrolled, may be with patients with lower risk the use of preoperative FOCUS might have yielded different results.
- Data regarding intraoperative hemodynamics were not collected, impact of step-up in monitoring in the FOCUS group could have been assessed.
- The application of preoperative FOCUS alone does not directly reflect a change in patient treatment.

■ REVIEWERS' VIEWPOINT

Although this trial was prematurely terminated due to the impact of COVID-19 pandemic, the primary outcome was numerical higher in the FOCUS group compared to control group (25% vs. 21%). Hence, it would be unrealistic to expect a change in the result even if the calculated sample size was achieved. They also identified new pathologies mostly pertaining to LVEF, aortic valve, and volume status in almost half of the patients. Despite these findings not translating to change in outcomes, these are important variables every perioperative team would be interested in. Moreover, for preoperative FOCUS to have significant effect on outcomes, these findings must lead to change in patient management. This change in management should further result in change in outcomes (10% vs. 10%). In this trial, however, the identification of new pathologies resulted in a step-up of monitoring (4% vs. 21%). Hence, considering the lack of harm and the logistic difficulty in obtaining echocardiography before emergency surgery, use of FOCUS as a potential preemptive tool to guide perioperative management cannot be disregarded.

IMPACT ON CURRENT PRACTICE AND TAKE HOME MESSAGE

Routine FOCUS in ASA 3 and 4 patients prior to noncardiac surgery does not seem to improve outcomes. Its utility in a different class of patients remains to be seen. FOCUS can detect new pathology in nearly half of the patients, which may or may not result in improved perioperative outcomes. However, the use of FOCUS despite lack of benefit in terms of improved perioperative outcomes still has a role, especially when obtaining a comprehensive echocardiography prior to emergency surgery becomes difficult. A larger multicentric trial involving different geographical locations is required before adopting or discouraging its role in the perioperative setting.

ARTICLE 45

The Impact of Thoracic Ultrasound on Clinical Management of Critically Ill Patients (UltraMan): An International Prospective Observational Study[5–8]

Heldeweg MLA, Lopez Matta JE, Pisani L, Slot S, Haaksma ME, Smit JM, et al. The Impact of thoracic ultrasound on clinical management of critically ill patients (UltraMan): An international prospective observational study.

Crit Care Med. 2023;51(3):357-64.

CLINICAL QUESTION OR PROBLEM

Does the usage of thoracic ultrasound (TUS) examination have an impact on the clinical management of the critically ill patients?

WHAT IS ALREADY KNOWN?

Patients admitted to the critical care unit have multiple concurrent issues and multi-organ failures. The treating physician might encounter diagnostic dilemmas at several points of time during the patient's ICU stay. The physician must rely on various invasive and noninvasive diagnostic modalities to diagnose and manage the issues. Point-of-care thoracic ultrasound (POC TUS) is routinely used by critical care physicians for rapid and repeatable noninvasive assessment of the heart, lungs, diaphragm, and vena cava, which provides reliable information on circulatory, respiratory, and volume status. Various studies showed significant improvements in diagnosis and management with the introduction of ultrasound technology into the bedside assessment of critically ill patients. Integration of POCUS into clinical practice reduces the time to diagnose and treat and reduces the need for costly and invasive modalities.

STUDY DESIGN

This is an international prospective multi-center observational study done in ICU of two academic and two large nonuniversity hospitals in the Netherlands and Italy. Cases were recruited from January 21, 2020 to February 1, 2022, and need for informed consent was waived off by the Ethical Committee, as bedside ultrasound examination performed by physician is a part of conventional clinical practice. A total of 725 TUS examinations were done across 534 patients during the study period, and 4 were excluded due to death within 8 hours by 111 distinct operators ranging from supervised and inexperienced to highly experienced and internationally certified physicians. In these 525 examinations, 72.4% were done for diagnostic purposes, 200 (27.6%) were for monitoring, and 399 (55% of the examinations) were respiratory examinations, 135 (18.6%) were cardiac examinations, 166 (22.9%) were volume status assessments, and 24 (3.3%) included other examinations.

POPULATION STUDIED INCLUDING DEMOGRAPHICS

All adult patients (>18 years) admitted to the ICU during the study period were included, and multiple times if an indication for TUS existed and the patients dying within 8 hours of TUS were excluded as they could not be followed-up appropriately. Baseline characteristics and demographics, including the admission disposition, reason, number of actual diagnoses, and medical history, were collected. The recorded variables consisted of severity of disease, arterial blood gas, partial pressure of arterial oxygen/fraction of inspired oxygen (P/F) ratio, Sequential Organ Failure Assessment (SOFA), and mechanical ventilation variables (when applicable). The cumulative fluid balance was collected at the time of TUS, 8 hours after, and difference between was the fluid balance change.

INTERVENTION(S) STUDIED

Thoracic ultrasound consisted of assessment of the cardiac, lung, diaphragm, and inferior vena cava as per clinical indication and was documented on a case report form. The case report form recorded the following: the details of the operator and their training level, reason for TUS, current diagnosis and treatment plan, TUS findings, clinical contribution of TUS, potential changes in diagnosis, and management's data. The data was transcribed to an electronic data capture system **(Flowchart 1)**.

OUTCOMES EVALUATED

Primary Outcome

A change in management is defined as a TUS-induced change in the clinician's treatment plan only if documented by the operator in the case reporter form (CRF). Out of the 725 examinations, 28 (3.8%) had no clinical contribution, 352 (48.6%) confirmed the clinical impression of the operator, and 345 (47.6%) changed the clinical impression of the operator. TUS changed or added a diagnosis in 156 examinations and changed the intended management in a total of 279 examinations. The most frequent TUS findings were atelectasis, pleural effusion, and pulmonary

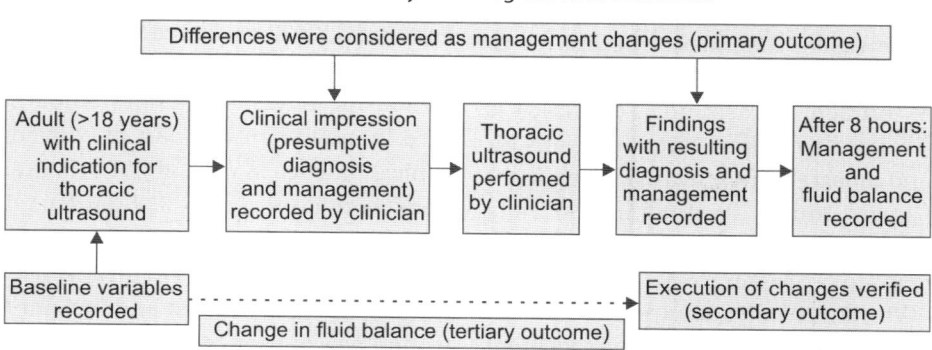

Flowchart 1: Study flow diagram with outcomes.

Flowchart 2: Diagnostic and management changes induced by thoracic ultrasound (TUS).

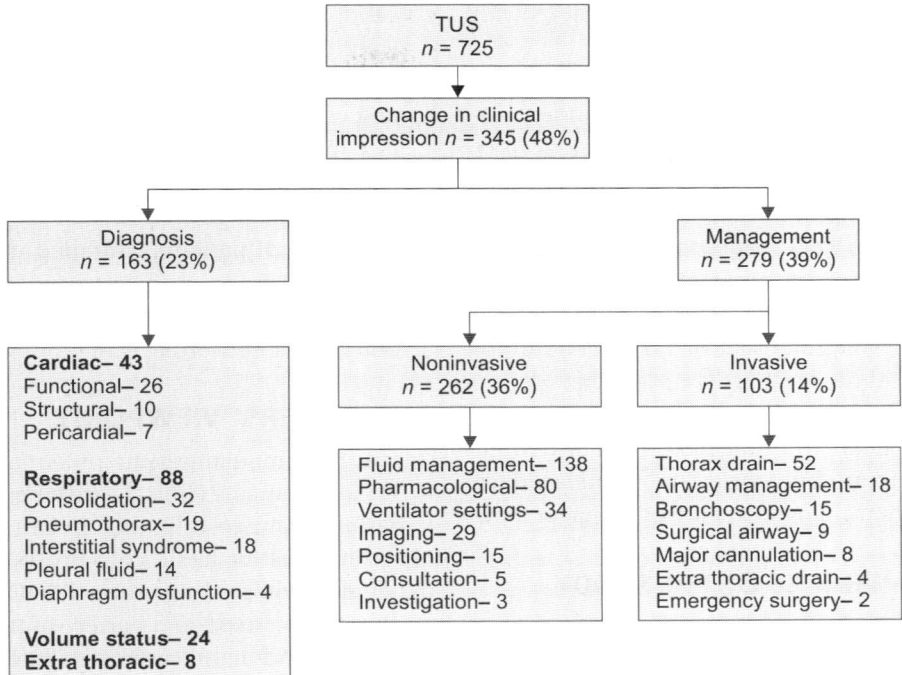

edema. The various diagnoses and planned management are shown in **Flowchart 2**.

Secondary Outcome

- The execution of CRF recorded changes in management within 8 hours after TUS. A total of 247 (88.5%) of all management changes were executed within 8 hours after TUS, out of which 55.1% had a component related to fluid management.
- The fluid balance changed between the TUS assessment and after 8 hours. There was a significant difference in fluid balance in the follow-up period between TUS-guided and unguided management.

■ AUTHORS' VIEWPOINT

The authors of this study are of the viewpoint that addition of POC TUS to the standard diagnostic pathway significantly increases the percentage of correct diagnoses, sensitivity, and specificity. They also found that timely intervention can also be carried out thereby improving the overall outcome in the critically ill patients. Even though it may be limited by relevance of diagnostic accuracy to clinical decision-making, the clinician also must consider the potential downstream health impact of erroneous and indeterminate findings, clinical context, and disease prevalence which may be particularly relevant in the complex and dynamic ICU environment.

■ STRENGTH OF THE STUDY

- Large multicenter study
- Largest study on this subject to date—sample size exceeds the cumulative sample size of all previous studies on this subject.

- High external validity—multicenter, international design, >100 operators with varying level of expertise.
- Rigorous registration on CRF and electronic data capture system decreases subjectivity and allows for robust conclusions.
- Corroborates the existing evidence and adds further evidence to bridge the gap between TUS-induced changes in clinical decision-making and verifiable patient centered changes.
- Only small number of TUS (4%) did not contribute to clinical impression.
- High yield compared to traditional routine diagnostic modalities—89% intended clinician behavior was translated to verified changed in patient management.

■ DRAWBACKS OF THE STUDY

- Non-RCT
- Relies on clinician reporting of management changes—leading to several forms of bias
  - Form bias—clinician inclined to select an answer provided on the CRF
  - Completion bias—the clinicians might only complete the CRF when the results were beneficial.
  - Confirmation bias—the pre-TUS impressions may influence the post-TUS CFR recordings.
  - Although preventive steps have been taken to overcome these bias, complete elimination of these bias cannot be ensured.
- Lack of feasibility—patient factors (acute change in therapeutic priorities); departmental factors (logistic or personal issues), TUS factors (erroneous interpretation)
- More respiratory findings than other system—cardiac ultrasound requires high level of expertise along with the availability of cardiac windows during suboptimal positioning.
- Failure to capture whether these changes would have occurred in the absence of TUS and whether these would trickle down to impact patient outcomes; conventional clinical parameters may have produced similar management decisions.
- Exclusion of patients who died within 8 hours of TUS—might have provided larger insights into the TUS decisions that affect outcome or end-of-life care.

■ REVIEWERS' VIEWPOINT

This study demonstrates the potential value of TUS in enhancing clinical care for critically ill patients, suggesting that it can be an important tool for healthcare professionals in their decision-making process. POCUS will continue to be used in a variety of medical disciplines and acute care settings. POCUS can supplement or completely replace advanced imaging in certain circumstances, reduce medical errors, and give a more effective real-time diagnosis. Additionally, POCUS might make it possible to be used as a screening tool for defined indications more widely and more affordably. Hence, routine implementation of the POC TUS can bring a change in clinical outcome especially in ICU involving multidisciplinary care. As a user-dependent technology, POCUS necessitates suitable training and quality assurance. POC TUS can induce substantial changes in the clinical decision-making. This can save the time of the clinician by providing a reliable bedside diagnostic tool, which would otherwise require a time-consuming, more invasive diagnostic modality. However, indiscriminate use of ultrasonography may result in extra testing that is not essential, pointless treatments in the event of falsely positive results, or insufficient investigation of falsely negative results. For effective utilization of POCUS these difficulties can be overcome by improving our knowledge of when and how to use it and also deciding on the training and evaluation. It will be necessary to guarantee the skillful usage of the technology, and establishing reimbursement and policy to promote suitable and efficient use.

IMPACT ON CURRENT PRACTICE AND TAKE HOME MESSAGE

The TUS will be more impactful by providing timely bedside diagnosis and can be helpful in implementing a timely intervention. Improvement in the quality of TUS by regular training and standardized protocols would improve the overall outcome of the patient. Further studies are to be conducted to bridge the gap between clinical decision-making and improved health outcome and to quantify the impact of TUS on the downstream outcome measures. TUS should be a part of the ICU armamentarium for its safe, reliable, repeatable noninvasive diagnostic modality. Steps to be taken for standardization of the training thereby improving the quality of image acquisition and reducing interobserver variability. Further clinical trials may pave a way for precision fluid management in the critically ill patients.

ARTICLE 46

Does Point-of-care Ultrasonography Improve Diagnostic Accuracy in Emergency Department Patients with Undifferentiated Hypotension? An International Randomized Controlled Trial from the SHOC-ED Investigators.[9–13]

Peach M, Milne J, Diegelmann L, Lamprecht H, Stander M, Lussier D, et al. Does point-of-care ultrasonography improve diagnostic accuracy in emergency department patients with undifferentiated hypotension? An international randomized controlled trial from the SHOC-ED investigators.
CJEM. 2023;25(1):48-56.

CLINICAL QUESTION

Does POCUS improve diagnostic accuracy in emergency department (ED) patients with undifferentiated hypotension?

WHAT IS ALREADY KNOWN?

Undifferentiated hypotension remains a formidable challenge in emergency medicine, demanding swift and accurate assessment to guide timely interventions. In this dynamic landscape, the integration of POCUS has emerged as a promising tool to augment diagnostic accuracy. This review delves into the existing body of knowledge surrounding the impact of POCUS on diagnostic precision in the context of undifferentiated hypotension within the ED setting. Over the past decades, the conventional approach to patients presenting with undifferentiated hypotension predominantly relied on clinical evaluation, laboratory studies, and invasive procedures. However, advancements in ultrasound technology have revolutionized the diagnostic process, allowing for real-time visualization of critical structures and hemodynamic parameters directly at the patient's bedside.

The existing body of knowledge points toward several key themes such as expedited diagnostic timelines, heightened accuracy in identifying underlying pathologies, refined risk stratification strategies, reduced dependency on invasive procedures, and most importantly, the potential for improved patient outcomes. These findings collectively underscore the potential of POCUS to revolutionize the approach to undifferentiated hypotension. Previous studies have shown that POCUS is helpful in narrowing diagnostic etiologies for nontraumatic hypotension. Previous studies showed that the early use of ultrasound for identification of nontraumatic hypotension increases the diagnostic accuracy by 25% and the use of POCUS in septic shock increases clinical diagnosis by 25%.

Building upon this foundation of knowledge, the SHOC-ED (Sonography in Hypotension and Cardiac Arrest in the Emergency Department) investigators have undertaken a pioneering international RCT to rigorously evaluate the impact of POCUS on diagnostic accuracy in this high-stakes clinical scenario. By leveraging a diverse patient population and a multinational approach, this study is poised to provide crucial insights into the effectiveness of POCUS across different healthcare settings and patient demographics. Although there are reported benefits with the use of POCUS in assessing hypotensive patients, evidence comparing the diagnostic accuracy of POCUS to that of standard care in the diagnosis of patients with undifferentiated shock is lacking.

STUDY DESIGN

- Multicenter RCT
- Block sampling stratified by site
- Software-based randomization was done to randomly assign either *"control"* (no POCUS protocol) or *"intervention"* (POCUS).
- Independent oversight committee ended the trial early due to lack of predicted meaningful difference between groups for the primary outcome of mortality.

POPULATION STUDIED AND DEMOGRAPHICS

Inclusion Criteria

- Age > 19 years
- ED presentation
- Systolic blood pressure (SBP) <100 mm Hg or Shock Index >1 [heart rate (HR)/SBP].

Exclusion Criteria

- Pregnancy (known at time of presentation or discovered during initial screening)
- Advanced life support interventions—CPR
- History of significant trauma in the past 24 hours
- Acute myocardial infarction (AMI)
- Clear mechanism or etiology for the hypotension or shock
- Vagal episode (as a cause for the hypotension)
- Nonpathologic hypotension—normal blood pressure for the patient.

Population

- A total of 347 were screened but 273 were randomized.
- *POCUS group*: 138
- *Control group (no POCUS)*: 135

Baseline Characteristics—Intervention versus Control Group

- *Age (years)*: 56 versus 58
- *Male*: 73 versus 65
- North America 90 versus 89
- South Africa 48 versus 46

- SBP *(mm Hg)*: 91 versus 91
- HR *(beats/min)*: 106 versus 111
- Respiratory rate *(RR) (breaths/min)*: 24.2 versus 23.7
- Temperature *(°C)*: 36.7 versus 36.9
- Category of shock:
  - Cardiogenic: 15 versus 13
  - Noncardiogenic: 121 versus 118
  - Both: 1 versus 0
  - Uncertain: 1 versus 4

INTERVENTIONS

- POCUS group was subjected to the popular RUSH (rapid ultrasound for shock and hypotension) and ACES (abdominal and cardiac evaluation with sonography in shock) protocol.
- Performed within 60 minutes of arrival to the ED, after an initial clinical assessment by a physician.
- *Control group*: Subjected to only clinical assessment
- Physicians had to document their first impression of category of shock as *cardiogenic* or *noncardiogenic* as well as a *suspected diagnosis*.
- In complex cases physicians may leave it blank, meaning uncertain, or may have suggest more than one suspected contributing etiology.
- At 60 minutes, physicians reevaluated participants and completed a secondary clinical impression, again documenting their perceived category of shock and suspected diagnosis, with the additional information provided in the POCUS protocol group.
- Additional information included complete blood count, electrolytes, creatinine, venous blood gas, and lactate.

COMPARATOR

Normal physician clinical assessment.

OUTCOMES STUDIED

- *Primary outcomes*: Diagnostic performance of POCUS protocol in terms of sensitivity, specificity, and positive and negative likelihood ratios.
- *Secondary outcomes*: Accuracy measures of subcategories of shock; rate of change of perceived shock category and diagnosis with the addition of a POCUS protocol.

OUTCOMES MEASURED

Primary Outcomes

- Specificity of POCUS was 95.5% [95% CI (89.9–98.5) vs. control 93.8% (87.7–97.5)].
- Sensitivity of POCUS was 80% (51.9–95.6) versus 91.7% (61.5–99.8).
- Positive likelihood ratio 17.92 (7.33–43.8) versus 14.80 (7.08–30.9).
- Negative likelihood ratio 0.21 (0.08–0.58) versus 0.09 (0.01–0.58).
- Overall diagnostic accuracy between the two approaches was similar [POCUS 93.7% (88–97.2) vs. control 93.6% (87.8–97.2)].

Secondary Outcomes

- Clinicians in the POCUS protocol group were more likely to change their perceived category of shock (17.39%) versus control (7.4%).
- However, were no more likely to change it to the correct category when compared with the control (59% vs. 70%).
- There was no important difference in rate of change of diagnosis between the POCUS protocol (35.0%) versus control group (26.7%) $p = 0.15$.

AUTHORS' POINT OF VIEW

In ED patients with undifferentiated hypotension, the addition of a POCUS protocol did not translate to additional benefit.

STRENGTH OF THE STUDY

- RCT
- Largest comparative study till date
- Blinding to the initial clinical and POCUS findings and the use of two reviewers and consensus reasoning.

DRAWBACKS

- The accuracy of interpretation of both POCUS and clinical findings in this study relied on the trained clinician at the bedside.
- Images were not recorded nor reviewed.
- Their reference standard of a chart review to determine the actual diagnosis and shock category is not a gold standard.
- Original study ended prior to recruitment of the initially planned 400 patients.

REVIEWERS' POINT OF VIEW

The results indicate that there were no significant differences in overall diagnostic accuracy between the POCUS and control groups. Both approaches demonstrated remarkably high levels of accuracy, with POCUS at 93.7% and the control group at 93.6%. This finding is noteworthy, as it suggests that while POCUS is a powerful diagnostic tool, it did not confer a substantial advantage over traditional clinical evaluation. The slight high specificity and positive likelihood ratio of POCUS confirm its valuable role in confirming specific diagnoses, especially in cases where the clinical picture is unclear. The slightly lower sensitivity of POCUS indicates that clinical assessment should not be neglected, as it remains vital in identifying true positives. The similarity in overall diagnostic accuracy between POCUS and the control group suggests that while POCUS offers significant advantages, it should be considered as a complementary tool rather than a replacement for traditional clinical evaluation. The integration of both approaches allows for a more comprehensive assessment, potentially leading to more accurate and timely interventions. In conclusion, the primary outcomes of this trial underscore the significant contribution of POCUS in improving diagnostic accuracy for patients with undifferentiated hypotension. By providing high specificity and positive likelihood ratios, POCUS enhances the confidence in positive findings. However, it is essential to recognize the continued importance of traditional clinical evaluation, as evidenced by the higher sensitivity in the control group. This study reinforces the value of a multimodal approach to patient assessment in the ED.

IMPACT ON CLINICAL PRACTICE

The findings from the international RCT conducted by the SHOC-ED investigators have the potential to significantly impact clinical practice in emergency medicine, particularly in the evaluation of patients with undifferentiated hypotension.

- *Incorporating POCUS into protocols:* The high specificity and positive likelihood ratios of POCUS suggest that it should be integrated into standard protocols for evaluating undifferentiated hypotension. Clinicians should consider incorporating POCUS as a routine part of their assessment to enhance diagnostic accuracy.
- *Complementary role:* POCUS should be viewed as a complementary tool to traditional clinical evaluation. While it excels in confirming specific diagnoses, clinicians should continue to rely on clinical judgment, especially to identify true positives.

- *Efficient resource utilization:* The use of POCUS can streamline patient management by reducing the need for invasive procedures and accelerating the diagnostic process. This can lead to more efficient resource utilization, shorter hospital stays, and reduced healthcare costs.
- *Training and standardization:* Hospitals and healthcare systems should invest in training programs to ensure that ED staff is proficient in POCUS techniques. Standardization of POCUS protocols and quality assurance measures should be implemented to maintain consistency and reliability.

TAKE HOME MESSAGE

The key take home message from this research is that POCUS is a valuable tool that can enhance diagnostic accuracy in ED patients with undifferentiated hypotension. Clinicians should recognize that POCUS is not a replacement for clinical judgment but rather a powerful adjunct that can aid in confirming specific diagnoses. While POCUS provides high specificity and positive likelihood ratios, it should be used in conjunction with traditional clinical evaluation to achieve the most accurate and comprehensive assessment. Its ability to expedite the diagnostic process, reduce the need for invasive procedures, and facilitate timely interventions can significantly improve patient outcomes. To implement POCUS effectively, healthcare systems should invest in training programs for their staff, standardize protocols, and establish quality assurance measures. By doing so, they can harness the full potential of POCUS in emergency medicine, ultimately benefiting patients by improving diagnostic accuracy and streamlining care.

REFERENCES

1. Boretsky KR, Kantor DB, DiNardo JA, Oren-Grinberg A. Focused Cardiac Ultrasound in the Pediatric Perioperative Setting. Anesth Analg. 2019;129(4):925-32.
2. Li L, Yong RJ, Kaye AD, Urman RD. Perioperative Point of Care Ultrasound (POCUS) for Anesthesiologists: An Overview. Curr Pain Headache Rep. 2020;24(5):20.
3. Via G, Hussain A, Wells M, Reardon R, ElBarbary M, Noble VE, et al. International Liaison Committee on Focused Cardiac UltraSound (ILC-FoCUS); International Conference on Focused Cardiac UltraSound (IC-FoCUS). International evidence-based recommendations for focused cardiac ultrasound. J Am Soc Echocardiogr. 2014; 27(7):683.
4. Byrne M, Singleton M, Kalagara H, Haskins SC. Perioperative Point-of-Care Ultrasound. Adv Anesth. 2021;39:189-213.
5. Hew M, Tay TR: The efficacy of bedside chest ultrasound: From accuracy to outcomes. Eur Respir Rev. 2016;25:230-46.
6. Bernstein E, Wang TY. Point-of-care ultrasonography: Visually satisfying medicine or evidence-based medicine? JAMA Intern Med. 2021;181:1558–9.
7. Robba C, Wong A, Poole D, et al. European Society of Intensive Care Medicine task force for critical care ultrasonography*: Basic ultrasound head-to-toe skills for intensivists in the general and neuro intensive care unit population: Consensus and expert recommendations of the European Society of Intensive Care Medicine. Intensive Care Med. 2021;47:1347-1367.
8. Heldeweg MLA, Vermue L, Kant M, et al. The impact of lung ultrasound on clinical-decision making across departments: a systematic review. Ultrasound J. 2022; 14:5
9. Stickles SP, Carpenter CR, Gekle R, Kraus CK, Scoville C, Theodoro D, et al. The diagnostic accu- racy of a point-of-care ultrasound protocol for shock etiology: a systematic review and meta-analysis. Canad J Emerg Med. 2019.

10. Cortellaro F, Ferrari L, Molteni F, Aseni P, Velati M, Guarnieri L, et al. Accuracy of point of care ultrasound to identify the source of infection in septic patients: a prospective study. Inter Emerg Med. 2017.
11. Rivers E, Nguyen B, Havstad S, Ressler J, Muzzin A, Knoblich B, et al. Early goal-directed therapy in the treatment of severe sepsis and septic shock. New Engl J Med. 2001.
12. ProCESS Investigators. A randomized trial of protocol-based care for early septic shock. N Engl J Med. 2014.
13. Atkinson PRT, McAuley DJ, Kendall RJ, Abeyakoon O, Reid CG, Connolly J, et al. Abdominal and cardiac evaluation with sonography in shock (ACES): an approach by emergency physicians for the use of ultrasound in patients with undifferentiated hypotension. Emerg Med J. 2009.

Section 10

Nutrition and Metabolic

Section Editor: *Sivakumar MN*
Associate Editor: *Lakshmikanthcharan S*

ARTICLE 47

Continued Enteral Nutrition until Extubation Compared with Fasting Before Extubation in Patients in the Intensive Care Unit: An Open-label, Cluster-Randomized, Parallel-group, Non-inferiority Trial

Landais M, Nay MA, Auchabie J, Hubert N, Frerou A, Yehia A, et al; Mercat REVA network and CRICS-TriggerSEP F-CRIN research network. Landais M, Nay MA, Auchabie J, Hubert N, Frerou A, Yehia A, Mercat REVA network and CRICS-TriggerSEP F-CRIN research network. Continued enteral nutrition until extubation compared with fasting before extubation in patients in the intensive care unit: an open-label, cluster-randomized, parallel-group, non-inferiority trial.
Lancet Respir Med. 2023;11(4):319-28.

CLINICAL QUESTION OR PROBLEM

Whether the pursuit of enteral nutrition until extubation is associated with an increased risk of failure compared with fasting prior to extubation. To compare continued enteral nutrition until fasting before extubation in patients in the intensive care unit (ICU).

WHAT IS ALREADY KNOWN?

Fasting is frequently practiced before extubation in patients in ICUs, with the aim to reduce risk of aspiration. This unevaluated practice might delay extubation, increase workload, and reduce caloric intake. Fasting and nutrition practice before extubation in ICUs and its effect on patient-centered outcomes had scarcely been evaluated. Three cohort studies in the past have shown a caloric intake deficit related to intubation or extubation procedures and showed that extubation and ventilator weaning represent a frequent cause of nutrition interruption among critically ill patients.[1] Two surveys among ICU practitioners showed high heterogeneity in nutritional practices before extubation, with patient fasting durations ranging from 2 to 12 hours.[2] Evaluation of the fasting practices on patient-centered outcomes had not been conducted and the topic is not covered by current guidelines.

STUDY DESIGN

It is an open-label, cluster randomized, parallel-group, noninferiority trial done in

22 ICUs in France. Patients aged 18 years or older were eligible for enrolment if they had received invasive mechanical ventilation for at least 48 hours in the ICU and received prepyloric enteral nutrition for at least 24 hours at the time of extubation decision. Centers were randomly assigned (1:1) to continued enteral nutrition until extubation or 6-hour fasting with concomitant gastric suctioning before extubation, to be applied for all patients within the unit.

Masking was not possible because of the nature of the trial. The primary outcome was extubation failure (composite criteria of reintubation or death) within 7 days after extubation, assessed in both the intention-to-treat and per-protocol populations. The noninferiority margin was set at 10%. Pneumonia within 14 days of extubation was a key secondary endpoint.

■ INTERVENTION

- *Maximal gastric vacuity strategy group*: Interruption of enteral nutrition at least 6 hours before extubation and concomitant continuous suctioning via the gastric tube whenever feasible for 6 hours before extubation.
- *Maintenance of caloric intake strategy group*: Maintenance of the enteral caloric supply at the same flow rate until extubation.

POPULATION STUDIED INCLUDING DEMOGRAPHICS

Adults who underwent invasive mechanical ventilation for no <48 hours in the ICU and prepyloric enteral nutrition for no <24 hours at the time of extubation decision from 22 ICUs in France between April 1, 2018 and October 31, 2019 were included. Out of 7,056 patients receiving enteral nutrition and mechanical ventilation admitted to the ICUs, 4,198 were assessed for eligibility. 1,130 patients were enrolled and included in the intention-to-treat population and 1,008 were included in the per-protocol population.

■ OUTCOMES EVALUATED
Primary Outcome

- In the intention-to-treat population, extubation failure occurred in 106 (17.2%) of 617 patients assigned to receive continued enteral nutrition until extubation versus 90 (17.5%) of 513 assigned to fasting, meeting the a priori defined noninferiority criterion [absolute difference—0.4%, 95% confidence interval (CI) 5.2–4.5].
- In the per-protocol population, extubation failure occurred in 101 (17.0%) of 595 patients assigned to receive continued enteral nutrition versus 74 (17.9%) of 413 assigned to fasting (absolute difference—0.9%, 95% CI 5.6–3.7).

Secondary Outcome

Pneumonia within 14 days of extubation occurred in 10 (1.6%) patients assigned to receive continued enteral nutrition and 13 (2.5%) assigned to fasting (rate ratio 0.77, 95% CI 0.22–2.69).

■ AUTHORS' VIEWPOINT

This study to their knowledge is the largest randomized clinical trial to evaluate continuation of enteral nutrition until extubation compared with fasting as part of a maximum gastric vacuity strategy, including gastric content suctioning when feasible, in the immediate timeframe before extubation in the critical care setting. This study shows the overall safety of pursuing enteral nutrition until extubation, given the noninferior rate of extubation failure—a patient-centered endpoint evaluating the overall safety of the procedure. These results support changes in clinical practice because extubation, as part of airway management, represents a very frequent cause of enteral nutrition interruption. Furthermore, continued enteral nutrition until extubation might reduce side effects and improve patient outcomes.

■ STRENGTH OF THE STUDY

The study design and the intention of the study is relevant. The power of the study and the number of patients included is quite high. The study being multicentric, randomized, and being a noninferiority trial adds strength to the results. Having both intention-to-treat arm and per-protocol arm helps us to analyze a good number of patients by avoiding omission of many of them for the minor breach in protocol.

■ DRAWBACK OF THE STUDY

The study was not blinded, due to the nature of the intervention and the pragmatic design with cluster randomization at the level of the ICU.

The primary composite outcome of extubation failure is in part influenced by the physicians' decision to intubate patients. However, the long observation period of 7 days decreases potential bias. The primary composite outcome is to be considered as objectively measured but potentially influenced by clinician judgement, which is associated with a low risk of bias.

The open-label, cluster randomized design might not fully control for all potential recruitment bias and confounding factors. Some potential confounders could have favored extubation failure in the fasting group.

Conversely, patients in the continued enteral nutrition group were more severely ill, as measured by the simplified acute physiology score, had more frequently failed their first spontaneous breathing trial, and had less frequently received steroids to prevent laryngeal edema, all of which might have favored extubation failure in this group. More frequent steroid administration in the fasting group might be due to the available time to administer the therapy before extubation because of the 6-hour fasting duration, but one cannot formally exclude a patient-related or unit-related bias given the potential heterogeneity in care in the periextubation period across centers.

The slight group imbalances, which in part counterbalance each other, should not distract from the pragmatic finding of the present large-scale study showing an equal risk of extubation failure among 1,130 patients whether they undergo fasting or not before extubation. Of note, the post hoc sensitivity analysis of the primary composite outcome adjusted for potential confounders, including, among others, steroid administration and cough effectiveness, confirmed the noninferiority of the continued enteral nutrition until extubation strategy in all cases.

■ REVIEWERS' VIEWPOINT

The fact that continued enteral nutrition was associated with faster discharge from the ICU is a patient-centered benefit and is surprising. Additionally, the fact that mortality was lower in the continued enteral nutrition group was unexpected and deserves further evaluation to understand potential mechanisms. If we negate the limitations mentioned before, the study finding is good enough to compel practice changes. Patients with high risk for reintubation have to be identified and may be a subgroup analysis of them is needed to know whether they have to be made an exception to this finding.

IMPACT ON CURRENT PRACTICE AND TAKE HOME MESSAGE

As medical practices continuously evolve based on new evidence, it might be prudent for healthcare providers to reevaluate the standard protocols regarding enteral feeding during the extubation process. The study's findings highlight the need to move away from the practice of holding enteral feeding prior to extubation with the fear of aspiration. Implementing a continuous enteral feeding approach may lead to improved patient outcomes and a more efficient use of resources within the ICU. However, it is crucial to consider each patient's unique circumstances and risk factors before making any changes to established protocols.

ARTICLE 48

A Randomized Trial of Enteral Glutamine for Treatment of Burn Injuries

Heyland DK, Wibbenmeyer L, Pollack JA, Friedman B, Turgeon AF, Eshraghi N, et al; RE-ENERGIZE Trial Team. A Randomized Trial of Enteral Glutamine for Treatment of Burn Injuries.
N Engl J Med. 2022;387:1001-10.

CLINICAL QUESTION OR PROBLEM

To evaluate the effect of supplemental enteral glutamine on the time to discharge alive in patients with severe burn injuries. The aim of the trial was to determine whether this inexpensive therapeutic strategy leads to lower morbidity and mortality or whether it should be abandoned.

WHAT IS ALREADY KNOWN?

Burn injuries represent a public health problem worldwide, are ranked fourth in all injuries, and are among the leading cause of disability adjusted life years in low- and middle-income countries. More than in any other injury, the inflammation and catabolism associated with severe burns can exacerbate nutrient deficiencies, thereby predisposing patients to impaired immune function and increased risk of developing infectious complications, organ dysfunction, and death. Numerous trials have evaluated the effect of different nutritional strategies in patients with severe burns. Glutamine is of particular interest because it is vital for numerous key stress response pathways in serious illness. Observational studies have shown that glutamine levels decrease rapidly after burn injury. In critically ill patients, low levels of glutamine are associated with increased morbidity and mortality. Several small, single-center, randomized controlled trials (RCTs), when statistically aggregated, suggest a dramatic reduction in mortality and length of hospital stay associated with enteral glutamine supplementation in patients with burns. In 2009, a systematic review of RCTs concluded that the administration of glutamine-enhanced enteral nutrition in patients with severe burns helped shorten the length of stay (LOS).[3] The existing randomized trials of glutamine supplementation in burns patients have suggested a significant reduction in mortality, infection, and hospital LOS. The European Society for Parenteral and Enteral Nutrition (ESPEN) guidelines in 2019 for severe burns included administering enteral glutamine (grade B recommendation—strong consensus 95% agreement).[4] A survey of 37 burn units worldwide showed that 47.7% of mechanically ventilated patients with burns received glutamine supplementation.

However, randomized, controlled trials involving other critically ill patient populations have suggested that glutamine administration may be ineffective or even harmful. Given these conflicting data, a higher level of evidence was needed to inform clinical recommendations regarding the use of glutamine in this unique population.

■ STUDY DESIGN

It is an international, double-blind, parallel-group, randomized, placebo-controlled trial. They assigned patients with deep second- or third-degree burns within 72 hours after hospital admission to receive 0.5 g/kg of body weight per day of enterally delivered glutamine or placebo. Trial agents were given every 4 hours through a feeding tube or three/four times a day by mouth until 7 days after the last skin grafting procedure, discharge from the acute care unit, or 3 months after admission, whichever came first.

■ POPULATION STUDIED INCLUDING DEMOGRAPHICS

About 1,200 burn patients from 54 burn units in 14 countries were included in this randomized trial, from May, 2011 through June, 2021. Investigators included 596 patients in the group given glutamine supplementation and 604 in the group given the placebo.

Inclusion Criteria

- Deep second- or third-degree burns requiring grafting
- Patients 18–59 years, without inhalation injury total burn surface area (TBSA) ≥20%
- Patients 18–59 years, with inhalation injury TBSA ≥ 15%
- Patients ≥ 60 years, (with or without inhalation injury) TBSA ≥ 10%.

Exclusion Criteria

- More than 72 hours from admission to ICU to time of consent
- Patients younger than 18 years of age
- In patients without known renal disease, renal dysfunction defined as a serum creatinine >171 µmol/L or a urine output of <500 mL per last 24 hours (or 80 mL per last 4 hours if a 24-hour period of observation is not available). In patients with acute on chronic renal failure (predialysis), an absolute increase of >80 µmol/L from baseline or preadmission creatinine or a urine output of <500 mL per last 24 hours (or 80 mL per last 4 hours) will be required. Patients with chronic renal failure on dialysis will be excluded.
- *Liver cirrhosis*: Child's class C liver disease
- Pregnancy
- *Absolute contraindication for enteral nutrition*: Intestinal occlusion or perforation and abdominal injury
- Patients with injuries from high-voltage electrical shock
- Patients who are moribund
- *Patients with extreme body sizes*: Body mass index (BMI) 50
- Enrolment in another industry sponsored ICU intervention study
- Received glutamine supplement for >24 hours prior to randomization
- Known allergy to maltodextrin, corn starch, corn, corn products or glutamine.

The trial groups had similar characteristics at baseline.

■ OUTCOMES EVALUATED

The primary outcome was the time to discharge alive from the hospital, with data till 90 days.

A total of 1,209 patients with severe burns (mean burn size, 33% of TBSA) underwent randomization, and 1,200 were included in the analysis (596 patients in the glutamine group and 604 in the placebo group).

The median time to discharge alive from the hospital was 40 days [interquartile range (IQR) 24–87] in the glutamine group and 38 days (IQR 22–75) in the placebo group (subdistribution hazard ratio for discharge alive, 0.91; 95% CI 0.80–1.04; $p = 0.17$). Their results did not differ when the data were adjusted according to either site or for covariates.

Mortality at 6 months was 17.2% in the glutamine group and 16.2% in the placebo group (hazard ratio for death, 1.06; 95% CI 0.80–1.41). No substantial between-group differences in serious adverse events were observed.

■ AUTHORS' VIEWPOINT

The results were unexpected given the magnitude of the signal from previous trials of supplemental glutamine in burn-injured patients. Authors felt that their trial differed from the previous trials in several important ways.

First, the previous randomized, controlled trials were small, single-center trials ranging from 30 to 48 patients each. This multicenter trial with a much larger sample showed no combined effect of reduced mortality and shorter hospital stay [95% CI for the subdistribution hazard ratio for discharge alive (0.80–1.04) ruled out a clinically meaning benefit]. Previous research has shown that the effect of intravenous glutamine was also subject to a single-center bias in which all the positive effects were seen in single-center, randomized, controlled trials, whereas larger, multicenter, randomized, controlled trials did not confirm a positive treatment effect. Others have shown how the results of single-center trials consistently overestimate the treatment effect as compared with larger multicenter trials. The practice of translating the results of single-center trials into clinical practice recommendations, as occurred with enteral glutamine supplementation, should be reexamined.

Second, the management of burn injury has evolved in the past decade since the publication of results of previous trials (from 2003 through 2009), and in most geographic areas worldwide, there has been a substantial decline in the mortality and morbidity associated with burn injury. With greater attention to initial resuscitation, wound management, and early surgical intervention, it may be unlikely that a single-nutrient replacement strategy will affect the underlying pathophysiological processes.

■ STRENGTH OF THE STUDY

The strengths of this trial include its robust scientific methods and high-fidelity implementation, which enhance the internal validity of the findings. The large number of diverse patients recruited across a large global network of burn units supports broad generalizability of the findings.

■ DRAWBACK OF THE STUDY

The major weakness of this trial is the low accumulation of patients that led to the alteration of the sample size and primary outcome. Although blinded sample size reestimation is widely accepted to have only trivial effects on type I error, we cannot rule out the possibility that the midtrial alterations could slightly distort the type I and II error rates.

An additional weakness is the low completion rate of 6-month survivor questionnaires, although the rate was similar to or higher than those in other burn care studies of this nature.

Finally, the trial statistician (who is on the steering committee) conducted the interim analysis, but this analysis included only baseline characteristics, adverse events, and deaths, and results were kept from the rest of the steering committee to avoid influence on decisions regarding trial changes.

■ REVIEWERS' VIEWPOINT

Studies on major burns typically only involve a small number of patients, nevertheless existing randomized trials have repeatedly shown that glutamine (and its precursor ornithine alpha-ketoglutarate) has positive effects on major burn injuries, lowering mortality as well as infectious complications (primarily gram-negative infections). This has been confirmed by multiple meta-analysis, and was included in the specific ESPEN burn guidelines 2019, but is now challenged by this largest RCT revealing no benefit from glutamine supplementation in burns. A higher glutamine requirement in burn patients is explained by exudative losses. Analysis of burn exudates shows that glutamine is lost in larger amounts than any other amino acid. As per the ESPEN guidelines 2023 that took this current study into consideration, they have still given a recommendation that "in patients with burns >20% body surface area, additional enteral doses of glutamine (0.3–0.5 g/kg/day) should be administered for 10–15 days as soon as enteral nutrition is commenced. (grade B, strong consensus, 95%)". Another systemic review and meta-analysis was conducted by Han-Yang Yue et al. in 2023 including six randomized controlled trials involving 1,398 patients (including this RE-ENERGIZE study).[5] It concluded that compared to the control group, enteral glutamine administration may not improve the mortality, although it may be associated with a shorter LOS, a lower LOS/TBSA, and may reduce the risk of wound infection in patients with severe burns.

■ IMPACT ON CURRENT PRACTICE AND TAKE HOME MESSAGE

At present, taking into consideration the most recent ESPEN guidelines recommendation, it is appropriate to continue supplementing severe burn patients with glutamine until additional substantial RCTs persuade the recommendations to be amended.

ARTICLE 49

Intravenous Vitamin C in Adults with Sepsis in the Intensive Care Unit

Lamontagne F, Masse MH, Menard J, Sprague S, Pinto R, Heyland DK, et al. LOVIT Investigators and the Canadian Critical Care Trials Group. Intravenous Vitamin C in Adults with Sepsis in the Intensive Care Unit.
N Engl J Med. 2022; 386:2387-98.

■ CLINICAL QUESTION OR PROBLEM

Does a high dose of vitamin C reduce the risk of death or persistent organ dysfunction at 28 days in adults with sepsis who are receiving vasopressor therapy in the ICU.

■ WHAT IS ALREADY KNOWN?

In sepsis, the antioxidant effects of vitamin C therapy may mitigate tissue injury induced by oxidative stress. Vitamin C cannot be synthesized by humans, and levels are low in many critically ill patients, which has increased the plausibility of benefit with supplementation. A single-center retrospective study by Marik et al. in 2017 spurred interest in the use of intravenous vitamin C, administered with hydrocortisone and thiamine.[6] Subsequently, the VICTAS randomized clinical trial by Sevransky et al. in 2021 and a systematic review and component network meta-analysis by Fujii et al. in 2022 evaluating this combination treatment did not show any benefits.[7,8] In contrast, in the CITRIS-ALI (Vitamin C Infusion for Treatment in Sepsis Induced Acute Lung Injury) trial, a randomized controlled trial by Fowler et al. in 2019, patients with sepsis and acute lung injury who received a higher dose of vitamin C (50 mg/kg of body weight every 6 hours) had a lower 28-day risk of death than those who received placebo.[9] Oral and intravenous vitamin C shortened the length of ICU stay on an average by 7.8% in a meta-analysis of 12 trials by Hemila et al. in 2019 with 1,766 patients. In another meta-analysis of eight trials by Hemila et al. again in 2020 with 685 patients,[10] vitamin C reduced the length of ventilation time, and meta-regression indicated that the effect was significantly greater in patients with more severe medical conditions.[11] However, recently two systematic meta-analyses by Fujii et al. and Patel et al. in 2022 suggest that the overall evidence supporting the use of vitamin C therapy in patients with sepsis is of low certainty.[12,13]

STUDY DESIGN

In this international trial, they enrolled patients in 35 adult medical–surgical ICUs in Canada, France, and New Zealand. It was a phase 3, international multicenter, concealed-allocation, parallel-group, blinded, randomized placebo-controlled trial. Patients were randomized 1:1 using centralized web-based system with permuted blocks of variable, undisclosed size, and stratified according to the site.

POPULATION STUDIED INCLUDING DEMOGRAPHICS

Patients were enrolled from November 14, 2018 to July 19, 2021.

Inclusion

- Patients ≥18 years old
- Admitted to ICU with proven or suspected infection as the main diagnosis
- Currently treated with a continuous intravenous infusion of vasopressors (norepinephrine, epinephrine, vasopressin, dopamine, phenylephrine).

Exclusion

- More than 24 hours of ICU admission
- Known glucose-6-phosphate dehydrogenase (G6PD) deficiency
- Pregnancy
- Known allergy to vitamin C
- Known kidney stones within the past 1 year
- Received any intravenous vitamin C during this hospitalization unless incorporated in parenteral nutrition
- Expected death or withdrawal of life-sustaining treatments within 48 hours
- Previously enrolled in this study
- Previously enrolled in a trial for which co-enrolment is not allowed
- 2,234 screened ≥872 randomized ≥8 patients further found to be ineligible ≥1 further withdrew consent
- The actual number of patients who completed follow-up at 28 days were:
  - 429 in vitamin C group
  - 434 in placebo group

- Comparing baseline characteristics of vitamin C versus placebo group:
  - Age (years): 65.0 versus 65.2
  - Female sex (%): 35.2 versus 40
  - Admission type:
    - Medical (%): 81.6 versus 85.2
    - Surgical (%): 18.4 versus 14.8
  - APACHE II (Acute Physiology and Chronic Health Evaluation) score: 24.2 versus 24.1
  - SOFA (Sequential Organ Failure Assessment) score: 10.2 versus 10.1
  - Primary site of infection (%)
    - Pulmonary: 33.8 versus 36.7
    - Gastrointestinal or intra-abdominal: 31 versus 25.9
  - Severe acute respiratory syndrome coronavirus 2 (SARS CoV-2) positive (%): 8.6 versus 6.0
  - Lactate mmol/L: 3.4 versus 3.0
  - Vitamin C level µmol/L: 20.6 versus 19.1
  - Septic shock (requirement for a vasopressor infusion and a lactate ≥2 mmol/L) (%): 59.6 versus 56.1
  - Time from ICU admission to randomization (hour): 12.9 versus 12.3
  - Treatment (%)
    - Glucocorticoids: 46.4 versus 45.4
    - Mechanical ventilation: 68.5 versus 65.4
    - Renal replacement therapy: 10.7 versus 9.7
    - Vasopressor infusion: 99.8 versus 100.

■ INTERVENTION(S) STUDIED

Patients in the intervention group received intravenous vitamin C in a bolus dose of 50 mg/kg mixed in a 50 mL solution of either dextrose 5% in water or normal saline. Doses were administered over 30–60 minutes every 6 hours for 96 hours (i.e., 200 mg/kg/day, with a maximum of 16 doses) as long as patients remained in the ICU.

■ COMPARATOR USED

In the control group, patients received a matching placebo infusion (dextrose 5% in water or normal saline) every 6 hours for up to 96 hours.

■ OUTCOMES EVALUATED

Primary Outcome

- Composite of death or persistent organ dysfunction (defined as receipt of vasopressors, invasive mechanical ventilation, or new renal replacement therapy) on trial day 28—significantly higher in vitamin C group.
- Vitamin C 191/429 (44.5%) versus placebo 167/434 (38.5%).
- Risk ratio (RR) 1.21; 95% CI, 1.04–1.40; $p = 0.01$.

Secondary Outcomes

- No significant difference in:
  - Median number of days without organ dysfunction in ICU at day 28 (vitamin C 17 vs. 19.5 placebo)
  - Death by 6 months number/total (%): 191/417(45.8) versus 185/426(43.4)
  - Health-related quality of life at 6 months
  - SOFA scores on day 1, 2, 3, 4, 7, 10, 14, 28
  - Markers of tissue dysoxia (lactate), inflammation, and endothelial injury at day 1, 3, and 7
- No significant difference in safety outcomes:
  - Stage 3 acute kidney injury (AKI)
  - Acute hemolysis
  - Hypoglycemia.

AUTHORS' VIEWPOINT

In adults with sepsis receiving vasopressor therapy in the ICU, those who received intravenous vitamin C had a higher risk of death or persistent organ dysfunction at 28 days than those who received placebo.

STRENGTH OF THE STUDY

- The largest study till date
- A well-designed international trial
- Blinded to limit ascertainment bias
- A median enrolment time of approximately 12 hours after ICU admission
- High protocol adherence
- Ascertainment of the renal replacement therapy component of the primary outcome in patients who were discharged from the hospital before day 28
- Assessment of biomarkers and baseline vitamin C levels.

DRAWBACK OF THE STUDY

- Nine patients who had undergone randomization did not contribute data to the primary analysis; of these patients, eight had not received either vitamin C or placebo and had met the prespecified criteria for exclusion after randomization. Only one patient who withdrew consent could not be included in the intention-to-treat analysis. Given the high number of events that were recorded in each group, the effect of these exclusions is probably small.
- Information regarding specific pathogens and the appropriateness of antimicrobial therapy was not collected; however, systematic differences in post-randomization care are less likely in blinded trials.
- Information to ascertain the presence of acute respiratory distress syndrome at baseline was not collected, so it remains unclear whether this subgroup had a different response to vitamin C.
- Although the patients were representative of those with sepsis being treated in the ICU in many high-income countries, the trial population differs substantially from patients in many low- and middle-income countries, where the incidence of sepsis and the associated case fatality rate are highest.
- Secondary analyses did not determine a possible mechanism for the worse outcome seen with intravenous vitamin C.
- In this trial, 25% of patients had baseline vitamin C levels <5.37 µM which is half the customary level for diagnosing vitamin C deficiency based on plasma level. The upper limit in the second plasma vitamin C level quartile of patients was 12.38 µM, which is barely higher than the usual limit for classifying vitamin C deficiency. Thus, nearly half the LOVIT (Lessening Organ Dysfunction with Vitamin C) patients had baseline vitamin C levels lower than the plasma level for considering scurvy, noting that scurvy symptoms often start before that plasma level has even been reached. Given that scurvy is a serious and potentially life-threatening disease it seems ethically inappropriate to randomize half the patients who have vitamin C levels <5.37 µM to a placebo group which is not administered vitamin C. There is no discussion in the LOVIT trial protocol or trial report, of how the diagnosis of scurvy was intended to be carried out, or what symptoms the authors considered relevant for concluding that a patient did or did not suffer from scurvy when the vitamin C plasma level was very low.

REVIEWERS' VIEWPOINT

The composite primary outcome (death or persistent organ dysfunction at trial day 28) occurred more frequently in patients who had received intravenous vitamin C than in those who had received placebo. This was an unexpected finding, and the secondary analyses which included the evaluation of five biomarkers of tissue dysoxia, inflammation, and endothelial injury measured up to day 7, did not provide an explanatory mechanism for harm.

The median ICU stay was 6 days, but interestingly vitamin C was administered for only 4 days. No discussion of the biological justification for the short vitamin C administration was provided. If there is increased consumption of vitamin C in critically ill patients, it seems important to administer vitamin C over the entire period of critical illness.

Furthermore, there has been concern about the possibility of harmful rebound effects if high-dose vitamin C is abruptly terminated, and such a phenomenon might be most evident in critically ill patients with very low initial vitamin C levels. Hence, a secondary analysis of LOVIT trial was done by Hemila et al. who used Cox regression with two time periods to model the distribution of deaths over the first 11 days in the LOVIT trial.[14] Compared with a uniform difference between vitamin C and placebo groups over the 11-day follow-up period, addition of a separate vitamin C effect starting from day 5 improved the fit of the Cox model ($p = 0.026$). There was no difference in mortality between the groups during the 4-day vitamin C administration with RR = 0.97 (95% CI 0.65–1.44). During the week after the sudden termination of vitamin C, there were 57 deaths in the vitamin C group, but only 32 deaths in the placebo group, with RR = 1.9 (95% CI 1.2–2.9; $p = 0.004$). They concluded that increased mortality in the vitamin C group in the LOVIT trial is not explained by ongoing vitamin C administration, but by the abrupt termination of vitamin C.

In a recent retrospective cohort study conducted in Korea by Jung et al. using propensity score matching, vitamin C administration was associated with lower mortality in sepsis patients who were treated for ≥5 days, but it was ineffective when treatment was shorter.[15] Thus, the 4-day administration of vitamin C in the LOVIT trial may have been too short for sepsis patients, one quarter of whom had ICU stays ≥12 days.

In spite of the above findings, because of the merits of the study design the findings of the study holds importance. If not for the increased mortality associated with vitamin C, at least the fact that there was no improvement in any of the primary and secondary outcome parameters has to be considered with due respect. Hence, there is no positive implication from the study for the use of high-dose vitamin C in patients with sepsis.

IMPACT ON CURRENT PRACTICE AND TAKE HOME MESSAGE

Theoretically, vitamin C has been established to protect cells from oxidative damage, reduce inflammatory response, maintain immune functions, and increase the hemodynamic reserve. All these physiological rationales may be beneficial in the management of sepsis and septic shock. However, in the aftermath of recent interests and several multi-center trials including LOVIT trial, it can be concluded that there is still a lack of strong evidence to prove its clinical benefits. Hence, routine use of high-dose vitamin C is presently not recommended in the management of sepsis or septic shock. We recommend that future studies should focus on finding the ideal dosage, timing, and length of treatment as well as which critically ill patient population may benefit most from this therapy through carefully designed RCTs.

ARTICLE 50

Effect of High-dose Selenium on Postoperative Organ Dysfunction and Mortality in Cardiac Surgery Patients: The SUSTAIN CSX Randomized Clinical Trial

Stoppe C, McDonald B, Meybohm P, Christopher KB, Fremes S, Whitlock R, et al. SUSTAIN CSX Study Collaborators. Effect of high-dose selenium on postoperative organ dysfunction and mortality in cardiac surgery patients: the SUSTAIN CSX randomized clinical trial.

JAMA Surg. 2023;158(3):235-44.

CLINICAL QUESTION OR PROBLEM

Does high-dose selenium therapy impact outcomes in patients at high risk of organ dysfunction and death after cardiac surgery?

WHAT IS ALREADY KNOWN?

Cardiac surgery is performed in 1 million patients worldwide annually. Death and morbidity requiring immediate postoperative life-supportive therapy currently occur in nearly 20% of cardiac surgery patients. Prolonged life-supportive therapies negatively impact longer-term survival and quality of life. Major morbidity in cardiac surgery occurs in the context of oxidative stress from ischemia–reperfusion injury following operative global ischemic cardioplegic arrest of the heart or embolic events. Such oxidative stress triggers an intense inflammatory response marked by endothelial dysfunction, microvascular thrombosis, and injury of all major organ systems resulting in prolonged ICU stay.

Novel therapies to reduce the morbidity and mortality associated with high-risk cardiac surgery are needed. A potential way to reduce organ dysfunction is supplementation with the essential trace element selenium, which contributes to anti-inflammatory and immunomodulatory pathways and is a constituent of the active site of multiple antioxidant enzymes. In cardiac surgery patients, low selenium levels are associated with postoperative multiorgan failure and several smaller studies suggested significant clinical benefits associated with a selenium supplementation in cardiac surgery patients.[16] Of these, some showed that perioperative supplementation of high-dose selenium prevents the dramatic intraoperative decrease of circulating selenium levels, which leads to less oxidative stress, reduced need of postoperative vasoactive support, less myocardial injury, fewer organ dysfunctions, and reduced hospital LOS.[17]

These findings strengthen the hypothesis that this key nutrient can ameliorate oxidative stress and improve outcomes. Yet, a higher level of evidence was needed to inform clinical guidelines regarding the use of selenium in cardiac surgery patients.

STUDY DESIGN

It is an international, prospective, double-blind, randomized, placebo-controlled trial conducted at 23 sites in Canada and Germany. Consolidated Standards of Reporting Trials (CONSORT) reporting guideline was followed. Each patient gave written informed consent to participate in the study before surgery. Patients were screened from January 14, 2015 to January 11, 2021.

The participants were randomly assigned in a 1:1 ratio to the intervention and placebo groups, respectively. Randomization was performed through a central, password-protected, web-based system with an audit trail that has been used for several prior international studies. Selenium and placebo were provided similar in appearance, consistency, volume, and smell; study researchers were blinded to the treatment assignment at the time of enrolment to exclude selection bias.

According to the group allocation, patients either received 2,000 μg/L of intravenous selenium (sodium selenite; Selenase) within 30 minutes after induction of anesthesia and prior to initiation of cardiopulmonary bypass (CPB), then 2,000 μg/L of intravenous selenium immediately on admission to the postoperative ICU, then 1,000 μg/L of intravenous selenium each successive morning while in ICU or placebo at the same time points for a maximum of 10 days.

POPULATION STUDIED INCLUDING DEMOGRAPHICS

Inclusion Criteria

Adult patients (>18 years of age) scheduled to undergo elective or urgent cardiac surgery with the use of CPB and cardioplegic arrest that exhibit a high perioperative risk profile as defined by the presence of one or more of the following:
- Planned valve surgery combined with coronary artery bypass grafting (CABG) or multiple valve replacement/repair surgeries or combined cardiac surgical procedures involving the thoracic aorta
- Any cardiac surgery with a high perioperative risk profile, defined as a predicted operative mortality of ≥5% [EuroSCORE II (European System for Cardiac Operative Risk Evaluation)].

Exclusion Criteria

- Isolated procedures (CABG only or valve only)
- Known hypersensitivity to sodium selenite or to any of the constituents of the solution.
- Severe renal dysfunction as evidenced by preoperative creatinine clearance <50 mL/min and/or preoperative value of serum creatinine level above 200 micromoles/L; renal failure requiring dialysis at the point of screening.
- Chronic liver disease as evidenced by a preoperative total bilirubin > 2 mg/dL
- Disabling neuropsychiatric disorders (severe dementia, severe Alzheimer's disease, advanced Parkinson's disease)
- Pregnancy or lactation period
- Selenium supplementation (open-label selenium), not related to the study
- Patients undergoing heart transplantation or preoperative planned LVAD insertion or complex congenital heart surgery.

OUTCOMES EVALUATED

Primary Outcome

Number of days alive and free of persistent organ dysfunction within the first 30 days after surgery; persistent organ dysfunction was defined daily as the need for life-sustaining therapies that developed postoperatively at any time during the day. Life-sustaining therapies included mechanical ventilation, noninvasive ventilation, any vasopressor therapy, mechanical circulatory support, continuous renal replacement therapy, or intermittent hemodialysis. Patients who died within 30 days after surgery were recorded as having zero persistent organ dysfunction-free days.

Secondary Outcomes

- 30-day mortality
- Hospital-acquired infections
- Cardiovascular complications
- Duration of mechanical ventilation
- Incidence of postoperative delirium (measured by the Confusion Assessment Method for the ICU)
- ICU LOS
- Hospital readmission rates
- Hospital LOS
- Six-month survival
- Quality of life
- After hospital discharge, follow-up was performed at 3 and 6 months after randomization.
- To assess the safety of the study medication, patients were monitored daily for the occurrence of unexpected serious adverse events until death or discharge.

This primary modified intent-to-treat analysis included 1,394 patients with 697 in each treatment group. The baseline demographics and operative characteristics of patients were found to be similar in the selenium and placebo group. The results were as follows:

- Selenium did not increase the number of persistent organ dysfunction-free and alive days over the first 30 postoperative days [median (IQR), 29 (28–30) vs. 29 (28–30); $p = 0.45$].
- The 30-day mortality rates were 4.2% in the selenium and 5.0% in the placebo group (odds ratio 0.82; 95% CI 0.50–1.36; $p = 0.44$).
- Safety outcomes did not differ between the groups.

■ AUTHORS' VIEWPOINT

Preliminary evidence received from smaller studies provided mixed results on whether intravenous selenium supplementation was beneficial. A potential explanation for these divergent findings on efficacy was that trials with nonsignificant effects used single-dose selenium at a lower concentration compared with trials that used a higher dose given multiple times. However, results in this study did not support the hypothesis that high-dose daily intravenous selenium improves major clinical outcomes in high-risk cardiac surgery patients.

There are several potential reasons identified by authors for this neutral trial result, which differs from previous studies. Notably, this trial was the first and only multinational and multicenter study with an adequate sample size to determine if differences existed. Although they demonstrate an increase in selenium levels in the selenium group relative to the placebo group, normalization of circulating levels alone may not alter the cardiac surgery-related inflammatory response to oxidative stress. The activity of glutathione peroxidase, which is capable of neutralizing reactive oxygen and nitrogen species, did not differ between the trial groups indicating inadequate transcription of selenoproteins and thus a poor biological response to high-dose selenium. Patients may not have been deficient enough, as measured by their plasma selenium levels, as previous studies demonstrated best correlations between selenium and glutathione peroxidase at lower levels.[18]

Further, systemic inflammatory response-related cytokines are known to decrease expression of selenoproteins or secretion, which may limit the effect of high-dose selenium on urgent acutely diseased high-risk cardiac surgery cases.[19] Therefore, the administration of selenium immediately before surgery may have been too late to provide intraoperative benefit in our trial as a significant increase in the antioxidant glutathione peroxidase can take 72 hours. The efficacy of a preoperative selenium supplementation strategy initiated 2 weeks prior to surgery showed clinical benefits and raises the hypothesis that the early introduction of selenium prior to cardiac surgery may be of benefit.

Furthermore, recent innovations in surgical myocardial preservation techniques, such as combined antegrade and retrograde myocardial perfusion alone during bypass, are associated with smaller perioperative myocardial injury, which makes it challenging to demonstrate additional clinical benefits.[20] Thus, speculatively, optimization of surgical techniques may have led to a progressively smaller periprocedural injury and postoperative complications in trial participants. Improvement in cardiac surgery management may diminish the potential benefits of any additional organ protective strategy. A subgroup analysis designed to identify these higher-risk subpopulations did not demonstrate any significant treatment benefit. While frail patients tended to favor selenium, patients with urgent procedures or patients with prolonged CPB time showed a trend favoring placebo, which is in contrast to the hypothesis. There exists currently no surrogate markers to help identify patients who are sick but not too sick to ultimately benefit from the intervention and may provide explanations for the observed findings. More personalized approaches based on the patient's illness severity and/or inflammatory status seem to represent future goals for successful interventions.

They further postulate that more strategic approaches for identification of patients at higher risk for complicated postoperative courses and/or in combination with earlier introduction of selenium may translate into improved clinical outcomes.

■ STRENGTH OF THE STUDY

The strengths of this study include its robust scientific methods and high-fidelity implementation, the randomized and blinded design, rigorous determination of selenium laboratory values, and intent-to-treat analysis, all of which augment the internal validity of the trial.

The high rate of adherence to trial interventions, large number of patients, and enrolment in ICUs in Canada and Germany underline the high degree of precision and external validity.

■ DRAWBACK OF THE STUDY

One limitation of the trial is the use of the EuroSCORE II as part of the inclusion criteria to identify patients at increased risk for postoperative complications. The inaccuracy of the EuroSCORE II for cardiac surgery preoperative risk assessment is demonstrated in the discordance between the observed and predicted EuroSCORE II. Although the elevated EuroSCORE II closely correlated with the observed CPB and total operation time, indicating increased risk, this did not translate into clinically meaningful effects and the majority of enrolled patients had a rather short ICU LOS. Future trials therefore need to consider how to identify and enroll patients at higher risk.

A second limitation is that the population was predominantly male. Biosynthesis of selenoenzymes and selenoproteins is sex-specific in a dose-dependent manner. Further, the trial participants were predominantly

White, which may limit the generalizability of the findings to populations of other races and ethnicities. Selenium measurements differ according to ethnicity with Black individuals having the lowest selenium levels. In addition, the low enrolment of female individuals, which is consistent with other cardiovascular trials, makes it difficult to understand and address the implications of potential sex-specific responses.

■ REVIEWERS' VIEWPOINT

Though the study methodology was robust there were some important limitations as mentioned by the authors themselves. The primary endpoints as well as the secondary outcomes are not significantly different between the groups. They tried doing subanalysis to see if it was beneficial in certain subgroups but was again not found to be significant. The baseline selenium levels were below normal in almost all the patients and even after supplementing a high dose of selenium, the levels were just in the low normal range. The rise in selenium levels did not translate into the increase in glutathione peroxidase 3 activity which is considered to reflect the level of antioxidant action. So, it is obvious that supplementing high-dose selenium is not enough to improve the antioxidant effect in the study group to prevent organ failure and death. This negative trial is similar to the current evidences on the other antioxidant of interest, vitamin C. As the authors suggested the risk assessment tool for the surgery must be more accurate, future studies can try to elucidate the combined effect of selenium with other antioxidants like vitamin C and started much earlier before surgery.

■ IMPACT ON CURRENT PRACTICE AND TAKEHOME MESSAGE

In high-risk cardiac surgery patients, perioperative administration of high-dose intravenous sodium selenite did not reduce morbidity or mortality. The present data do not support the routine perioperative use of selenium for patients undergoing cardiac surgery.

ARTICLE 51

Parenteral Vitamin C in Patients with Severe Infection: A Systematic Review

Agarwal A, Basmaji J, Fernando SM, Ge FZ, Xiao Y, Faisal H, et al. Parenteral vitamin C in patients with severe infection: a systematic review.
NEJM Evid. 2022;1(9).

■ CLINICAL QUESTION OR PROBLEM

The efficacy and safety of parenteral vitamin C administration, as monotherapy or in combination with other therapies, in adult patients with severe infections, including coronavirus disease 2019 (COVID-19).

■ WHAT IS ALREADY KNOWN?

Severe infections manifest with inflammation and oxidative damage. Vitamin C (ascorbic acid) deficiency has been reported in patients with severe infection.[21] Preclinical evidence suggests that vitamin C supplementation may reduce endothelial injury in the pulmonary and systemic vasculature, oxidative damage, and harmful inflammation.[22] Critically ill patients and those with SARS-CoV-2 infection have low plasma vitamin C levels, and the World Health Organization (WHO) has included vitamin C among candidate therapies for COVID-19.[23,24]

Randomized controlled trials evaluating the effectiveness of vitamin C supplementation for severe infections, either alone or in combination with other therapies such as glucocorticoids and thiamine, have yielded varied results.[25] Systematic reviews have also shown variable effects.[26] The recent publication of results from LOVIT, the largest trial to date addressing this question, justifies a comprehensive reexamination of the evidence.

▪ STUDY DESIGN

A systematic review of RCTs of parenteral vitamin C as combined therapy or monotherapy versus no parenteral vitamin C administered to adults hospitalized with severe infection.

▪ POPULATION STUDIED INCLUDING DEMOGRAPHICS

Ovid MEDLINE, Embase, CINAHL, the Centers for Disease Control and Prevention COVID-19 database, Cochrane Central Register of Controlled Trials, and ClinicalTrials.gov from inception to March 30, 2021, were searched for randomized controlled trials evaluating parenteral vitamin C versus no parenteral vitamin C in hospitalized adults with severe infection. Eligible studies included at least one arm involving any dose of parenteral vitamin C alone or in combination with other cointerventions and at least one arm not involving parenteral vitamin C. Of 1,547 citations, 41 RCTs (n = 4,915 patients) were eligible for inclusion.

Among studies with data, the median patient age was 60 years (range 37–71) and the median proportion of female patients was 54%. Twenty-six studies reported baseline use of vasopressors, invasive ventilation, or other organ support. Six studies included patients exclusively with COVID-19. Nine trials evaluated low-dose therapy, 25 evaluated moderate-dose therapy, six evaluated high-dose therapy, and two did not report doses evaluated. One trial evaluated both low and high doses. Eleven trials used a weight-based regimen.

The most common daily dose was 6 g (21 studies). Of 22 trials evaluating combination therapy, 16 evaluated vitamin C therapy combined with hydrocortisone and thiamine. The control arm was placebo or usual care without vitamin C in 36 trials. In three trials, both vitamin C and control groups received an additional treatment as part of the regimen. In three trials, patients in the control group received hydrocortisone and in one trial each, they received ulinastatin and oral vitamin C.

▪ OUTCOMES EVALUATED

The primary outcomes of interest included inhospital, 30-day, and 90-day mortality. Because hospital discharge and 30 days were both considered to represent similar time points for mortality measurement after an intervention for an acute condition, they conducted a post hoc analysis of "early" mortality by adding 30-day mortality data to the meta-analysis of hospital mortality for studies not reporting the latter.

Secondary outcomes included use of and duration of ICU admission and invasive mechanical ventilation, duration of hospitalization, time to clinical improvement using change in WHO 7-point ordinal scale scores for clinical status or other severity measures, 72-hour change in SOFA score from baseline, stage 3 AKI based on Kidney Disease: Improving Global Outcomes (KDIGO) criteria, use of renal replacement therapy, serious adverse events leading to discontinuation of vitamin C, and specific prespecified adverse events (hemolysis, nephrolithiasis, and hypoglycemia). The time point of interest for all secondary outcomes was 30 days (except 72 hours or 3 days for SOFA scores), or the closest available.

Low-certainty evidence suggested that vitamin C may reduce:
- Inhospital mortality [21 RCTs, 2,762 patients; RR 0.88 (95% CI 0.73–1.06)].
- 30-day mortality [24 RCTs, 3,436 patients; RR 0.83 (95% CI 0.71–0.98)].
- Early mortality [before hospital discharge or 30 days; 34 RCTs, 4,366 patients; RR 0.80 (95% CI 0.68–0.93)].
- For 90-day mortality, all trials had low risk of bias; moderate-certainty evidence suggested harm [five RCTs, 1,722 patients; RR 1.07 (95% CI, 0.94–1.21)].

Moderate-certainty evidence suggested: An increased risk of hypoglycemia [RR 1.20 (95% CI, 0.69–2.08)]

Effects on other secondary outcomes were mixed and informed by low-certainty evidence. No credible subgroup effects were observed for mortality related to cointerventions (monotherapy vs. combined therapy), dose, or type of infection (COVID-19 vs. other).

■ AUTHORS' VIEWPOINT

Current international guidelines provide no recommendations for use of parenteral vitamin C for patients with COVID-19, a large group of acutely ill hospitalized patients for which even a small benefit of vitamin C would be of clinical relevance. They did not observe a differential effect of vitamin C in hospitalized patients with COVID-19 compared with other severe infections, but few vitamin C-treated patients with COVID-19 have been included in published trials. In contrast, guidelines provide a weak recommendation against the use of vitamin C in patients with sepsis or septic shock based on seven trials evaluating mortality, one trial evaluating organ failure, and one trial evaluating vasopressor use. This systematic review provides more compelling evidence to support this recommendation, informed by a larger and recent body of evidence.

■ STRENGTH OF THE STUDY

The study design of systematic review and meta-analysis adhered to the PRISMA (Preferred Reporting Items for Systematic Reviews and Meta-Analyses) reporting guidelines and the review protocol was publicly available. They used a comprehensive search strategy to incorporate all trials and conducted sensitivity and subgroup analyses to explore heterogeneity.

■ DRAWBACK OF THE STUDY

The main limitation is unexplained inconsistency of effects on early mortality. Although blinded low risk of bias published trials showed no statistically significant effects on mortality at any time point, the point estimates differed, with corresponding changes in interpretation as informed by a minimally contextualized GRADE approach. For this review, they did not adopt a fully contextualized GRADE approach used by guideline panels, which defines thresholds for trivial, small, moderate, and large effects and considers all critical outcomes, along with explicit statements of values and preferences.

REVIEWERS' VIEWPOINT

Though the study design was good and it tried to include all possible studies where vitamin C was used, there was a lot of variability in the trials included. The dose of vitamin C used was varying, the control arm was very different in many of the trials and the coadministration of other study drugs was also not uniform. Though all efforts were taken by the authors to subanalyze the study to see the effect of these confounders, it was not very convincing. The use of certainty of evidence and risk of bias to explain the results obtained may not be clearly understood by the readers. Effect of vitamin C in causing hypoglycemia is not obvious. There was low certainty of evidence in improvement in short-term mortality, but it was found to be harmful with moderate certainty of evidence when long-term mortality was taken into consideration. The reason for long-term mortality whether it can be attributed to vitamin C is anyhow questionable. Finally, it can be pronounced based on this review that vitamin C might not be beneficial and can be harmful when used in severe sepsis including COVID-19.

IMPACT ON CURRENT PRACTICE AND TAKE HOME MESSAGE

This meta-analysis has further reinforced the findings from earlier studies, such as the LOVIT trial, that vitamin C is no longer advised for the treatment of severe sepsis, including COVID-19.

REFERENCES

1. O'Meara D, Mireles-Cabodevila E, Frame F, Hummell AC, Hammel J, Dweik RA, et al. Evaluation of delivery of enteral nutrition in critically ill patients receiving mechanical ventilation. Am J Crit Care. 2008;17(1):53-61.
2. Schneider JA, Lee YJ, Grubb WR, Denny J, Hunter C. Institutional practices of withholding enteral feeding from intubated patients. Crit Care Med. 2009;37(7):2299-302.
3. Jiang Hua, Chen Wei, Hu Wen, et al. Effects of glutamine-enhanced enteral nutrition on clinical outcomes in critically ill patients: a systematic review of randomized controlled trials [J]. Chinese Journal of Burns. 2009; 25(5):325-30.
4. Singer P, Blaser AR, Berger MM, Alhazzani W, Calder PC, Casaer MP, et al. ESPEN guideline on clinical nutrition in the intensive care unit. Clin Nutr. 2019;38:48-79.
5. Yue HY, Wang Y, Zeng J, Jiang H, Li W. Enteral glutamine supplements for patients with severe burns: a systematic review and meta-analysis. Chinese Journal of Traumatology. 2023; ISSN 1008-1275.
6. Marik PE, Khangoora V, Rivera R, Hooper MH, Catravas J. Hydrocortisone, vitamin C, and thiamine for the treatment of severe sepsis and septic shock: a retrospective before-after study. Chest. 2017;151:1229-38.
7. Sevransky JE, Rothman RE, Hager DN, et al. Effect of vitamin C, thiamine, and hydrocortisone on ventilator- and vasopressor-free days in patients with sepsis:the VICTAS randomized clinical trial. JAMA. 2021;325:742-50.
8. Fujii T, Salanti G, Belletti A, et al. Effect of adjunctive vitamin C, glucocorticoids, and vitamin B1 on longer-term mortality in adults with sepsis or septic shock: a systematic review and a component network meta-analysis. Intensive Care Med. 2022;48:16-24.
9. Fowler AA III, Truwit JD, Hite RD, et al. Effect of vitamin C infusion on organ failure and biomarkers of inflammation and vascular injury in patients with sepsis and severe acute respiratory failure: the CITRIS-ALI randomized clinical trial. JAMA. 2019;322(13):1261-70.
10. Hemilä H, Chalker E. Vitamin C can shorten the length of stay in the ICU: a meta-analysis. Nutrients. 2019;11(4):708.
11. Hemilä H, Chalker E. Vitamin C may reduce the duration of mechanical ventilation in critically ill patients: a meta-regression analysis. J Intensive Care. 2020;8:15.

12. Fujii T, Salanti G, Belletti A, Bellomo R, Carr A, Furukawa TA, et al. Effect of adjunctive vitamin C, glucocorticoids, and vitamin B1 on longer-term mortality in adults with sepsis or septic shock: a systematic review and a component network meta-analysis. Intensive Care Med. 2022;48(1):16-24.
13. Patel JJ, Ortiz-Reyes A, Dhaliwal R, et al. IV vitamin C in critically ill patients: a systematic review and meta-analysis. Crit Care Med. 2022;50(3): e304-e12.
14. Hemilä H, Chalker E. Abrupt termination of vitamin C from ICU patients may increase mortality: secondary analysis of the LOVIT trial. Eur J Clin Nutr. 2023;77(4):490-4.
15. Jung SY, Lee MT, Baek MS, Kim WY. Vitamin C for ≥ 5 days is associated with decreased hospital mortality in sepsis subgroups: a nationwide cohort study. Crit Care. 2022; 26(1):3.
16. Stoppe C, Spillner J, Rossaint R, et al. Selenium blood concentrations in patients undergoing elective cardiac surgery and receiving perioperative sodium selenite. Nutrition. 2013;29(1):158-65.
17. Schmidt T, Pargger H, Seeberger E, Eckhart F, Felten S von, Haberthur C. Effect of high-dose sodium selenite in cardiac surgery patients: a randomized controlled bi-center trial. Clin Nutr. 2018;37(4):1172-80.
18. Demircan K, Bengtsson Y, Sun Q, et al. Serumselenium, selenoprotein P and glutathione peroxidase 3 as predictors of mortality and recurrence following breast cancer diagnosis:a multicentre cohort study. Redox Biol. 2021;47:102145.
19. Dreher I, Jakobs TC, Kohrle J. Cloning and characterization of the human selenoprotein P promoter: response of selenoprotein P expression to cytokines in liver cells. J Biol Chem. 1997;272(46):29364-71.
20. Candilio L, Malik A, Ariti C, et al. A retrospective analysis ofmyocardial preservation techniques during coronary artery bypass graft surgery: are we protecting the heart? J Cardiothorac Surg. 2014;9:184.
21. Moskowitz A, Andersen LW, Huang DT, et al. Ascorbic acid, corticosteroids, and thiamine in sepsis: a review of the biologic rationale and the present state of clinical evaluation. Crit Care. 2018;22:283.
22. Oudemans-van Straaten HM, Spoelstra-de Man AM, de Waard MC. Vitamin C revisited. Crit Care. 2014;18:460.
23. Galley HF, Davies MJ, Webster NR. Ascorbyl radical formation inpatients with sepsis: effect of ascorbate loading. Free Radic BiolMed. 1996;20:139–43.
24. World Health Organization. A coordinated global research roadmap: 2019 novel coronavirus. Geneva: World Health Organization, 2020 (https://www.who.int/publications/m/item/a-coordinatedglobal-research-roadmap).
25. Fujii T, Luethi N, Young PJ, et al. Effect of vitamin C, hydrocortisone, and thiamine vs. hydrocortisone alone on time alive and free of vasopressor support among patients with septic shock: the VITAMINS randomized clinical trial. JAMA. 2020;323:423–31.
26. Assouline B, Faivre A, Verissimo T, et al. Thiamine, ascorbic acid, and hydrocortisone as a metabolic resuscitation cocktail in sepsis: a meta-analysis of randomized controlled trials with trial sequential analysis. Crit Care Med. 2021;49:2112–20.

Section 11

Guidelines

Section Editors: Gunjan Chanchalani, Ranajit Chatterjee
Associate Editors: Lalit Gupta, Seema S Tekwani

ARTICLE 52

Analysis: ARDS Clinical Practice Guideline 2021

Tasaka S, Ohshimo S, Takeuchi M, Yasuda H, Ichikado K, Tsushima K, et al; ARDS Clinical Practice Guideline 2021 committee from the Japanese Society of Intensive Care Medicine; the Japanese Respiratory Society; the Japanese Society of Respiratory Care Medicine. ARDS Clinical Practice Guideline 2021.
J Intensive Care. 2022;10(1):32.

■ INTRODUCTION

The guidelines have been created with the joint effort of the Japanese Society of Intensive Care Medicine/Japanese Respiratory Society/Japanese Society of Respiratory Care Medicine, which covers clinical questions related to adults and to children with acute respiratory distress syndrome (ARDS).

■ CLINICAL QUESTION OR PROBLEM

Despite various advances, the mortality in ARDS continues to remain high at 25–40%. Much research is advanced in the same, with inconclusive results.

■ WHAT IS KNOWN?

Acute respiratory distress syndrome has varied etiology and very few strategies seem to improve morbidity and mortality.

■ POPULATION

Both adults and children with ARDS, for diagnosis and prognosis prediction, use of noninvasive and invasive respiratory support, adjunctive treatment, and use of drug and nondrug therapy.

■ INTERVENTION/METHOD USED

A systemic review method with the GRADE (Grading of Recommendations, Assessment, Development and Evaluation) system and a degree of recommendation determination method has been used.

Various steering and governing committees, support teams, and guideline consultants worked in collaboration to create clinical questions and evidence profiles, and thus finalize the clinical practice recommendations.

Five core areas were identified, and key clinical issues in these areas were identified and PICO (Population, Intervention, Comparator, Outcome) sheets created, followed by literature search, data extraction, evaluation, and integration to create recommendations. Modified Delphi method was used for consensus building at the panel meetings. Recommendations were graded as per the GRADE system.

■ NEW ISSUES ADDRESSED

The guideline gives a good practice statement to have a high suspicion for ARDS in patients with ARDS and shares weak recommendations on use of respective diagnostic tests and identification of cause of ARDS for pneumococcal pneumonia, *Legionella* pneumonia, cytomegalovirus (CMV) pneumonia, invasive pulmonary aspergillosis, and also use of blood brain natriuretic peptide (BNP) and NT-proBNP levels for identifying cardiogenic pulmonary edema. However, it recommended against using C-reactive protein (CRP) and procalcitonin (PCT) levels be used for identifying bacterial pneumonia as the underlying cause, and against use of antigen tests of the pharyngeal/nasopharyngeal swabs and PCR tests of the bronchoalveolar lavage fluid be used for identifying influenza pneumonia.

For prognostication, it recommends only considering tests for lung pathology for the same by use of imaging or PF [partial pressure of oxygen in arterial blood (PaO_2) to the fraction of inspiratory oxygen concentration (FiO_2)] ratio.

Weak recommendation is provided for doing early tracheostomy in adult patients with ARDS, with no objective criteria provided for the decision-making of the same. A weak recommendation to start rehabilitation in 72 hours has been provided. A weak recommendation to give high omega-3 fatty acids in enteral nutrition is suggested.

■ CHANGES FROM CURRENT GUIDELINES

Weak recommendation to use noninvasive positive pressure ventilation (NPPV)/high-flow nasal cannula (HFNC) over conventional oxygen or tracheal intubation, if no contraindications for the same; however, it stresses on avoiding a delay in tracheal intubation, as it worsens mortality.

Strong recommendation for low tidal volume (TV) ventilation is continued, however the range of TV mentioned is 4–8 mL/kg. A high positive end-expiratory pressure (PEEP) is recommended in mechanically ventilated patients, with limiting plateau pressures. No recommendation for any specific mode of ventilation has been provided [pressure-controlled ventilation (PCV)/volume-controlled ventilation (VCV)/airway pressure release ventilation (APRV)/high frequency oscillatory ventilation (HFOV)], and suggest it to choose the mode as per common practice.

No reference range to mild permissive hypoxemia is suggested, however suggests against excessively low PaO_2 levels. It suggests use of neuromuscular (NM) blockers in early phase of moderate-to-severe ARDS, for no longer than 48 hours, however, no mention of use by infusion or bolus or monitoring has been provided.

The guidelines suggest use of prone positioning in moderate-to-severe ARDS, and extracorporeal membrane oxygenation (ECMO) in severe ARDS, lacking objective criteria of PF ratio. There is a strong recommendation for use of low-dose corticosteroids, 1–2 mg/kg of methylprednisolone. A weak recommendation to use minimal or no sedation in mechanically ventilated adult ARDS patients.

The guidelines suggest against the use of nitric oxide inhalation and high-dose corticosteroids.

Strengths

- A joint effort of various societies of respiratory and intensive care.

- A detailed recommendation covering from diagnosis to respiratory management, drug therapy, and physical therapy, to allow use by healthcare professionals from multiple disciples, including non-specialist physicians.
- Includes recommendations for pediatric patients with ARDS.
- Emphasis is laid on diagnosing the cause for ARDS.

Weaknesses

- Originally written for Japanese healthcare professionals
- Excluded coronavirus disease 2019 (COVID-19) ARDS in view of insufficient evidence
- TV limits have been mentioned 4–8 mL/kg with no mention of using the predicted body weight/ideal body weight has been suggested.
- No upper limit for plateau pressures have been provided, and no recommendation or even good practice statement for use of driving pressure has been provided.
- No mention for permissive hypercapnia has been made.
- Lacks objective criteria to use of prone positioning and ECMO.
- Though it gives a strong recommendation for low-dose corticosteroids, it stays silent about the time of initiation and duration.

REVIEWERS' OPINION

The guidelines have summarized the recommendations about the care of adult and pediatric patients with ARDS, in the current review we have analyzed only the recommendations for adult ARDS patients.

Though the guidelines outlines the management of ARDS, it does not provide objective criteria to use various modalities - the accuracy in defining use of predicted body weight, use of steroids, and acceptable targets of oxygenation and ventilation. No mention for targets of plateau pressure and no recommendations for driving pressure make them incomplete. Prone positioning continues to give a weak recommendation.

Some recommendations appear quite vague such as use of early tracheostomy and rehabilitation in 72 hours and use of omega 3 fatty acids.

Overall, a poor guideline to refer to, by intensive care professionals, as it lacks precision.

ARTICLE 53

Analysis: Awake Proning in Patients with COVID-19-related Hypoxemic Acute Respiratory Failure: A Rapid Practice Guideline

Myatra SN, Alhazzani W, Belley-Cote E, Møller MH, Arabi YM, Chawla R, et al. Awake proning in patients with COVID-19-related hypoxemic acute respiratory failure: A rapid practice guideline.
Acta Anaesthesiol Scand. 2023;67(5):569-75.

CLINICAL QUESTION OR PROBLEM

Coronavirus disease 2019 pandemic has been a challenge and resource limitation, led to use of awake proning in hypoxemic patients. However, various studies used different protocols and no recommendations have been available till date.

WHAT IS KNOWN?

Awake proning is a simple maneuver that can intubation and invasive ventilation in some patients. This should be protocolized and requires efforts by the medical team and meticulous monitoring, to detect failure and prevent delay in ventilation in such a case.

POPULATION

All COVID-19 patients with acute hypoxemic respiratory failure, who are not intubated.

INTERVENTION/METHOD USED

A panel of 20 experts from 12 countries, including one patient representative, along with methodological support from Guidelines in Intensive Care, Development, and Evaluation (GUIDE) group, evaluated the evidence using the GRADE method and thus developed recommendations using the Evidence to Decision framework.

NEW ISSUES ADDRESSED

The panel recommends a trial of awake prone positioning in patients with acute hypoxemic respiratory failure due to COVID-19, if feasible. The target should be at least 4–6 hours per day, and higher if tolerated.

These patients should be monitored in an area where there is availability of experienced staff who can rapidly detect deterioration and are knowledgeable to manage them.

CHANGES FROM CURRENT GUIDELINES

No clear previous guidelines are available on this condition.

Strengths

- Experts from 12 countries were included in the panel.
- A patient representative was also included, as the technique involves patient cooperation and tolerability.

Weaknesses

- Awake proning may not be feasible in some patients and some patients may not tolerate it.
- Trial of awake proning may not be feasible in many patients with contraindications and most trials on awake proning have excluded such patients.

REVIEWERS' OPINION

All hypoxemic COVID-19 patients should be given a trial of awake proning. Awake proning if well tolerated, reduces the risk of trachea intubation, although it may not reduce mortality.

ARTICLE 54
Analysis: Practice Update to Optimise the Performance and Interpretation of Blood Cultures: 2022

Papavarnavas N S, Brink A J, Dlamini S, Wasserman S, Whitelaw A, Ntusi N A B, et al. Practice update to optimise the performance and interpretation of blood cultures: 2022.
S Afr Med J. 2022;112(6).

■ CLINICAL QUESTION OR PROBLEM

Blood cultures are essential for diagnostic stewardship in patients with infection and can change outcomes.

■ WHAT IS KNOWN?

Collecting blood cultures during the febrile phase and prior to antibiotic administration, collection of higher volume and use of two sets (each set includes aerobic and anaerobic culture bottle), can increase the yield of the culture and thus influence outcomes in patients with infection.

■ POPULATION

All patients with suspected infection and intermediate to high likelihood of having a positive blood culture.

■ INTERVENTION/METHOD USED

Literature search and evaluation of the evidence has been discussed in the document. Details on the panel involved in formulating the guidelines and the process used have not been documented in the article.

■ NEW ISSUES ADDRESSED

In resource-limited settings, standard culture bottles are defined sufficient for use in suspected candidemia.

If suspicion of tuberculosis and systemic nontuberculous mycobacterial infections, obtaining at least one *Mycobacterium tuberculosis* (MTB) blood culture, and if resources permit, obtaining two is suggested for the investigation of disseminated tuberculosis in hospitalized patients. This culture is in addition to other diagnostic tests for mycobacteria.

Follow-up blood culture is recommended for methicillin-resistant *Staphylococcus aureus* (MRSA) bloodstream infection (BSI) and *Staphylococcus lugdunensis* BSI at 2–4 days' interval.

■ CHANGES FROM CURRENT GUIDELINES

Septic patients who need urgent antibiotic administration, blood cultures should be collected preferential, or within 45 minutes of before antibiotic administration.

Usually, two bottles per set of blood cultures and two sets of blood cultures, which equates to blood volume of 40 mL to be collected; the current article recommends taking two bottles be taken as two separate procedures in settings with resource limitations.

Both anaerobic and aerobic blood culture bottles are to be used and in such a scenario, anaerobic blood culture bottles should be inoculated first.

In resource-limited settings with suspected infective endocarditis (IE), three aerobic blood culture bottles from different peripheral sites, each separated in time, ~30 minutes prior to antibiotic administration should be taken. Whereas, for other infections, two aerobic blood cultures taken at the same time from two different sites can be taken.

The guidelines recommend against use of double-needle technique for blood collection.

70% alcohol/0.5% chlorhexidine gluconate solution can be used for skin preparation in adults, prior to blood collection.

Follow-up blood culture for candida BSI should preferably be done daily or three times per week if daily is not feasible.

Strengths

- The guidelines are quite crisp and clear, based on evidence search.
- Recommendations have been drafted keeping in mind the resource-limited conditions of Africa, and thus can be used for many other such resource-limited countries.

Weaknesses

- The process of formulating the guidelines has not been described.
- No grading of the recommendations have been done.

■ REVIEWERS' OPINION

Blood cultures are an important tool for diagnostic stewardship in critically ill infected patients, and if used properly can help in antibiotic stewardship, thus reducing development of antibiotic resistance. Following the simple principles, as defined in the guidelines and tailored as per individual patient and hospital setup, these can improve the yield of the test.

Further research is needed in understanding the use of PCR-based identification of infection, along with the resistance parents to improve patient outcomes.

ARTICLE 55

Analysis: Canadian Stroke Best Practice Recommendations: Acute Stroke Management, 7th Edition Practice Guidelines Update, 2022

Heran M, Lindsay P, Gubitz G, Yu A, Ganesh A, Lund R, et al. Canadian stroke best practice recommendations: Acute stroke management, 7th edition practice guidelines update, 2022.

Can J Neurol Sci. 2022:1-94.

■ CLINICAL QUESTION OR PROBLEM

Appropriate management of acute stroke has great implications in the quality of life of the patients. With the wealth of data available recently from various clinical trials on reperfusion therapies in acute ischemic stroke, stroke guidelines are possibly one of the rapidly changing guidelines in critical care medicine.

■ WHAT IS KNOWN?

Awareness and early recognition of stroke, and thrombolysis of ischemic within the window period under close monitoring and BP control, has been a game changer for the patients presenting with symptoms of acute stroke of transient ischemic attack (TIA). The use of mechanical methods of thrombectomy and treatment of wake up stroke has been an advancement to further management of stroke, with improved outcomes. The approval of use of tenecteplase as a thrombolytic agent, has been a boon for low-income countries.

POPULATION

Initial section pertains to awareness, triaging, and emergency management of all patients with acute stroke or TIA. The later sections are specific for management of patients with acute ischemic stroke or TIA.

INTERVENTION/METHOD USED

An interdisciplinary group of experts along with seven people with stroke and one caregiver participated in the process of guideline formulation. Peer-reviewed literature search was done, and reviewed and after discussing and debating the evidence, GRADE system was used to develop a final set of recommendations.

NEW ISSUES ADDRESSED

A strong recommendation has been provided for use of virtual care for secondary stroke prevention.

Use of tenecteplase for thrombolysis has been given a strong recommendation, along with alteplase. A clinical decision to use thrombolysis versus endovascular therapy (EVT) in an eligible patient should be based on the principle of "time is brain" and the anticipated time for door-to-needle versus door-to-puncture.

A detailed section on the management of intracerebral hemorrhage (ICH) or extracranial hemorrhage following thrombolysis, has been included, with strong recommendations on doing an immediate NCCT (noncontrast computed tomography) head, and conditional recommendation for the use of fibrinogen concentrates, fresh frozen plasma, cryoprecipitate, tranexamic acid, and against use of prothrombin complex concentrates, platelet transfusions, and factor VIIa.

Another important aspect covered is the pre- and postoperative care of patients undergoing EVT.

CHANGES FROM CURRENT GUIDELINES

A detailed section on evaluation of patients with acute stroke, including recommendations on use of blood work, echocardiography, and acute brain imaging has been discussed. A strong recommendation has been laid on screening of stroke on-scene by the paramedic and rapid mobilization, with special emphasis to look for signs of large-vessel occlusion and referring this group of patients for early EVT. A prenotification while en route to the emergency medical service (EMS) with activation of a "Code Stroke" is strongly recommended.

A strong recommendation has been evaluation of need for intravenous (IV) thrombolysis or EVT, in patients with disabling within 6 hours of onset of symptoms, after consultation with a stroke specialist onsite or virtually.

Strengths

- Every aspect of management of acute ischemic stroke has been covered, in detail with precise recommendation statements.
- Meticulous literature search and grading for all recommendations has been done.

Weaknesses

- Country-specific guidelines and cannot be applied globally, especially to low-income countries.

- No recommendation has been made on use of mobile stroke units to improve outcomes, when other countries like Australia, USA, and Germany have already proven its benefit in randomized trials.

REVIEWERS' OPINION

Very clear and comprehensive guidelines, with detailed review of latest evidence and advances in the management of acute stroke.

The guidelines are extensive and precise, looking into every minute aspect of management of a patient with acute stroke, including early investigations needed, early evaluation including assessment of swallowing and also monitoring with clear targets and even recommendations of performance of minor procedures like use of urethral catheters.

However, more changes in the evidence and recommendations are expected faster, more so on the topic of use of EVT, with or without thrombolysis, and in posterior circulation stroke, as clinical trials are underway. It is important to stay updated with the latest research on the management of acute stroke to provide the best evidence-based practice to the patients.

ARTICLE 56

Analysis: Expert Consensus on the Glycemic Management of Critically Ill Patients

Wu Z, Liu J, Zhang D, Kang K, Zuo X, Xu Q, et al. Expert consensus on the glycemic management of critically ill patients.
J Intensive Med. 2022;2(3):131-45.

An expert working group on glycemic management composed of Chinese experts in critical medicine, conducted five rounds on discussions to strengthen the glycemic management of critically ill patients, and issued 26 statements for providing guidance and reference opinions for the same, using the GRADE approach.

CLINICAL QUESTION OR PROBLEM

The ideal target glucose in critically ill is unknown, with a disagreement among guideline recommendations.

Society of Critical Care Medicine recommends a target blood glucose 140–180 mg/dL,[1] whereas the American College of Physicians recommends a target of 140–200 mg/dL.[2]

WHAT IS KNOWN?

Glycemic variability plays a significant contribution to increased mortality in the critically ill patients. Hyperglycemia, relative hyperglycemia, and more so hypoglycemia are associated with increased mortality in the intensive care unit (ICU).

POPULATION

The guidelines are for adult critically ill patient, irrespective of their diabetic status preadmission to the ICU.

INTERVENTION/METHOD USED

A group of Chinese experts on glycemic management in critical medicine conducted five rounds of discussion to create recommendations on 26 important statements about glycemic management in critically ill patients. The research progress worldwide, along with the current situation in China, was taken into consideration and a consensus established. Using the PICO principles, clinical issues were identified and recommendations developed using the GRADE approach. Each recommendation was included after detailed collective discussion and only if there was sustained agreement to the same ≥80%.

■ NEW ISSUES ADDRESSED

A weak recommendation in favor of more accurate measurement by arterial blood gas analyzers overuse of glucometers.

A weak recommendation to monitor coefficient of variation of blood glucose, and adjust insulin levels to minimize glycemic swings and thus reduce fatality.

Metformin is suggested in combination with insulin, if there is suspicion of insulin resistance.

There is a detailed section of identification and management of hypoglycemia and expert opinion in use of clinical signs of unexplainable tachycardia, sweating, drop in blood pressure and wide pulse pressure be taken as a sign of hypoglycemia in sedated patients.

A suggestion to closely monitor blood glucose level every 15 minutes, after an episode of hypoglycemia until stabilization and every 1–2 hours in patients at high risk of hypoglycemia. While correcting iatrogenic hypoglycemia, a weak recommendation is made to stop insulin infusion and 15–20 g of glucose be administered and repeated until the target range is achieved and also avoid over administration of glucose and avoidance of iatrogenic hyperglycemia.

■ CHANGES FROM CURRENT GUIDELINES

A weak recommendation to monitoring period not longer than 1 hour in admitted critically ill patients or those who are critically ill and on continuous insulin infusion until glucose levels and the rate of insulin injection are stabilized.

A suggestion was made to prefer arterial blood sample over venous blood for glucose monitoring, and to use continuous glucose monitoring (CGM) in patients with huge blood glucose fluctuations.

Recommendation on sugar control in hyperglycemic patients while using parenteral nutrition for critically ill patients are all based on expert opinion, with suggestion to limit that the rate of glucose infusion to not exceed 5 mg/kg/min, and using IV insulin alone.

Target blood sugar levels in various clinical situations is defined, with a weak recommendation and at places where evidence is lacking as an expert opinion **(Table 1)**.

Strengths

- These are evidence-based guidelines with an attempt to deal into every aspect of glucose control.
- A section of monitoring and control of hypoglycemia in critically ill has been included.

Weaknesses

While these guidelines provide valuable insights, they have a few limitations, given as follows:
1. Most recommendations are weak with low level of evidence and expert opinion. Only three strong recommendations have been made and this points toward lack of high-quality research in the topic.

TABLE 1: The target range of blood sugar levels in various disease conditions.

Disease condition	Low target limit (mg/dL)	High target limit (mg/dL)	Level of recommendation
Nondiabetic critically ill	110	140	Weak
Diabetic critically ill	110	200	Weak
Severe brain injury*	110	200	Weak
Septic	70–80	180–200	Weak
Severe acute pancreatitis	140	180	Expert opinion
Postoperative major surgery —nondiabetic	140	180	Strong
Severe burn patients	*Avoid glycemic variability		Strong
For inpatients receiving glucocorticoids	*Less strict blood glucose goals		Expert opinion

* In severe brain patients, it is strongly recommended against an intensive regimen of 80–106 mg/dL.

2. The authors suggest that they have been tailored to the Chinese population.
3. Lack of blood sugar targets in various conditions like burns and acute pancreatitis.

■ REVIEWERS' OPINION

Limited by the available evidence, these guidelines have covered the subjected from all aspects, right from the source of blood sampling, frequency of sampling, the method of sugar measurement and blood sugar targets in numerous subpopulations, to detection and correction of hypoglycemia. However, "one size does not fit all" and the therapy should be individualized and tailored.

The management of glucose levels in stable ICU patients has not been discussed, and use of subcutaneous insulin administration may be considered in this group of population.

More prospective RCTs are needed in various populations and subpopulations, to have stronger recommendations to management of blood sugar levels in the critically ill.

ARTICLE 57

Analysis: ERS/ESICM/ESCMID/ALAT Guidelines for the Management of Severe Community-acquired Pneumonia

Martin-Loeches I, Torres A, Nagavci B, Aliberti S, Antonelli M, Bassetti M, et al. ERS/ESICM/ESCMID/ALAT guidelines for the management of severe community-acquired pneumonia.
Intensive Care Med. 2023;49(6):615-32.

■ INTRODUCTION

The European Respiratory Society (ERS), European Society of Intensive Care Medicine (ESICM), European Society of Clinical Microbiology and Infectious Diseases (ESCMID), and Latin American Thoracic Association (ALAT) collaborated to create the first international guidelines for severe community-acquired pneumonia (sCAP). The guidelines, developed by a multidisciplinary team of experts from Europe and North America, address eight clinical questions related to sCAP diagnosis and treatment.

They aim to offer guidance on effective treatments and management strategies for adult sCAP patients admitted to the ICU, primarily for healthcare professionals in respiratory and intensive care medicine, but also relevant to general internists, infectious disease specialists, pharmacists, microbiologists, and policymakers.

The critical analysis of these guidelines provides a deeper understanding and evaluation of its content, ensuring that the information is reliable and relevant.

■ WHAT IS KNOWN?

The guidelines commence by outlining the existing knowledge pertaining to sCAP. This initial section is vital because it provides a foundational understanding for the recommendations that ensue. It underscores the need for precise definitions and criteria for sCAP, an imperative step in ensuring consistent clinical practices, acknowledging that existing knowledge helps an insight in the evolving field of pneumonia management.

■ POPULATION

A significant emphasis is placed on the patient population affected by sCAP. The guidelines underscore the urgency of early recognition and intervention, particularly in critically ill patients. This encompasses individuals with severe respiratory failure, sepsis, and shock. Notably, the guidelines advocate for clear risk factors and criteria to identify these patients accurately, ensuring timely, and appropriate care.

■ INTERVENTION

A substantial portion of the guidelines is devoted to the topic of intervention, specifically antibiotic therapy for sCAP. Rapid administration of suitable antibiotics is highlighted as a cornerstone of management. Beta-lactam antibiotics are recommended as the primary therapy, with guidance provided on antibiotic selection based on patient-specific factors, including comorbidities and local epidemiology. The guidelines emphasize the urgency of the appropriate antibiotic regimen to combat the underlying infection.

■ CONTROL

Control measures are discussed comprehensively, with a strong emphasis on the importance of early empirical antibiotic therapy. This is crucial for mitigating the progression of sCAP and reducing morbidity and mortality. Moreover, the guidelines advocate for continuous monitoring of clinical responses with an agile approach to therapy adjustment based on these responses. The control measures are dynamic, reflecting the evolving nature of the patient's condition.

■ OUTCOMES

The guidelines place considerable importance on various outcome measures. These encompass parameters such as mortality rates, length of hospital stay, and clinical stability. These outcome metrics are not only used for evaluating the effectiveness of interventions but also serve as benchmarks for quality of care in sCAP management. Regular assessment of these outcomes informs clinical decision-making and helps fine-tune treatment strategies.

■ STRENGTH

The strengths of these guidelines for the management of sCAP lie in their comprehensive approach to addressing a complex and critical medical condition.
- *Evidence-based recommendations*: One of the primary strengths of these guidelines is their reliance on existing evidence and systematic reviews. They draw from a vast body of clinical research to form

recommendations. This evidence-based approach enhances the credibility of the guidelines, providing a solid foundation for clinical decision-making.

- *Clear differentiation of recommendations*: The guidelines effectively differentiate between strong and conditional recommendations. This distinction is vital as it reflects the varying levels of confidence in the evidence supporting each recommendation. Strong recommendations are based on high-quality, consistent evidence, instilling confidence in clinicians to follow them as best practices. In contrast, conditional recommendations are made when the evidence base is less robust or when patient-specific factors should influence the decision-making process. This flexibility acknowledges the complexity of sCAP management.
- *Multidisciplinary collaboration*: The guidelines stress the importance of a multidisciplinary approach to sCAP management. They emphasize collaboration among various healthcare providers, including emergency physicians, pulmonologists, intensivists, and infectious disease specialists. This collaborative approach fosters a holistic and well-rounded perspective on patient care, ensuring that all aspects of the patient's condition are addressed effectively.
- *Patient-centered care*: These guidelines underscore the significance of tailoring treatment to individual patient characteristics. They acknowledge that not all sCAP cases are the same and encourage clinicians to consider comorbidities, local epidemiology, and patient preferences when making treatment decisions. This patient-centered approach aligns with the broader shift in healthcare toward personalized medicine, recognizing that a one-size-fits-all approach may not be suitable for complex conditions like sCAP.
- *Monitoring and adaptability*: The guidelines highlight the importance of continuous monitoring of clinical responses to therapy. This dynamic approach allows for real-time adjustments in treatment plans based on a patient's progress or deterioration. It aligns with the concept of "patient response-guided therapy", ensuring that care remains tailored to the evolving needs of the individual.
- *Bridge between research and practice*: These guidelines serve as a bridge between the latest research findings and clinical practice. They take into account the challenges of implementing research findings in real-world settings and offer practical recommendations. By doing so, they aim to close the gap between evidence generation and application, ultimately improving patient outcomes.

■ WEAKNESS

While these guidelines provide valuable insights into the management of sCAP, they are not without their limitations.

- *Limited high-quality evidence*: A significant challenge in developing these guidelines is the paucity of high-quality evidence in certain areas of sCAP management. Clinical trials involving critically ill patients, especially those with sCAP, are challenging to conduct due to ethical and logistical issues. As a result, some recommendations are based on lower-quality evidence or expert consensus, which may limit their applicability and robustness.
- *Heterogeneity in sCAP cases*: sCAP is not a homogeneous condition. Patients can present with varying degrees of severity, underlying comorbidities, and causative pathogens. These guidelines

acknowledge the heterogeneity of sCAP but may not provide specific guidance for every unique scenario. Clinicians must exercise clinical judgment in applying the recommendations to individual cases.
- *Resource and setting variability*: The guidelines do not extensively address resource and setting variability. The management of sCAP can differ significantly between high-resource settings with access to advanced diagnostic tools and low-resource settings with limited healthcare infrastructure. Tailoring recommendations to different resource settings would enhance their global applicability.
- *Limited discussion of pediatric sCAP*: These guidelines primarily focus on adult patients with sCAP. The management of sCAP in pediatric populations may involve distinct considerations and challenges. A dedicated section addressing pediatric sCAP management would have been valuable for clinicians who care for children with this condition.
- *Timing of updates*: Medical knowledge and research are continually evolving. These guidelines are based on the evidence available up to a specific point in time. As such, they may not reflect the latest developments in sCAP management. Regular updates to guidelines are crucial to incorporate emerging evidence and ensure that clinicians have access to the most current recommendations.
- *Lack of cost considerations*: The guidelines do not explore into cost considerations associated with sCAP management. While clinical effectiveness is paramount, healthcare systems worldwide are increasingly concerned with the cost-effectiveness of interventions. Integrating cost considerations into future iterations of the guidelines would provide a more comprehensive perspective.

■ CHANGE IN PRACTICE

A key objective of the guidelines is to facilitate changes in clinical practice. They provide evidence-based recommendations and advocate for a multidisciplinary approach involving collaboration among healthcare providers. By doing so, the guidelines aim to bridge the gap between research findings and bedside care, ultimately improving patient outcomes.

■ SUGGESTED RESEARCH PRIORITIES

The guidelines play a pivotal role in shaping research priorities in the field of sCAP management. They pinpoint areas necessitating further investigation, including the need for well-designed international multicenter, RCTs. These RCTs are envisioned to evaluate various facets of sCAP management, including antibiotic therapy, biomarker-guided therapy, antiviral therapy, corticosteroid use, and the utility of prediction scores in guiding treatment decisions. This forward-looking approach is instrumental in advancing the field.

■ OVERALL ASSESSMENT

In summation, these guidelines offer a comprehensive roadmap for managing sCAP, from diagnosis to treatment. They acknowledge the limitations of the current evidence base while providing recommendations with varying levels of strength to guide clinical practice. The emphasis on research priorities underscores the commitment to continually enhance the care of sCAP patients. Clinicians should regard these guidelines as an indispensable resource in their decision-making process when managing patients with sCAP. They offer not only a synthesis of existing knowledge but also a forward-looking perspective on areas requiring further exploration, ultimately contributing to improved patient care and outcomes.

ARTICLE 58

Analysis: Atrial Fibrillation Occurring During Acute Hospitalization: A Scientific Statement From the American Heart Association

Chyou JY, Barkoudah E, Dukes JW, Goldstein LB, Joglar JA, Lee AM, et al; American Heart Association Acute Cardiac Care and General Cardiology Committee, Electrocardiography and Arrhythmias Committee, and Clinical Pharmacology Committee of the Council on Clinical Cardiology; Council on Cardiovascular Surgery and Anesthesia; Council on Cardiopulmonary, Critical Care, Perioperative and Resuscitation; Council on Cardiovascular and Stroke Nursing; and Stroke Council. Atrial fibrillation occurring during acute hospitalization: A scientific statement from the American Heart Association.

Circulation. 2023;147:e676-e698.

CLINICAL QUESTION OR PROBLEM

Atrial fibrillation (AF) can manifest acutely in various medical and surgical conditions and warrants specific guidelines for its acute management as well as long-term follow-up.

WHAT IS KNOWN?

Atrial fibrillation, which develops in the context of acute illness, is associated with increased morbidity and greater mortality and a high risk of chronic AF.

POPULATION

Acutely ill patients develop AF, and it can manifest in both medical and surgical conditions.

INTERVENTION/METHOD USED

The writing group consisted of the association of cardiology, acute care, electrophysiologists, clinical pharmacologists, cardiovascular surgery and anesthesia, cardiopulmonary (CP), critical care, perioperative and resuscitation, and stroke and stroke nursing. Data was reviewed from randomized clinical trials, registries, and observational studies to form the guidelines.

NEW ISSUES ADDRESSED

A new terminology "acute AF" has been introduced for AF developing in acute care settings or during an acute illness.

Use of predicting scores (CHA_2DS_2-VASc score) and additional factors like type of surgery, elevated brain natriuretic peptide (BNP) is suggested. A multipronged approach needs to be used for management, with multidisciplinary involvement, identifying triggers, and substrates for the same.

Individualized approach to choice of rate versus rhythm control and management of anticoagulation needs to be considered. The document also covers the detailed management of acute AF in specific areas like emergency room (ER), intensive care units (ICUs), and also in specific conditions like coronavirus disease 2019 (COVID-19) disease, hyperthyroidism, stroke, cardiac, and noncardiac surgery.

CHANGES FROM CURRENT GUIDELINES

No such specific guidelines have been made in the past. However, the long-term management is similar to long-term management of AF. Long-term management involves monitoring, lifestyle, and risk factor modification, in addition to rate and rhythm control and anticoagulation.

Strengths
- Specific guidelines for acute AF
- Management in various settings and conditions has been covered.
- Multidisciplinary involvement in the formation of the scientific statement.

Weaknesses
Acute AF is a new terminology with gaps in the current knowledge and there are large gaps in the current knowledge, and limited research.

■ REVIEWERS' OPINION
Acute AF and is not benign and the current guideline has covered the scope of the topic in detail, with management in various settings and conditions. It will be useful at various settings in the hospital and involvement of authors from various disciplines, has made it very comprehensive.

The scientific statement covers a very important topic, however with the current gaps in the knowledge on the subject, makes the statement volatile and demands further research on this topic. The authors have also defined the scope for the future research.

ARTICLE 59

Analysis: Organ Donation after Circulatory Determination of Death in India: A Joint Position Paper

Seth AK, Mohanka R, Navin S, Gokhale AG, Sharma A, Kumar A, et al. Organ donation after circulatory determination of death in India: A joint position paper.

Indian J Crit Care Med. 2022;26(4):421-38.

■ CLINICAL QUESTION OR PROBLEM
The organ donation in India is mainly donation after brainstem death, and the donation rate has been very low, <1 per million population. The Transplantation of Human Organs Act, 1994 defines a "deceased person" as one in whom permanent disappearance of all evidence of life occurs, by reason of brain stem death or in a CP sense at any time after live birth has taken place.

Donation after brain death and living organ donations are unable to fill the rising demand for organs for transplant.

■ WHAT IS KNOWN?
Brain death accounts for only 2% of all deaths after devastating brain injury due to trauma, stroke, or hypoxia. Organ donation after circulatory determination of death (DCDD) is authorized or planned when death is anticipated and such donation before death or after death poses new challenges—medical, procedural, ethical, legal, and economical.

■ POPULATION
Patients with futile available treatment options, with options of do not attempt resuscitation (DNAR), withdrawal of life-sustaining treatment (WLST), end-of-life-care (EOLC), and palliative care.

■ INTERVENTION/METHOD USED
Various professional societies with expertise in various fields including legal and Indian

Ministry compiled this document, keeping in mind the existing international best practices, tailored as per Indian population. Various rounds of virtual interactions, due to imposed restrictions by the COVID pandemic, were conducted and written inputs and write-ups of all authors were compiled, edited, and finalized to form a joint position station for furthering DCDD in India.

■ NEW ISSUES ADDRESSED

Modified Maastricht classification was chosen relevant to India, to classify DCDD based on the circumstances of death.

Legislations, guidelines, procedures, protocols for declaration of death, consent, no-touch period, antemortem interventions, and organ preservation methods are discussed as per unique ethical, social, cultural, legal, and economic factors in India.

A checklist with importance on documentation has been made, along with specifications as per organ considered for retrieval.

■ CHANGES FROM CURRENT GUIDELINES

No such guidelines/position statements on DCDD have been published previously.

Strengths

- Multidisciplinary panel—including intensive care physicians, transplant surgeons, palliative care physicians, members of NGOs on organ donation and legal policy, from Indian Ministry of Health and Family Welfare.
- Various professional bodies—Indian Society of Organ Transplantation (ISOT), Indian Society of Critical Care Medicine (ISCCM), Society of Neurocritical Care (SNCC), Indian Academy of Neurology (IAN), Indian Association of Palliative Care (IAPC), Liver Transplantation Society of India (LTSI), Indian Society for Heart and Lung Transplantation (INSHLT), Indian Academy of Pediatrics (IAP), and Critical Care Chapter were represented.

Weaknesses

- The recommendations have been made as per international best practice statements and experiences.
- Very limited available data on DCDD in India and hence possibly practical recommendations as per local scenario has not been provided.

■ REVIEWERS' OPINION

Acceptance and increase of DCDD can significantly increase the available organ pool in India, and the detailed position statement will help increase its success.

Initial selection of centers and undertaking pilot projects of DCDD at several transplant centers will further help understand logistic difficulties and other ethical and economic factors involved and thus further modification of the recommendations on the subject.

However, it is a difficult journey, understanding the limited awareness of EOLC and WLST in the country. Improving awareness about the same and positive changes to perimortem procedures, and legislation may greatly change future practices in DCDD in India.

ARTICLE 60

Analysis: EASL Clinical Practice Guidelines on the Management of Hepatic Encephalopathy

European Association for the Study of the Liver. EASL clinical practice guidelines on the management of hepatic encephalopathy.

J Hepatol. 2022;77:807-24.

■ CLINICAL QUESTION OR PROBLEM

Hepatic encephalopathy (HE) is a frequent and debilitating complication of liver disease, and leading to cognitive impairment, and increased morbidity and poor outcomes.

■ WHAT IS KNOWN?

The previous guidelines have divided the treatment of HE as per the cause of the cirrhosis. Also with the fast advances in the field, and including liver transplantation, the guidelines were formulated.

■ POPULATION

Patients with cirrhosis with risk of HE.

■ INTERVENTION/METHOD USED

A panel of experts were selected by the European Association for the study of the Liver (EASL) governing board, which later identified 36 reviewers to form a Delphi panel. The reviewers consisted of gastroenterologists, hepatologists, internists, nurses, neurologists, methodologists, neurologist, neurophysiologist, neuroradiologist, neuroscientist, and a patient with a background in psychology. The panelists identified topics in the form of 31 questions, by Delphi.

An extensive literature search was also performed using MeSH (Medical Subject Headings) terms, and evidence was evaluated and scored to formulate the recommendations, and a Delphi panel approval was sought, with consensus of >75%.

■ NEW ISSUES ADDRESSED

Strongly recommends screening of patients with cirrhosis for covert HE, with the experience and tests available locally. Early referral to a liver transplantation center after the first episode of overt HE, and those with recurrent or persistent HE should be considered for transplantation.

Recommends rapid removal of blood from the gastrointestinal (GI) tract, in patients presenting with GI bleeding, and obliteration of portosystemic shunts in recurrent or persistent HE in stable patients with a MELD (Model for End-stage Liver Disease) score < 11.

A strong recommendation to consider early liver transplantation in hepatic myelopathy. Provides driving safety instructions and neurological workup required for nonurgent TIPS (transjugular intrahepatic portosystemic shunt).

■ CHANGES FROM CURRENT GUIDELINES

A strong recommendation to label as "acute encephalopathy" in the context of acute on chronic liver failure, and not to classify HE based on the etiology of their underlying liver disease.

The current guidelines recommend identifying HE as an alternative or additional cause of neuropsychiatric impairment, to improve the prognosis, as against the previous guidelines[3] which recommended HE as a diagnosis of exclusion.

The guidelines recommend against the use of zinc supplementation, and to treat only demonstrated vitamin/micronutrient deficiency. Replacement of animal protein, with vegetable and dairy protein, maintaining the overall protein intake is given a weak recommendation.

Strengths

- Formulated by a multidisciplinary team
- Recommendations provide flexible and detailed approaches to the screening, diagnosis, and management of HE.

Weaknesses

Lacks mention of the emergency management of airway and hemodynamic factors in the management of severe HE.

■ REVIEWERS' OPINION

Hepatic encephalopathy has a complex pathogenesis and there is no clear diagnostic test available for its diagnosis, or an effective treatment modality. The guidelines provide recommendations on the clinical management of HE, irrespective of the cause of the cirrhosis. They also recommend the management of HE, post TIPS.

The guidelines are well detailed and can be used by physicians, gastroenterologists, neurologists, intensivists. However, they lack the management of a critical patient with severe HE.

ARTICLE 61

Analysis: The Association of Obstetric Anesthesiologists, India—An Expert Committee Consensus Statement and Recommendations for the Management of Maternal Cardiac Arrest

Pandya ST, Jain K, Grewal A, Parikh K, Sharma K, Gupta A, et al. The Association of Obstetric Anesthesiologists, India—An expert committee consensus statement and recommendations for the management of maternal cardiac arrest.

J Obstet Anaesth Crit Care. 2022;12(2):85-93.

■ CLINICAL QUESTION OR PROBLEM

Maternal mortality is a major health issue globally and in India. In India, we largely lack a registry on the incidence of maternal cardiac arrest (MCA) and its outcomes.

■ WHAT IS KNOWN?

Managing maternal cardiac is complex and challenging, with two patients at risk, needing two specialized teams to work simultaneously and in a coordinated manner, to improve both maternal and fetal outcomes.

■ POPULATION

All pregnant patients with cardiac arrest.

■ INTERVENTION/METHOD USED

The committee members did an electronic search on articles on MCA using PubMed, EMBASE, Google scholar database, Ovid, and Cochrane Library. They also deliberated on guidelines by various international bodies (American Heart Association, Society of Obstetric Anesthesia and Perinatology, Obstetric Anesthesia Association UK, European Resuscitation Council guidelines, and Royal College of Obstetricians and Gynecologists guidelines. Thus, the consensus statement was formulated to improve outcomes in cases of MCA.

■ NEW ISSUES ADDRESSED

The guidelines mention about activating the "maternal code blue team", which is a special trained team for the management of maternal emergencies, consisting of an adult resuscitation team, an obstetric resuscitation team and a neonatal team, with specific roles.

A recommendation for use of extracorporeal membrane oxygenation (ECMO) or CP bypass, if available, in patients with refractory local anesthetic systemic toxicity is given. And also ECMO CPR is recommended to stabilize the obstetric patients.

Mention of supplementary medications as a part of advanced cardiac life support (ACLS) protocol has been done—naloxone, tranexamic acid.

It has expanded the role of resuscitative uterine interventions beyond perimortem cesarean delivery, to include uterine compression sutures, hysterectomy, or other additional interventions commensurate to the underlying cause, expertise, and facilities available at the healthcare setting.

■ CHANGES FROM CURRENT GUIDELINES

A special mention to consider specific obstetric causes of uterine rupture and abnormal placentation, and sepsis, oxytocin use, and opioids.

A few recommendations have been provided on what should not be done like no tilt of bed to the left to increase venous return, not to delay defibrillation due to removal of fetal monitors, and not to be give cricoid pressure routinely.

Emphasis is laid on real-time documentation, incident reporting, debriefing, and training.

Strengths

- Clear recommendations, including mention of what should not be done.
- A common guideline for all obstetricians, physicians, neonatologists, intensivists dealing with this group of patients—as all the respective guidelines were deliberated in the process.
- Mentions various obstetric causes as the cause of arrest and how to correct them.

Weaknesses

Not clear and detailed about ethical aspects faced while resuscitating a pregnant patient.

■ REVIEWERS' OPINION

Although rare, managing MCA is more complex than a nonpregnant woman in cardiac arrest. Both the mother and the fetus require special considerations and also have different challenges, though maternal survival is the priority. These guidelines emphasize on forming a special "maternal code blue team", for coordinated efforts and improved outcomes.

The cause for arrest includes the mnemonic ABCDE-UPS (A: anaphylaxis; anesthetic causes; B: bleeding; C: cardiovascular causes; D: drugs; E: eclampsia, embolism (amniotic/air); U: uterine causes (placenta accreta spectrum, abruptio, rupture); P: pulmonary causes; S: sepsis), with additional obstetric causes to consider and additional medications to be used. The recommendations have been formed using latest science and deliberating on the available guidelines, which makes them comprehensive.

ARTICLE 62

Analysis: Sepsis-associated Acute Kidney Injury: Consensus Report of the 28th Acute Disease Quality Initiative Workgroup

Zarbock A, Nadim MK, Pickkers P, Gomez H, Bell S, Joannidis M, et al. Sepsis-associated acute kidney injury: Consensus report of the 28th Acute Disease Quality Initiative workgroup.
Nat Rev Nephrol. 2023;19:401-17.

■ CLINICAL QUESTION OR PROBLEM

Sepsis-associated acute kidney injury (SA-AKI) is common in the ICU, and is associated with high morbidity and mortality. Also, many aspects of SA-AKI are poorly understood.

■ WHAT IS KNOWN?

Management of SA-AKI is challenging, and early identification of patients at risk of developing AKI or severe/persistent AKI is crucial needing timely intervention with various measures.

■ POPULATION

Patients with clinical or subclinical SA-AKI.

■ INTERVENTION/METHOD USED

A diverse panel of clinicians and researchers from various relevant disciples, including intensivists, anesthetists, nephrologists, and pharmacologists from various countries were convened by the Acute Dialysis Quality Initiative (ADQI) consensus committee. A modified Delphi process was followed and a combination of expert panel and evidence appraisal was used to formulate the practice guidelines and to propose the research questions to be addressed in the future.

■ NEW ISSUES ADDRESSED

The statement has proposed the definition and the distinction between SA-AKI and SI-AKI.

■ CHANGES FROM CURRENT GUIDELINES

Along with source control and treatment of sepsis, fluid and vasopressor optimization are the key strategies to manage SA-AKI, with a net fluid-sparing effect. There is a grade 2B recommendation on the choice of vasopressor (vasopressin or angiotensin 2) in some subtypes of SA-AKI. Grade 1C recommendation has been given to the possible benefit of albumin and bicarbonate in SA-AKI.

Grade 1A recommendation has given to the use of extracorporeal blood purification techniques (EBP) to remove pathogens, microbial toxins, inflammatory mediators, and metabolites.

Strengths

A combination of expert panel consensus with appraisal of evidence has been used to formulate the consensus statements.

Weaknesses

- SA-AKI involves a lot of heterogenicity, with various phenotypes and subphenotypes, and endotypes, thus using a single consensus statement, without the ease of identification of the same at the bedside, has its limitations.
- The consensus statements are graded, however they lack the objective targets of management.
- Early identification of SA-AKI at the subclinical point, with the available

biomarkers is challenging and thus with limited management strategies.

■ REVIEWERS' OPINION

The consensus statements will help the clinicians in understanding the underlying pathophysiology crucial for the early identification, and treatment of SA-AKI.

Despite the growing knowledge on the pathophysiology of the disease, the strategies for management of SA-AKI are nonspecific and focus on hemodynamic management and treatment of sepsis, with preventing further insult to the kidney. The preventive strategy with removal of inflammatory metabolites and microbial toxins with extracorporeal therapies is recommended in this consensus statement.

ARTICLE 63

Analysis: New International Guidelines and Consensus on the Use of Lung Ultrasound

Demi L, Wolfram F, Klersy C, De Silvestri A, Ferretti VV, Muller M, et al. New international guidelines and consensus on the use of lung ultrasound.
J Ultrasound Med. 2023;42:309-44.

■ CLINICAL QUESTION OR PROBLEM

Lung ultrasound (LUS) has become a part of the daily examination in the ER, ICUs, operation rooms (OR) and even the general medical and surgical wards. However, with this frequently used modality, standardized protocols for diagnosis, understanding the artifacts, and standardized reporting need to be developed.

■ WHAT IS KNOWN?

Lung ultrasound has various advantages, especially for the unstable ICU patients, especially the portability and real-time imaging. It is being widely used for diagnostic and therapeutic purposes in an emergency situation.

Population

Clinicians using LUS for diagnostic and therapeutic purposes.

■ INTERVENTION/METHOD USED

A core group selected with LUS experts with >10 years of experience, from various countries and medical specialities, along with physicists and engineers was formed. Further up to 60 panel members were included as per the area of expertise. Each member of the core group performed a careful literature review in their area of expertise and then a two-step modified Delphi method was used and statements with >80% of more experts agreement was considered to achieve content validity. A second round on practical aspects with addition of suggestions for future development were added after achieving consensus.

■ NEW ISSUES ADDRESSED

Inputs from engineers and physicists expert in this modality have been included along with the clinical view point to cover the aspects of essential elements for image formation and processing as well as the safety aspects.

Clinical aspects on standardization of imaging protocols and analysis for the differential diagnosis and reporting of various patterns, the extent of study, and the considerations for qualitative and quantitative diagnosis of a disease process, have been discussed and recommendations stated.

Technical aspects to improve reproducibility of the LUS studies, and safety statements have also been provided about the concerns of pulmonary capillary hemorrhage. The need for adequate training before its implementation is recommended, and remote mentoring can be considered and also recommends to include the basics of ultrasound in student's curriculum.

Each statement also discusses the future developments expected, in this rapidly developing modality.

CHANGES FROM CURRENT GUIDELINES

The last guidelines were made a decade back in 2012, and after that the use of LUS saw a huge boost over the last 10 years, especially after the COVID pandemic. The current guidelines report the use of LUS in various conditions, with highlighting the differential diagnosis for various findings in the LUS.

The guidelines also recommend the use of the LUS in prehospital, emergency medicine, general/family medicine, over and above its use as a "point-of-care" assessment for dyspnea, chest pain, and desaturation. It also recommends integrating functional assessment of the diaphragm to complete the evaluation for respiratory failure.

Strengths

- Multidisciplinary clinical experts have been in the panel—pneumologists, intensivists, radiologists, cardiologists and internal medicine, from Europe, Canada, and the United States.

- The consensus includes inputs from the clinicians as well as from the engineers and physicists—this has complemented the clinical view to the understanding of the physics of image formation and processing as well as the safety aspects.
- The guidelines also stress on the importance of extensive training of the user.

Weaknesses

Unlike previous guidelines of 2012, these statements do not give a grade recommendation.

REVIEWERS' OPINION

These guidelines are unique as they have covered not only the clinical uses and protocols of LUS, but also gives position statements on technical, safety, and training aspects. The future developments discussed in the document may be a beginning for new research projects and international collaborations.

Though the document lacks the grading of the recommendations, it does guide its clinical application in everyday practice. Use of LUS in medicine has huge potential for wider applicability and acceptability.

REFERENCES

1. Jacobi J, Bircher N, Krinsley J, Agus M, Braithwaite SS, Deutschman C, et al. Guidelines for the use of an insulin infusion for the management of hyperglycemia in critically ill patients. Crit Care Med. 2012;40(12):3251-76.
2. Qaseem A, Chou R, Humphrey LL, Shekelle P. Clinical Guidelines Committee of the American College of Physicians. Inpatient glycemic control: best practice advice from the Clinical Guidelines Committee of the American College of Physicians. Am J Med Qual. 2014;29(2):95-8.
3. Vilstrup H, Amodio P, Bajaj J, Cordoba J, Ferenci P, Mullen KD, et al. Hepatic encephalopathy in chronic liver disease: 2014 Practice Guideline by the American Association for the Study Of Liver Diseases and the European Association for the Study of the Liver. Hepatology. 2014;60(2):715-35.

Index

A

Abscess
 epidural 120
 intra-abdominal 120
Acid-base
 imbalances 85
 parameters must 84
Acidemia, severe 95
Acidosis, metabolic 85
Acquired coagulation factor deficiency 156
Acute dialysis quality initiative 214
Acute hypoxemic respiratory failure 198
Acute kidney injury 57, 79, 87, 90, 100, 103, 110, 111
 group 91
 sepsis associated 214
 severe 107
Acute lung injury
 network, early treatment of 18
 sepsis induced 182
Acute physiology and chronic health evaluation 80, 98
Acute renal failure trial 95
Acute respiratory distress syndrome 33, 51
Acute stroke 201
 management of 200
Adjunctive therapy 49
Advanced cardiac life support 213
Aerobic blood culture bottles 199
Aggressive resuscitation group 8
Airway
 emergency management of 212
 pressure release ventilation 196
Albumin 54, 56, 59, 60, 63, 71
 administration 141, 142
 binds 55
 dialysis circuit, anticoagulation of 84
 efficacy of 141
 indications of 141
 infusion
  randomized trial of 54
  time of 141
  use of 70
 Italian Outcome Sepsis trial 57
 levels 56
 use of 142

Alkalosis, metabolic 84, 113
Allergy 138
Alzheimer's disease, severe 187
Amalgamation 142
American College of Gastroenterology 59
American College of Physicians 202
American Gastroenterology Association 69
American Heart Association 208, 212
American Society of Anesthesiologists 161
American Thoracic Society 33, 119
Amino acid 181
Analgesics 40
Anesthesia 163, 208
Anesthetics 40
Angiotensin 214
Animal protein, replacement of 212
Antibiotics 116, 129
 administration 132
 empirical 140
 resistance 129
  development of 200
  risk of 130
 therapy 139
Anticoagulants 79, 149
 use of 114
Anticoagulation use, association of 112
Anti-inflammatory and immunomodulatory effects 33
 pathways 186
Antimicrobial susceptibility testing 140
Anuria 108
Aortic valve pathology 163
Arabinitol 129
Arterial oxygen partial pressure 166
 ratio of 12
Arterial perfusion pressure 112
Arterial pressure 25
Arterial spin labeling 91
Articular infection 120
Ascites 73
 worsening of 56
Atrial fibrillation 208

B

Bacteremia 72, 120
 clearance rate 121
 persistent 120
Bacteria
 drug-resistant 124
 gram-negative 126
Bacterial infection 54
 type of 72
Beta-lactam 123
Bicarbonate concentration, low 84
Bile acids, concentration of 129
Bill and Melinda gates foundation 132
Bleeding 147, 213
 complications, risk of 70
 elevated risk of 155
 exacerbates 144
 grade 156
 incidence of 159
 procedures 148
 uncontrolled 80
Blood
 brain natriuretic peptide, use of 196
 consumption score, assessment of 150
 cultures 15, 121, 123, 127, 131, 132, 199
  contraindication for 131
  interpretation of 199
  performance of 199
 flow, microcirculatory 87
 gas parameters 44
 management 67, 69
 oxygen level dependent 92
 pressure 17
  control 39
  higher 87
  systolic 145
  uncontrolled 104
 product 145
  consumption 153
 sugar levels, target range of 204
 transfusions 51, 155
  massive 150, 154
 urea nitrogen 111
 volume 59
  appropriate 101

Bloodstream infection 199
Blunt trauma 151
Body mass index 162, 179
Body's albumin 54
Bone infection 120
Brain
   death 209
   injury, acute 39
   natriuretic peptide,
      elevated 208
Burn
   analysis of 181
   injury 178
      management of 180
      treatment of 178

C

Calcium
   substitution needs 85
   supplementation 85, 86
   systemic ionized 84
   total 85
Caloric intake strategy group,
      maintenance of 176
Capillary hydrostatic pressure 104
Capillary refill time 1
Cardiac arrest 170
Cardiac index 25
Cardiac output 17, 62
Cardiomyopathy, cirrhotic 61
Cardiopulmonary bypass,
      initiation of 187
Cardiopulmonary dysfunction 61
Cardiovascular complications 188
Cardiovascular dysfunction
      leading 72
Catecholamine index 28
Catheter
   site 156
   type 156
Ceftobiprole 120-122
   group 121
Ceftriaxone 127
Central venous catheter 156
   placement 154
Central venous pressure 2, 101
Cephalosporin 120
Cerebral
   abscess 120
   perfusion pressure 39
Cerebrospinal fluid drainage 40
Chemoembolization,
      transarterial 68

Chest
   injury, major 145
   tube 145
   X- 34
Child-Pugh score 63
Chlorhexidine gluconate
      solution 200
Chloride 11
   load 11, 13
Chronic obstructive pulmonary
      disease 119
Ciprofloxacin 127
Circulation, systemic 64
Circulatory dysfunction 71
Cirrhosis 54, 55, 63, 69, 71-73
   complication of 72
   decompensated 57
   etiology 65
   liver 141, 142, 179
   related complications 142
   underlying cause of 59
Citrate
   accumulation 82, 85
      rate of 82
   anticoagulation 83
   concentration solutions, low 83
   fluid 81
   level exceeds 85
   load 84
   metabolism 86
   net overload 85
   toxicity 85, 113
   use of 83
Clostridioides difficile 127
Coagulation, standard tests of 67
Coagulopathy, trauma-induced
      144, 145, 149, 150
Colistin 127
Colloid oncotic pressure,
      reduced 141
Comparative vasoactive therapies
      efficacy 63
Comprehensive literature
      search 52
Computed tomography scan 34
Congenital coagulation factor
      deficiency 156
Consciousness, altered level of 40
Continuous kidney replacement
      therapy 112
Continuous renal replacement
      therapy 79, 96-98, 100,
      112, 187
Continuous venovenous
      hemofiltration 79, 80

Coronary artery bypass grafting 187
Coronavirus disease 2019
      (COVID-19) 90, 94, 164,
      190, 192, 197
   disease 208
   hypoxemic 198
   infection 93
   pandemic 23, 138
      impact of 164
   severe 116
Corticosteroids, low-dose 196
COX regression analysis 3
Craniotomy, decompressive 40
C-reactive protein 196
Cryoprecipitate 69, 201
Crystalloid 135
   isotonic 13
Customized citrate
      anticoagulation 79
   group 80
Custom-made calcium-free
      trisodium citrate
      replacement fluid 80
Cystic fibrosis 34
Cytokine 138
   secretion of 54
Cytomegalovirus 196

D

Daptomycin 120-122
   group 121
Data and Safety Monitoring
      Committee 145
Death 55, 61, 147, 157
   circulatory determination
      of 209
   high risk of 1-9, 118, 139, 184
Decompression 145
Delirium, postoperative 188
Delphi method, modified 195
Dementia, severe 187
Deoxyhemoglobin 92
Diarrheal disease, acute 133
Digestive tract 126, 128
   selective decontamination of
      126-128
Digital ischemia, incidence of 29
Double-Blind Prospective
      Intervention Cohort
      Study 100
Dynamic albumin
      administration 142
   prognosis of 141

E

Echocardiography, formal 163
Eclampsia 213
Edema
    acute overload pulmonary 108
    interstitial 104
    peripheral 135
    pulmonary 61, 95
Eicosanoid prostaglandin E2 54
Ejection fraction 62
Electrolyte disturbances 86
Electronic healthcare records 142
Embolism 213
    pulmonary 101
Emergency medical
        service 136, 201
End-expiratory occlusion
        maneuver 27
Endocarditis
    infective 199
    right sided native valve 120
Endotracheal intubation 117
Endovascular therapy 201
End-stage liver disease score,
        model for 55, 142
Enteral glutamine, randomized
        trial of 178
Enteral nutrition
    absolute contraindication
        for 179
    interruption, cause of 177
    pursuit of 175
Enteric fever 130
    incidence of 130
    surveillance for 130
European Association for Study of
        Liver 211
European Committee on
        Antimicrobial
        Susceptibility
        Testing 123
European Respiratory Society 204
European Resuscitation Council
        Guidelines 212
European Society for Parenteral
        and Enteral Nutrition
        Guidelines 178
European Society of Intensive
        Care Medicine 33
European System for Cardiac
        Operative Risk
        Evaluation 187
Extracorporeal blood purification
        techniques, use of 214
Extracorporeal carbon dioxide
        removal 84
Extracorporeal life support organi-
        zation guidelines 84
Extracorporeal membrane
        oxygenation 84, 110, 196
    use of 213
Extracorporeal organ support
        systems 84
Extravascular space 54
Extubation failure 176

F

Feces, chemical composition of 129
Fetal monitors, removal of 213
Fever
    enteric 130
    paratyphoid 130
Fibrinogen concentrates, use of 201
Fibrinolytic activity,
        augmented 149
Fischer's exact test 138, 141
Fluid 1, 11, 21
    accumulation,
        life-threatening 103
    administration of 16, 136
    balance 97, 99, 167
    boluses 14, 16
    categorization of 12
    creep 12, 13
        role of 13
    overload 9, 135
        presence of 136
    prehospital administration
        of 136
    restriction protocol 17
    resuscitation 10
        moderate 7
    therapy data 12
French Guidelines
        Monotherapy 139
Fresh frozen plasma 67, 150
    consumption, median 152
Fungal infection 34
Furosemide
    stress testing 100-103
    use of 99

G

Gastric suctioning, concomitant 176
Gastroenterology 54
Glasgow coma scale 40, 46, 51, 145
    score 43
Glasgow outcome scale 51, 147, 153
Glucocorticoids 183
    role of 116
Glucose-6-phosphate
        dehydrogenase
        deficiency 138
Glutamine supplementation 179
Glutathione peroxidase 3
    activity 190
Glycemic management 202

H

Heart
    catheterization 107
    disease, ischemic 37, 61
    failure, chronic 7
    rate 25
    transplantation 187
Hematology 144
    ward 158
Hematoma 157
Hemodialysis 120
    intermittent 94, 113
Hemodynamic
    factors 212
    instability 101, 112, 141
    parameters 169
    variables 28
Hemolysis, acute 183
Hemorrhage 149
    extracranial 201
    intracerebral 201
    intracranial 39
    pulmonary capillary 216
    subarachnoid 39
Heparin
    low-molecular-weight 113
    systemic unfractionated 84
    unfractionated 113
Hepatic Doppler 105
Hepatic encephalopathy 57, 211
    management of 211
Hepatitis, active viral 34
Hepatocellular carcinoma,
        advanced 55
Hepatorenal syndrome 55, 59, 63
Herpes virus 34
Heterogeneity 99
High frequency oscillatory
        ventilation 196
High positive end-expiratory
        pressure 196
Higher illness severity scores 81
High-flow nasal cannula 34
    use of 117

Human albumin 70
 associated adverse events 73
 infusion 71
  use of 72
 solution 55
Human immunodeficiency virus
 presence of 130
 risk of 130
Human microbiome 129
Hydrocortisone 33, 34, 116, 118
 continuous infusion of 117
 use of 33
Hyperkalemia, refractory 80
Hypernatremia, risk of 84
Hyperosmolar therapy 40
Hypersensitivity 187
Hypertension
 intracranial 39
 portal 64
Hyperthyroidism 208
Hypertonic citrate solutions 84
Hyperventilation therapy 40
Hypoalbuminemia 141
Hypocalcemia 113
 persistent symptomatic 80
 stringent monitoring for 85
 systemic 84, 85
Hypoglycemia 183
Hypotension 98, 136, 169, 170
 sepsis induced 17, 135, 137
 severe 18
Hypothermia, prophylactic 39
Hypoxemic respiratory failure 13, 197
Hypoxia 209

I

Illness, severity of 7
Immunosuppression 54
Indian Academy of Neurology 210
Indian Academy of Pediatrics 210
Indian Association of Palliative Care 210
Indian Society for Heart and Lung Transplantation 210
Indian Society of Critical Care Medicine 210
Indian Society of Organ Transplantation 210
Infarction, myocardial 37
Infections 51, 55, 116
 bacterial 54
 extrapulmonary 140
 hospital-acquired 188
 primary site of 183

severe 190
type of 192
Infectious Diseases Society of America 33, 116, 119
Inflammation 185
 systemic 61
Influenza 34, 117
Injuries, severe traumatic 145, 149
Inotropes, use of 2
Inspired oxygen, fraction of 12, 34, 117, 166, 196
Integrated systems, anticoagulation of 84
Intensive care unit 1, 33, 54, 79, 103, 127, 136, 155, 175, 181, 198, 208
 length of 117
Interlobular renal veins 105
International Prospective Observational Study 165
Intra-abdominal pressure 25
Intracranial hemorrhage 39
 presence of 46
Intracranial hypertension 39
 treatment of 42
Intracranial pressure, management of 42
Intravenous fluid
 boluses 4
 restriction of 4
 therapy 11
Intravoxel incoherent motion 92
Intubation 198
Invasive pulmonary aspergillosis 196
Ionized calcium 85
Irritable bowel syndrome 129
Ischemia
 cardiac 29
 mesenteric 60

J

Japanese Healthcare Professionals 197
Japanese Respiratory Society 195
Japanese Society of Intensive Care Medicine 195
Japanese Society of Respiratory Care Medicine 195

K

Kaplan-Meier
 90-day mortality point 136
 survival curves 68, 140

Kidney
 disease improving global outcome 87
  classification system 101
  criteria 192
 disease, chronic 7, 101, 108
 function 109
  universal real-time marker of 98
 injury, acute 57, 79, 87, 90, 100, 103, 110, 111
 perfusion pressure 89
Krebs' cycle 85

L

Lactate, serum 142
Large volume intravenous fluids, administration of 17
Left ventricular
 assist device 84
 ejection fraction 163
Legionella pneumonia 196
Leukopenia 122
Linezolid 122
Liver
 cirrhosis 141, 142, 179
 disease 179
  chronic 55, 187
  cirrhotic 55
  severity of 65
 failure, acute-on-chronic 54, 59
 osmoreceptors 61
 support systems 84
 transplantation 60
Liver Transplantation Society of India 210
Logistic regression analysis 114
Low tidal volume ventilation 24, 196
Lung
 compliance, low 27
 ultrasound 215

M

Maastricht classification, modified 210
Macrophages 54
Magnesium, loss of 86
Magnetic resonance imaging 90
 phase contrast 91
Mann-Whitney U test 141
Maquet servo-i MR-conditional ventilator 91

Massive transfusion, risk of 149
Maternal cardiac arrest,
　　management of 212
Maximal gastric vacuity strategy
　　group 176
Mean arterial pressure 87, 136
Mechanical ventilation 36, 117,
　　126, 183, 187
　　duration of 43
Mental health disorders 129
Meropenem 124
　intermittent infusion of 124
Mesenteric ischemia 60
　rates of 29
Metabolome, altered 129
Meta-regression models 88
Metformin 203
Methemoglobin saturation 138
Methylene blue 21, 24, 138, 139
Methylprednisolone 33, 196
Microbial gene 129
Microbiome, imbalance of 129
Microcirculation 1
　direct assessment of 1
　sublingual measurements of 2, 4
Microflora 129
Midodrine 65, 66, 71
Minimum inhibitory
　　concentration 123
Mitochondrial dysfunction 84
Mitral valve pathology 163
Monotherapy 139, 140
Monte Carlo simulation 131
Mortality 68
Mottling score 1
Multicenter cohort study,
　　post-hoc analysis of 11
Multidisciplinary
　　collaboration 206
Multidrug-resistant organisms
　　pathogens, acquisition
　　of 140
Multiple organ dysfunction
　　syndrome 33
Mycobacterium tuberculosis 199
Myocardial injury 98, 186
Myopathy 121

N

Nafamostat mesylate 113
Nasopharyngeal swabs, antigen
　　tests of 196
National Institutes of Health
　　Stroke Scale Score 48

National Surveillance System for
　　Enteric Fever in India
　　Study 130
Nephrology 79
Nephrotoxic drugs 59
Neurocritical care 39, 42
Neurologic function 47
Neuromuscular blockers, use of 196
Neuroprotection 48
Neuropsychiatric disorders 187
Nitrate 138
　serum levels 138
Noninvasive multiparametric
　　magnetic resonance
　　imaging techniques 93
Noninvasive positive pressure
　　ventilation 196
Noradrenaline equivalent score 98
Norepinephrine 5, 64
Novel state-of-the-art
　　techniques 93
Nutrition 175
Nystatin, units of 127

O

Obesity 129
Octreotide 65, 66
Oliguria 108
　post-continuous renal
　　replacement therapy
　　commencement 99
Opioids 213
Optimal oxygenation target 36
Organ
　donation 209
　dysfunction 112, 184
　　persistent 184, 187
　　postoperative 186
　failure 135
Oropharynx 128
Oxygen saturation
　peripheral 36
　targets 36
Oxygenation 46
　index 110
　relative measure of 92
Oxytocin use 213

P

P value 118, 152
Packed red blood cell transfusion
　　69, 150
Pancreatitis, acute 7

Parkinson's disease, advanced 187
Pelvic injury 145
Percutaneous acetic acid
　　injection 68
Peripheral intravascular catheter,
　　epidemiology of 11
Peritoneal dialysis 113
Pharyngeal swabs, antigen
　　tests of 196
Phenothiazines 138
Phosphate depletion 86
Physiological citrate metabolic
　　rate 84
Piperacillin 123
Placenta accreta spectrum 213
Plasma
　expander 72
　neutrophil gelatinase-
　　associated lipocalin 101
　vasopressin concentration 27
Platelet
　concentrate consumption,
　　median 152
　count 157
　transfusion 69, 154-156, 201
Pneumonia 72, 120, 122, 176, 196
　community-acquired 116
　eosinophilic 121
　pneumococcal 196
　ventilator-associated 139
Point-of-care ultrasound 165
　beaubien-souligny used 104
Polymerase chain reaction 34, 91
Positive blood cultures 128
Positive end-expiratory
　　pressure 24, 117
　effect of 24
　test 24
Post-hoc analysis 12, 19
Postoperative vasoactive
　　support 186
Post-paracentesis circulatory
　　dysfunction 72
Postrenal obstruction factors,
　　presence of 101
Potassium chloride 80
Potential citrate toxicity, vigilant
　　monitoring for 86
Pragmatic inclusion criteria 153
Preexisting end stage renal
　　disease 113
Pregnancy 179
Prehospital, emergency
　　medicine 216

Pressure-controlled ventilation 196
Procalcitonin levels 196
Prognostication 196
Proinflammatory cytokine
    levels 116
Prophylactic fluid administration,
    role of 14
Prophylactic platelet concentrate
    transfusion 157
Prothrombin complex
    concentrates, use of 201
Proton pump inhibitors, use of 130
Pseudomonas aeruginosa 139
Public health problem 132
Pulmonary severity index score 34
Pulse pressure 25

R

Randomised-controlled
    multicenter study 1
    trial 21, 161
Rankin scale, modified 48
Rapid shallow breathing index 44
Red blood cell consumption,
    median 152
Refractory metabolic acidosis 80
Regional citrate anticoagulation
    82, 83, 86
Regional renal
    oxygenation 94
    tissue perfusion 92
Renal cortex 93
Renal dysfunction 55, 56
Renal failure, rate of 58
Renal function 62, 91
Renal hypoperfusion 72
Renal perfusion pressure 64, 87
Renal replacement therapy 5, 60,
    82, 83, 94, 105, 183
Renal resistive index 92
Renal water diffusion, calculate
    measures of 92
Renin-angiotensin-aldosterone 59
Rescue vasopressors 19, 136
Respiratory rate 46, 171
Respiratory secretions 122
Respiratory triggered gradient-
    and spin-echo 92
Restrictive fluid 14
    strategy 136
Resuscitation 208
    strategies 1
Rigorous double-blinding 125

Rigorous methodology 48
Ringer's solution 9

S

Salmonella
    paratyphi 130
    typhi 130
Sedatives 40
Seizure
    late posttraumatic 40
    prophylaxis 40
Selective serotonin reuptake
    inhibitors 138
Selenium
    high-dose 186
    measurements 190
    supplementation 187
Selenoenzyme, biosynthesis
    of 189
Selenoproteins 189
Sepsis 14, 15, 123, 135, 142, 181,
    213
    management 142
    resuscitation 18, 21
Septic pulmonary embolism 120
Septic shock 4, 7, 14, 21, 35, 72, 117,
    123, 137, 138, 142, 183
    absence of 116
    diagnosis 23
    moment of 138
    vasopressor for 34
Sequential organ failure
    assessment 166, 183
    scores of 58
Serum albumin level 57, 142
Serum creatinine 62
    concentration 108
Serum potassium concentration 108
Serum urea concentration 108
Severe community-acquired
    pneumonia 33, 116
    management of 204
Severe trauma score,
    coagulopathy of 145
Shock 1, 33
    category of 171
    hypovolemic 138
    management of 3
    obstructive 138
    refractory septic 27, 139
    septic 4, 7, 14, 21, 35, 72, 117,
        123, 137, 138, 142, 183
Sidestream dark field cameras 1

Single-center non-blinded
    randomized controlled
    trial 82
Society of Critical Care Medicine 33
    guidelines 69
    recommends 202
Society of Neurocritical Care 210
Society of Obstetric Anesthesia
    and Perinatology 212
Sodium 11, 59, 83
    chloride solution 22
    low 84
    selenite 187
Soft tissue source 120
Sonography 161, 170
Standard sodium concentration
    replacement fluid, use
    of 84
Staphylococcus aureus
    bacteremia 120
    methicillin-resistant 120, 199
    methicillin-sensitive 120
Staphylococcus lugdunensis 199
Steroids 40, 116
    duration of 117
    qualified for 119
    use of 35
Stroke 208, 209
    acute 201
        ischemic 47-49, 201
    management guidelines 49
    nursing 208
    prevention, secondary 201
    volume variation 25
Student's T-test 141
Subclavian vein 158
Subphenotypes 20
Supplemental enteral glutamine,
    effect of 178
Support hypoperfusion-induced
    renal hypoxia 94
Surgery
    cardiac 88, 186
    cardiovascular 208
Swachh Bharat Mission 133
Systemic inflammatory response
    syndrome
    absence of 8
    presence of 8
Systemic venous
    congestion, prevalence of 103
    pressure 104
Systolic pulse variation 27

T

Tachycardia 136
Target arterial oxygen saturation 36
Tazobactam 123
Tenecteplase, use of 201
Terlipressin 60, 63, 64, 66
    plus albumin group 59, 62
    therapy 61
Thai Clinical Trials Registry 80
Therapy intensity level 39
Thermodilution, transpulmonary 25
Thoracic ultrasound 166, 167
    impact of 165
    usage of 165
Thrombocytopenia 154
    heparin-induced 113
    severe 156
Thromboelastography 67
    guided therapy 67
Thrombolysis 201
Thrombolytic agent 201
Tidal volume 25
Tissue
    dysoxia, biomarkers of 185
    hypoxia 84
Tobramycin 127
Total antibiotic use 127
Total blood product consumption, median 152
Toxic aggression 108
Toxins, microbial 214
Tranexamic acid 144, 146, 147, 157, 201
    prehospital 144
Transfusion
    hemoglobin 51
    status 52
    timing of 50

Transjugular intrahepatic portosystemic shunt 60, 68
Transplant free survival 63
Trauma 144, 149
    severe 144
    systems, advanced 147
Traumatic brain injury 39, 50, 51
    management of 53
Tuberculosis, active 34
Tubular necrosis, acute 95
Typhoid
    burden of 130
    conjugate vaccine 130
    fever 130
        incidence of 132
        prevention of 132

U

Uremic symptom 80
Urinary tract infections 72
Urine output 81, 98, 99

V

Vascular occlusion 147
Vasoactive drug index 110
Vasoactive inotrope score 98
Vasoconstrictor medications 64
Vasodilator drugs, use of 2
Vasopressin 27, 28, 59, 214
    dose 29
    loading 27, 29
Vasopressor 5, 15, 21, 34, 37, 136, 137
    choice of 214
    dose of 142
    infusion 183
    therapy 117, 187
    use 19

Vena cava, inferior 105
Venous congestion 105, 107
    moderate-to-severe 106, 107
    severity of 107
Venous excess ultrasound
    grading system 103, 105
    score 103, 104
Ventilation
    invasive 198
    volume-controlled 196
Ventilator-associated pneumonia 139
    risk of 126
Ventilatory parameters 25
Vitamin
    C 184, 190, 192
        administration 185
        dose of 193
        effect of 193
        high-dose 181, 182, 185
        infusion 182
        intravenous 181
        level 183, 184

W

Weaknesses 197, 198, 200, 201, 203, 206, 209, 210, 212-214, 216
Web-based system 187
Whole body microcirculation 1

X

X2 test 141

Z

Zinc supplementation, use of 212